Concise Clinical Pharmacology: CNS Therapeutics

Notice

Concise Clinical Pharmacology: CNS Therapeutics

John P. Blass, MD, PhD
Winifred Masterson Burke Professor of Neurology, Neuroscience, and Medicine
Weill Medical College of Cornell University
New York, New York

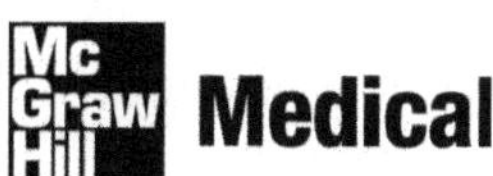

New York Chicago San Francisco Lisbon London Madrid Mexico City Milan New Delhi San Juan Seoul Singapore Sydney Toronto

The McGraw·Hill Companies

Concise Clinical Pharmacology: CNS Therapeutics

1 2 3 4 5 6 7 8 9 0 DOC DOC 0 9 8 7 6

ISBN-13: 978-0-07-144036-3
ISBN-10: 0-07-144036-4

This book was set in Times Roman by International Typesetting and Composition.
The editors were James F. Shanahan, Maya Barahona, and Lester A. Sheinis.
The production supervisor was Sherri Souffrance.
The cover designer was Anthony Landi.
Project management was provided by International Typesetting and Composition.
The index was prepared by Robert Swanson.
RR Donnelley was printer and binder.
This book is printed on acid-free paper.

Library of Congress Cataloging-in-Publication Data

Blass, John P.
Concise clinical pharmacology : CNS therapeutics / John P. Blass.
p. ; cm.
Includes bibliographical references and index.
ISBN-13: 978-0-07-144036-3 (softcover : alk. paper)
ISBN-10: 0-07-144036-4 (softcover : alk. paper)
1. Neuropharmacology—Handbooks, manuals, etc. 2. Neuropsychopharmacology—Handbooks, manuals, etc. I. Title.
[DNLM: 1. Central Nervous System Diseases—drug therapy. WL 300 B644c 2007]
RM315.B753 2007
615'.78—dc22

2006027954

International Edition ISBN-13: 978-0-07-110511-8, ISBN-10: 0-07-110511-5

Contents

Preface ix

CHAPTER ONE
Introduction **1**

CHAPTER TWO
General Principles **9**

Medications as Chemicals 9
Classification of Medications Acting on the Nervous System 10
Blood-Brain Barrier 11
Pharmacokinetics and Pharmacodynamics 13
Drug Action and Human Variation 18
Talk Therapy and Drug Therapy 20

CHAPTER THREE
Mood Disorders: Depression and Mania **25**

Depression 26
Mania 35
Manic-Depressive Disease 36
Suicide 38
Medications for Depression 42
Medications for Mania and Manic-Depressive Illness 60

Treatment of Acute Psychosis by the General Clinician 69
Nonpharmacological Treatments 70

CHAPTER FOUR
Thought Disorders: Including Schizophrenias and Related Psychoses 75

Classification and Diagnosis 78
Neurobiology 81
Treatment 86
Treatment of Acute Psychotic Emergencies 99
Nonpharmacological Treatments 100

CHAPTER FIVE
Cognitive Disorders: Delirium and Dementia 105

Incidence and Prevalence 106
Classification and Diagnosis 107
Neurobiology of Delirium and Dementia: General Considerations 127
Pathophysiology of Specific Forms of Dementia 131
Treatment 136

CHAPTER SIX
Anxiety 163

Classification and Diagnosis 164
Neurobiology 173
Treatment 174

CHAPTER SEVEN
Pain 185

Classification and Diagnosis 185
Neurobiology 195
Treatment 197

CHAPTER EIGHT
Sleep 225

Classification and Diagnosis 226

Neurobiology 235
Treatments 240

CHAPTER NINE
Cerebrovascular Disorders 255

Classification and Diagnosis 256
Neurobiology 266
Treatment 267

CHAPTER TEN
Disorders of Awareness: Dizziness, Fainting, Fits, Stupor, and Coma and Related Conditions 283

Dizziness 284
Fainting 286
Fits (Seizures) 289
Stupor 303
Coma 303
Brain Stem Compression (Herniation, "Coning") 309
Other Conditions 313

CHAPTER ELEVEN
Disorders of Motility: Including Parkinson Disease and Other Movement Disorders 319

Classification and Diagnosis 320
Diagnostic Considerations for Disorders of Motility Involve both Questions of Mechanism and Recognition of Certain Common Syndromes (Clinical Entities) 331
Neurobiology 341
Treatment 348

CHAPTER TWELVE
Disorders of Sensation 371

Classification and Diagnosis 371
Disorders of Special Sensations 372
Neurobiology 383
Treatment 385

CHAPTER THIRTEEN
Disorders of Both Sensation and Motility: Multiple Sclerosis and Related Disorders; Neuropathies 391

Multiple Sclerosis (MS) 392
Other Disorders of Myelin 401
Motor-Sensory Neuropathies 403
Neurobiology 410

CHAPTER FOURTEEN
Disorders of Conduct 415

Learned Maladaptive Behavior 415
Somatoform Disorders 417
Sexual Disorders 422
Personality Disorders 428
Adjustment Disorders and Posttraumatic Stress Disorder 435
Impulse Control Disorders 436
Addiction/Substance Abuse 438

Index 469

Preface

This book was written in response to a request by James Shanahan, an editor at McGraw-Hill, who saw a need for a book about medicines that act on the nervous system and that was relatively short, down-to-earth, scientifically sound, written as much as possible in English rather than jargon, and useful for general clinicians, trainees, and medical students. How well this monograph achieves those aims is for the reader to decide.

A longer-term origin of this book goes back to the mid-1950s, when I arrived in London to do a PhD in Neurochemistry with Professor Henry McIlwain. He had recently written a book entitled *Chemotherapy and the Central Nervous System.* In it he suggested that if a problem in biology were stated in chemical terms, the power of chemistry was such that it would probably be solved—and solved within a reasonable amount of time. English physiologists resented this "hubris," and I believe Henry eventually came to regret having written this idea down with his characteristic clarity. However, that insight of his has guided my professional lifetime, both clinically and in research.

Medications that act on the nervous system are of course chemicals. Their direct action is on other molecules in the body. Even when those other molecules are parts of "receptor complexes," the interactions between drug and receptor remain chemical interactions. So do the interactions of the chemicals we call drugs with other biological molecules.

Both in prescribing drugs to individual patients and in trying to develop new treatments, it has been useful for me to try to state the clinical problem to myself in as "chemical" terms as possible. That theme runs through this monograph. The publishers and I hope that the result is a succinct, clear description of the pharmacological and clinical principles of the use of drugs acting on the nervous system.

Thanks are due to many people who helped with this effort. They are not responsible for the failures of the text but deserve credit for whatever virtues it has. James Shanahan at McGraw-Hill first proposed that I write this book and encouraged—nay, prodded—me to get it finished. Maya Barahona and Lester A. Sheinis at McGraw-Hill have skillfully, firmly, and gently carried the text from manuscript to printed word. Several colleagues read the text and made extraordinarily useful comments. John Caronna, MD, Vice-Chairman of Neurology at NY Hospital–Weill Cornell Medical Center, went to the trouble of reading the whole thing and making appropriate comments, particularly where my knowledge of neurology was inadequate. Lady Judith (Milne) English, MBBCh, Principal of St. Hilda's College Oxford, went carefully through the chapters on psychiatric illnesses. The elegance of her thought and prose clarified issues whose muddiness in my own mind had led to confused redundancies in the text. Judith—a former colleague at the Maudsley Hospital in London—again pointed out the relation between disease classifications and diagnoses, as she did over twenty-five years ago when she and I were writing on this subject. George Alexopoulos, MD, of the Department of Psychiatry at Weill–Cornell Medical School, carefully edited the chapters on mood disorders and on anxiety, correcting many errors and bringing me up to steam on current concepts, classifications, and terminology. Michael Reding, MD, who directs the Stroke Service at the Burke Rehabilitation Hospital, went through the chapter on vascular disease meticulously and brought the information up to date, including current, cutting-edge practice.

Many thanks also go to my wife. She edited much of the text, and her ability to jump on ambiguities in wording does credit to her graduate training in Linguistics. During the nearly fifty years we have been together, including of course the writing of this monograph, she has continually encouraged me to worry about patients and science rather than "career." The writing of this book consumed many wonderful days while I pecked away at the word processor while she was painting in her studio, across our loft from my home office. Those days exemplified what my father taught was the aim of treating abnormalities of the nervous system: to help people to enjoy

Daily work,
Social evenings,
Lovely days,
Joyous holidays.*

John P. Blass, MD, PhD

*In my father's native German, "Tages Arbeit, Abends Gäste, Schöne Tage, Frohe Feste."

CHAPTER ONE

Introduction

Extensive information documents that about half of the people who seek the attention of a physician have problems related to the nervous system. The problems may appear to be primarily "psychiatric" or primarily "neurological," although careful examination of these patients often reveals both types of disability. This monograph emphasizes practical knowledge for the generalist clinician who will inevitably see patients with diseases of the nervous system. The descriptions of syndromes and of differential diagnoses in this book focus on deciding which medicine to use. Basic neurobiology is included only where it clarifies clinical decision making.

Classification and diagnosis are discussed together in this monograph because they are two sides of the same coin. Clinical classifications are lists of diagnostic categories. The diagnoses they list are a useful way to organize medical knowledge. Diagnostic groupings are, however, artificial, since every patient is different from every other patient.[1] It is important to remember that diagnoses are only useful abstractions, not material things like the organs of the body. Classifications of disease and the resulting diagnostic terminology change as new knowledge becomes available. For instance, *phthisis* was a useful diagnostic term for inflammation of the lungs before the development of bacteriology.

However, it is important to recognize that new techniques, and the new knowledge they generate, promise to revolutionize the way we classify diseases of the nervous system. Molecular genetics has documented that mutations of a single gene often lead to a variety of clinically distinct syndromes that are currently thought to be biologically distinct. For instance, the *HEXA* gene responsible for classic infantile Tay-Sachs disease has also been associated with at least seven other syndromes, including patients indistinguishable clinically from those with classic schizophrenia. Defects (mutations) of the *DRD4* gene are associated with several clinical entities: schizophrenia, bipolar disorder, abuse of alcohol and other drugs, and most recently with attention-deficit/hyperactivity disorders. The neuregulin 1 (*NRG1*) gene appears to predispose to both schizophrenia and bipolar disease. So do mutations in the dysbindin (*DTNBP1*) gene.

The association of mutations in a single gene with a variety of clinical syndromes is not limited to diseases of the nervous system. This problem, of "varying clinical phenotypes for the same genotype," is also true for disorders of other organs.[2] For instance, genetic disorders of the main protein of red blood cells (hemoglobinopathies), which are among the best studied genetic diseases of humans, show "remarkable phenotypic [clinical] diversity."[3] Recent studies are beginning to identify not only environmental causes of such variation but also effects of other *modifier* genes on the clinical expression of a *primary* gene defect. These studies raise the question of whether any disease, when fully understood, will turn out to result from a single gene rather than from a variety of genes. (Put technically, the question is whether *monogenetic* disorders actually exist or whether all clinical disorders with a major genetic component are in some sense *polygenetic*.) A full discussion of these issues is beyond the scope of this monograph, but they are likely to have major effects on the classification of diseases including diseases of the nervous system in the coming decades.[2,3] The rate of technological advance with these techniques is already thrilling and likely to become even faster.[4]

Intuitively, it seems likely that future pharmacological treatments will be directed more to underlying biological abnormalities than to symptom complexes. Again, to draw an analogy with bacteriology, clinicians' choices of antibiotics derive mainly from the susceptibility of the germs that cause an infection, and only in minor ways from the amount of pain, shortness of breath, or other symptoms that a specific infection causes. For diseases of the nervous system including psychiatric disorders, classifications based on genetics, brain imaging, and other biological techniques are likely to replace descriptions of symptom complexes. That is not so much because neurobiological classifications are more *accurate* but because they are likely to be better guides to choice of treatment.

Despite their theoretical attractiveness, these developments have not reached the level of most medical practice, including treatment of diseases of the nervous system. This monograph uses standard diagnostic categories and labels. That is the current state of the art, and this book tries to be useful for the current practice of medicine.

The organization of this book is by major complaints rather than by disease mechanisms. For instance, there is no chapter on infections of the nervous system, since patients seldom if ever present to a clinician complaining, "My nervous system is infected." (Those that do are more likely to be psychotic than to be suffering from a treatable infection.) Similarly, there is no chapter on nervous system malignancies. The exception to this generalization is the chapter on cerebrovascular disease. That exception is for convenience. Circulatory disorders, including strokes, are the most common cause of disease of the nervous system in developed countries. They can take so many different clinical forms that repetitive discussions of the same vascular disorders would have to be included in most of the chapters, were there not a separate chapter on cerebrovascular disease.

This monograph is written as much as possible in plain English. Technical terms are usually either inside double quotes or italicized in the text. Technical jargon has advantages. It can provide succinct terms to describe complex phenomena that otherwise require many more words. Jargon can thereby help with efficient communication among the professionals who have learned it; their use of it also helps them to recognize each other as trained professionals. However, jargon also has disadvantages. To those who do not know it, jargon communicates nothing except perhaps a sense of inferiority. To those who understand it only partially, jargon can be misleading. It can give the unfortunate impression that one understands a process simply because one can name it. For instance, describing a patient who complains of coughing up blood as having hemoptysis just restates what the patient has already said in English in a mixture of bad Latin and bad Greek. Neurology and psychiatry are full of complex terms that are simply descriptors derived from classic languages. Expert clinicians recognize that using one of these terms as a diagnosis does not necessarily help in treating the patient. (Of course, the use of an erudite term may convince a patient of how knowledgeable the physician is. That may help to comfort a patient, particularly a frightened one.)

In practice, a general clinician caring for patients with disease of the nervous system faces two sets of problems: (1) whether or not to refer, and if so, to whom; (2) whether or not to treat, and if so, how.

In regard to referral, the general rule is *if you think of referring, do so.* At least get a consultation. Diseases of the nervous system, if misdiagnosed or mistreated, can have catastrophic consequences including long term, expensive disability and death. The consequences can be catastrophic not only for the patient and the family but also for the physician—personally, professionally, and medicolegally. The specialist in neurology or psychiatry who provides a consultation may not do any more for the patient than the generalist can. However, the consultation/referral ensures that the generalist gives the patient the best care he or she can, and documents in the patient's medical records that a serious attempt was made to give the best possible state-of-the-art care.

In the United States in the new millennium, consultation and referral with a neurologist or psychiatrist is effectively always available. Rural areas where the specialist may be some distance away almost always have good enough transportation systems to allow a visit to a physician with formal specialty qualifications. If the family is unavailable to drive the patient to the appointment, a neighbor will often do so. Most jurisdictions also have publicly funded health transportation for those who need it. In more urban settings, clinics are available even for people with little money. Ethnic or other factors may present barriers to referral, but in most big American cities, hospitals and particularly the teaching hospitals have mechanisms in place to overcome such barriers. These institutions typically have staff who speak the necessary language. They also usually have staff who are concerned with providing diagnosis and care in a way that is comfortable for people of the particular ethnicity involved (i.e., are "ethnically sensitive").

Whether to refer a patient to a neurologist, psychiatrist, or neurosurgeon obviously depends on the major clinical manifestations in that patient and the relative clinical skills of the consultants available. The distinction between psychiatric disease and neurological disease is widely recognized to be artificial, even by those with specialty qualifications in one or the other. Brain disease usually although not always involves clinical manifestations of both types, even if one or the other may dominate. That is the reason this monograph is not divided into *psychiatric diseases* and *neurological diseases*.

In regard to treatment, there are two situations in which the generalist clinician has to treat diseases of the nervous system himself or herself. One is a neurological and/or psychiatric emergency, where immediate treatment is necessary. For instance, brain swelling that threatens to compress the brain stem (coning) requires immediate treatment. Transferring the patient to the care of a neurosurgeon or neurologist is desirable, but if the specialist does not arrive almost immediately to take over the care of the patient, the physician on the spot needs to start treatment. Other examples of conditions that require prompt treatment even if a consultant is not available include continuous seizure activity (status epilepticus), which can itself cause progressive brain damage; acute thiamin deficiency (Wernicke-Korsakoff syndrome), where prompt treatment prevents further—and permanent—brain damage; and acute psychosis, when patients are an active danger to themselves or to those around them. The second set of circumstances where generalists will have to care for patients with diseases of the nervous system is in the management of diseases that are very common, particularly if the diseases are chronic. The logistics of our medical care system require that most of the patients with common disorders of the nervous system will be under the care of a generalist, frequently in consultation with a specialist. Essentially all general clinicians will have to take care of patients with delirium and dementia. General medical practices can be predicted to include patients with other common diseases of the nervous system such as depression, cerebrovascular disease (strokes), and seizures.

As always in medical practice, knowing when not to treat is as important as knowing when to do so. Good clinical judgment includes the ability to leave well enough alone. One of the oldest and still best rules in medicine is, "first do no harm" (*primum non nocere*). A lighter version of the same thought is, "Don't just do something, doctor; stand there." That clinical principle is nowhere more true than for diseases of the nervous system, which typically lead to abnormalities of behavior. Sometimes the need to treat is obvious—for instance, for meningitis, or status epilepticus, or for life-threatening, suicidal depression. Even when a disorder is not life threatening, we did not go to medical school to withhold treatment from patients who need it out of a misplaced sense of tolerance for their behavior.[5] On the other hand, there are disorders that alter life but do not necessarily interfere with it. The extent to which people should be treated because they are "not normal" depends not only on how "not normal" they are but also on the degree of eccentricity that their society is prepared to accept. Behavior is life-threatening if it leads to the equivalent of people being thrown to the lions by the society in which they live, even if their behavior would be acceptable in another society. The distinction between "mad" and "odd" is difficult and is inherently influenced by societal norms.[6]

At one extreme, medicalization of the enforcement of conformity leads to such perversions as the Soviet Communist diagnosis of "Reformist Delusions."[7] In the decades before Russian Communism collapsed, people who thought they could improve the system were defined as *crazy* and incarcerated under intentionally unpleasant conditions. If, when they came out, they still tried to improve the system, they had obviously relapsed and required further unpleasant psychiatric hospitalization. They were considered "cured" when they quit trying to improve the political system.

The Maudsley Hospital in London, where the author of this monograph had an important part of his training, instilled quite a different view. Two examples are illustrative.

> A single lady with a responsible job in a financial institution not only talked to the walls when she went home but also perceived that the walls were talking back to her. She was followed relatively closely but not treated with antipsychotics. The consultant's reasoning was, "People have died from the side effects of psychiatric medications; they have not died from having quite pleasant conversations with the walls."

> A patient with florid Tourette's syndrome who did not respond to medication had developed a lifestyle well adapted to his illness. He worked in a foundry, had a girlfriend, good mates at the local pub, and so on. He was not treated neurosurgically. The consultant surgeon's comment was, "Why do you think this young man will be better off if I make a hole in his head?"

Medicine can be practiced the same way in the United States, but only if the patient and the family agree to the approach. The following examples are illustrative.

> An older gentleman with both parkinsonism and dementia (presumably with Lewy Body disease) required treatment with L-dopa to maintain his bodily functions within the safe range. However, he hallucinated on the minimal dose necessary to control his secretions. For many years, he and his wife had watched television in the evening, sitting in the same two chairs. On L-dopa, he hallucinated a beautiful young woman in his wife's chair. The wife, a sensible woman who loved her husband and knew he loved her, moved a third chair into the room. The husband, wife, and the hallucination watched TV together, without any need to change his medications.

> Another older man with mild to moderate Alzheimer disease paid his home health aide to have sex with him. There was no indication that the aide minded.[8] However, the patient's daughters minded terribly. They pleaded with the physician to "give him something to stop him." The American physicians with whom this issue was discussed had mixed opinions. On the whole, they tended to think that some treatment was indicated to calm the family if for no other reason. English and Danish physicians, on the other hand, tended to see nothing significantly wrong with the patient's relationship to the aide. A typical comment from that side of the Atlantic was, "Are the daughters that Oedipal?" Or, "If both he and the aide enjoy it and he

> can afford the money, why not?" In the end, the family solved the problem by finding a physician who was as appalled at the man's sexual behavior as they were. That physician identified and prescribed an antipsychotic that more or less shut down the old man's sex drive, although at the price of significant other side effects.[8]

The decision of when to use medicines to alter troubling behavior is often not trivial. This monograph does not attempt to offer precise rules. Rigid principles involve assumptions—often, unrecognized assumptions. The best guideline may be to respect the patient's humanity as well as your own. Being consistently humane to all the people involved is more important than being logically consistent.

REFERENCES

1. Kendall R. *The Role of Diagnosis in Psychiatry.* Oxford, UK, Blackwell Scientific Publications, 1975.
2. Weatherall DJ. From genotype to phenotype: genetics and medical practice in the new millennium. *Philos Trans R Soc Lond A.* 1999;354:1995–2010.
3. Weatherall DJ. Phenotype-genotype relationships in monogenic disease: lessons from the thalassaemias. *Nat Rev Genet.* 2001;2:246–255.
4. The development of DNA sequencing on chips is one of these advances. See Margulies M, Egholm M, Altman WE, et al. Genome sequencing in microfabricated high-density picolitre reactors. *Nature.* 2005;437:376–380.
5. Some years ago, an English psychiatrist decided that schizophrenia was a disease of a rigid society rather than of the afflicted patients. He established a shelter in London, where unmedicated schizophrenics could live. One of the residents poured kerosene over herself, lighted it, and died of horrible burns. Her father wrote a short letter to the journal *Lancet* telling that story. He concluded (my paraphrase), "I do not know whether schizophrenia is a disease of a person or of the society. I do know that my daughter is dead."
6. During the 1950s, it was seriously argued by some American pundits that a young woman's willingness to lose her virginity before she married was a clear sign of her psychological imbalance. The dull, whirring sound heard at that time was Sigmund Freud spinning in his grave.
7. This sorry story raises the question of who truly belonged in the asylum—those with reformist delusions or the psychiatrists treating them. This question is particularly pointed since the Communist system collapsed not too long thereafter, proving the prescience and, therefore, mental health of those who had been incarcerated with reformist delusions. A sad footnote is

that a former Soviet region, Uzbekistan, has recently been charged with re-instituting this perversion of medical practice.

8. Paying for sex is illegal even if common in many parts of the United States, and the point of this example is not to recommend the practice but to examine the medical issues that can arise at the interface of medical practice and conventional morality. These "ethical" issues and how they are handled in different societies go beyond the scope of this monograph.

CHAPTER TWO

General Principles

This chapter outlines some general principles of clinical neuropharmacology. The discussion is limited to aspects that are directly relevant to clinical practice. Excellent, more detailed, and neurobiologically oriented review articles and books are available on neuropharmacology.[1]

MEDICATIONS AS CHEMICALS

Drugs are chemicals. That holds as true for drugs that act on the nervous system as for other medications. The direct actions of drugs are on other chemicals. Those can include large molecules such as proteins (e.g., receptors), nucleic acids (e.g., genes), lipids (e.g., membrane structures), and smaller molecules (e.g., signal compounds including free radicals). Since the molecules on which drugs act mediate cellular processes, medications can be thought of as acting on cellular mechanisms. Since cellular processes, particularly in the nervous system, are the biological basis of behavior, drugs that act on the human nervous system typically alter how humans behave. That includes motor and sensory behavior as well as "higher functions" such as memory and the organization of thoughts and emotions. However, when thinking of drugs as agents that act on cellular mechanisms or on behaviors, it is important to remember that these mechanisms or behaviors are themselves indirect results of chemical interactions between exogenous therapeutic agents and endogenous chemicals in the body.

Using medications to influence higher order biological processes involves considerably more assumptions than thinking of drugs in terms of their chemical actions. For instance, selective serotonin reuptake inhibitors (SSRIs) like Prozac do not treat depressed mood directly nor do they directly treat such manifestations of depression as early morning wakening. They treat central serotonin deficiency. The question of whether or not to prescribe an SSRI is, scientifically and clinically, a decision about whether the patient in question suffers from a central serotonergic deficiency. If so, there is a good chance the appropriate drug of this class will help. If the patient's difficulties do not involve a central serotonergic deficiency, such a drug is unlikely to be useful. This issue is discussed in more detail in the discussion of treatment of mood disorders in Chap. 3 (Mood Disorders).

CLASSIFICATION OF MEDICATIONS ACTING ON THE NERVOUS SYSTEM

Medications prescribed for disease of the nervous system fall into three broad categories.

In the first are agents that have similar actions in all tissues, but are used to treat diseases of the nervous system because that is the tissue that happens to be diseased in the person being treated. One example is antibiotics to treat infections of the nervous system. The same antibiotic or combination of antibiotics used to treat meningitis is used to treat infections of other organs by the same microorganisms. The same antiviral agents that are used to treat herpes of the brain are used against manifestations of herpes virus in the skin or genitalia. Another example is anti-inflammatories. These are used to reduce excessive manifestations of inflammation in the brain the same way they are used to reduce excessive manifestations of inflammation in other tissues. Prednisone or other steroids are used to reduce swelling in the brain. They also reduce swelling in other tissues, where edema is not as life threatening as it can be inside the rigid box formed by the skull. To act directly on diseases of the brain, a drug must get into the brain. The ability of a medication to cross the *blood-brain barrier*, which is discussed below, can therefore determine which among a group of medications is chosen to treat disease of the central nervous system (CNS).

A second group of medications appears to act selectively on the brain because of the specific biological properties of that organ, even though at the chemical level these agents act more or less equally on all cells. An example is general anesthetics. Anesthetic gases typically have the same biological effects on all tissues, including cells in culture. They suppress responses in cellular membranes to a variety of stimuli. In practice, in living people or other animals, that effect is clinically useful because of its consequences for brain function. When neurons become markedly less responsive to intercellular signals, neurotransmission is reduced and people become unconscious. As far as we know, they also cease to lay down available memories, notably memory of pain. But the anesthetic gases do also affect other tissues. A striking example is halothane's ability to induce acute, sometimes fatal, atrophy of the liver.[2]

The third group of medications acts on molecules that are found primarily in the nervous system. More accurately, they act on molecules that are found in much higher concentrations in the nervous system than in other tissues. Most of the molecules in the nervous system are identical to molecules in other tissues. Put in genetic terms, most of the genes expressed in quantitatively meaningful levels[3] in the nervous system are also expressed in other tissues. Some of these are expressed widely in other tissues, and are often referred to as *housekeeping enzymes*. Others, like many neurotransmitter receptor systems, occur in meaningful amounts in only a relatively few places outside the nervous system. Such *extra neural* expression can be responsible for *physiological side effects*. For instance, the cholinesterase inhibitors such as donepezil are used to increase the activity of the deficient acetylcholine-mediated circuits in Alzheimer brain. However, they inherently also stimulate acetylcholine-mediated systems in the gut. In some patients, the effects on the gut are clinically unimportant. In other patients, gastrointestinal symptoms, such as diarrhea or nausea and vomiting, become so prominent that these remedies have to be discontinued.[4] The majority of the medications discussed in this monograph fall into this third category; medications designed to work primarily on the nervous system, that is, to interact with molecules that are much more common in the nervous system than in other tissues.

BLOOD-BRAIN BARRIER

Some chemicals, including some drugs, readily enter the nervous system from the general circulation. Others do not. The ability of the brain to exclude some compounds effectively is referred to as the blood-brain barrier. The term is unfortunate. It can be misunderstood to imply that the barrier is a rigid entity. In fact, of course, the blood-brain barrier is a biological entity and therefore operates stochastically (i.e., by changing the odds that a particular molecule will enter the brain). It is more like a patrolled international border than like a brick wall. Its importance for treatment is that it reduces the number of drugs that can be used conveniently to treat diseases of the central nervous system. Of course, medications that do not readily cross the blood-brain barrier can be introduced directly into the brain through a hole in the skull. They can also enter the brain where brain damage has led to at least local breakdown of the barrier.

The discovery of the blood-brain barrier occurred over a hundred years ago. An investigator injected a rat with a blue dye, and found on autopsy that all the tissues were blue except the brain. Peripheral nerves were as blue as the rest of the body. The dye was water soluble and carried a charge (i.e., was a polar molecule). Later experiments showed that if a fat-soluble dye was used, the brain would take on color as well. Thus, the barrier is selective. Recent studies have identified the structures responsible for the blood-brain barrier as the processes surrounding small blood vessels in the central nervous system. These processes are derived from a particular type of brain cell (astrocytes, a type of glia).

The normal physiological function of the blood-brain barrier is to keep out molecules that would interfere with brain function if they got into the brain. Most such substances would probably be harmful. The evolutionary usefulness of the blood-brain barrier is to limit the likelihood that we will poison our brains if we eat or drink something we shouldn't. As humans spread out of Africa and encountered new plants and other potential foods, the protection given by the blood-brain barrier had an obvious evolutionary advantage. It may still, given current concerns about food additives. However, our species has been ingenious in finding natural substances that do cross the barrier readily and alter brain function. When used therapeutically, we call such substances medicines. When used for pleasure, we call them recreational drugs. When used to harm people, we call them poisons or, more formally, neurotoxins.

When the brain is damaged, the blood-brain barrier can break down. For instance, it typically breaks down in an area damaged by a stroke or tumor. Sometimes this can be deleterious, by letting in molecules better kept out. Sometimes it may be useful therapeutically, by allowing local entry of medications that would otherwise be effectively excluded. In treating diseases of the nervous system, it is important to remember the existence of the blood-brain barrier, and neither to overestimate nor to underestimate its importance.

PHARMACOKINETICS AND PHARMACODYNAMICS

In using a drug to treat an illness, it is important to have information about both how the drug gets to the site where it acts and what it does when it gets there. *Pharmacokinetics* deals with the first issue, *pharmacodynamics* with the second. Another way to describe the distinction is that pharmacokinetics deals with what the body does to the drug, and pharmacodynamics deals with what the drug does to the body.

Pharmacokinetics includes absorption, distribution, metabolism, and excretion of pharmaceutical agents. Pharmacokinetic properties are obviously more or less specific for each drug. This discussion will focus on questions directly relevant to clinical decision making. Detailed discussions of basic mechanisms of pharmacokinetics are available elsewhere. (See especially Goodman and Gilman.[1])

A basic clinical issue related to pharmacokinetics is how the drug can be given. Can it be absorbed effectively from the digestive tract, and therefore given orally? If not, where can it be injected safely (under the skin, into muscle, or directly into the blood stream)? Can a medicine that is normally used orally also be injected, for instance in patients who are unable or unwilling to take oral medication (e.g., unconscious or psychotic), or in whom a rapid onset of action is important? As every clinician knows, the fastest but usually most risky way to get a medication into the blood stream is to inject it directly into the blood stream (i.e., intravenously). The slowest but usually safest method is to give it orally. The rate of absorption after subcutaneous or intramuscular injections falls between that of oral and intravenous administration.

Whether or not the patient actually takes the medicine more or less as prescribed is usually more important than pharmacokinetic niceties about what time of day to take it or whether or not it should be taken with food. Formally, this is referred to as "the vexatious problem of compliance." We referred to it on my clinical service as "the contraceptive principle—nothing works in the bureau drawer." In practice, issues of compliance are usually quantitatively overwhelming compared to purportedly more "scientific" concerns. For instance, if taking a medicine on an empty stomach nauseates a patient, it is more useful for the patient to take the medicine with food than not to take it at all. That typically holds even if the PDR (physicians' desk reference)[5] or the package insert recommends that the medication be taken on an empty stomach. It is also important to remember that patients may be embarrassed to admit to a physician that they are not taking a medicine as prescribed. In eliciting this information, it is important not to be so judgmental as to turn the patient off. It is hard to know what to prescribe in the face of an apparent treatment failure without having information on what the patient has actually been ingesting. This information can be hard to get from some psychiatric patients. It can be a severe and dangerous problem in the community treatment of those psychotics who can become violent when they are off their medications. Sometimes a relative can provide important information, but relatives also have emotional needs that are inevitably reflected in their reports.

An unfortunately frequent problem in compliance among older people has been described as the "child from the other coast syndrome." The description of this syndrome resulted from events in an older woman referred for dementia. The patient had mild hypertension, perhaps related in part to recent geographical separation from a daughter who had remarried and moved to a distant state with her new husband and two children from a previous marriage. The patient doted on those grandchildren, and developed mild hypertension after their departure. The patient's internist carefully prescribed a mild antihypertensive, which the patient (in her grief and suppressed anger) did not take. However, she did not want to tell the nice doctor that she wasn't taking the pills he had prescribed. The internist carefully titrated up her medication, but even strong combinations of antihypertensives did not affect the patient's blood pressure because she did not take them. Among other reasons, she did not like the side effects of the stronger antihypertensives. However, she continued to assure her devoted doctor that she was faithfully taking all her medications just as he had prescribed. The daughter arrived back in New York to visit, and was appalled and guilty that her mother had not been taking the medicines the doctor had recommended. After several days on the carefully prescribed medication, the mother was delivered confused and moderately hypotensive to a hospital emergency room. She was treated effectively by discontinuation of all but the initial, mild antihypertensive and strong encouragement to tell the truth to her private physician.

Once absorbed, a drug is distributed in the body. How it is distributed depends on its chemical properties. Drugs that dissolve better in fats than in water tend to concentrate in tissues with high levels of fat, namely, the brain and adipose tissue. Fat-soluble drugs also tend to cross the blood-brain barrier more readily than water-soluble medications, as discussed above. A term used to refer to the distribution of a medication among tissues is the drug's *physiological volume of distribution*. Another important determinant of how a drug moves from the blood to the tissues is the amount of it that is free in the blood. Some drugs bind relatively effectively to plasma proteins and are thus partially sequestered within the blood stream. The dose of such a drug may have to be adjusted downward if the level of plasma proteins is reduced, for instance from liver disease or severe malnutrition. The dose may also have to be reduced if the drug in question is displaced from plasma protein by another necessary medication or other compound. Even some foods can displace certain drugs from plasma proteins. These effects of foods can be important in using standard medications for a number of psychiatric diseases. Finally, specific carrier mechanisms can concentrate some drugs into certain locations. The carrier mechanisms have evolved to move physiological materials, but drugs that are similar enough to the natural materials can be carried by the same mechanisms. Unfortunately, that may be true for some toxins as well. For instance, carrier mechanisms have been proposed to be responsible in part for MPTP's (1-Methyl-4-Phenyl-1,2,3,6-Tetrahydropyridine) relatively selective damage to the substantia nigra *pars compacta* with subsequent severe variants of Parkinson disease. (See Chap. 11, Disorders of Motility.)

Many but not all drugs are acted on by body metabolism. Sometimes that increases their effectiveness by the formation of more active metabolites. Often it leads to their conversion to forms that are less active and/or more readily excreted into the urine or stool, bile, or sweat. Often but not always, metabolism of drugs leads to their being made more water soluble (polar) and therefore more easily excreted into the urine. Of course, active metabolites can be formed on a pathway to inactivation. The pathways by which a drug is inactivated depend on the chemical structure of the drug and are more or less drug-specific.

Some general principles of drug inactivation do, however, impinge on clinical decision making. Many drugs are metabolized primarily in the liver, and doses of these drugs may need to be reduced in people with significant liver disease. Many drugs are excreted into the urine, and doses may need to be lowered in people with significant kidney disease. A large number of medications including many drugs used in psychiatry are inactivated by oxidation, specifically in the CYP (cytochrome P450) system. This system occurs in the cytoplasm of liver cells and to a lesser extent in the intestine. It utilizes a specific type of oxidizing molecule (cytochrome P-450), for which the system is named. The complexities of the CYP system have been elucidated in detail.[1] In clinical practice, it is important to remember: (1) that drugs and other chemicals can compete for this system, and (2) that some drugs can increase the level of the system (i.e., induce CYP). The rate at which a medication is acted on by the CYP system therefore depends significantly on what other medications or other compounds the patient is being exposed to. This is a prime example of drug interactions at the pharmacokinetic level.

Often obtaining the level of a drug in the blood of a patient provides a single measure that summarizes pharmacokinetic mechanisms for that drug in that patient. However, blood levels can also be misleading clinically. They are usually assumed to reflect the level of the drug when the rate of removal is equal to the rate at which the drug is being absorbed into the body, that is, the "steady-state" level reached when a "dynamic equilibrium" has been achieved. Measurement of a blood level of a medication when that level is either rising or falling does not provide a summary of the pharmacokinetics of the drug in that patient. Such "nonsteady state" measures can sometimes provide clinically useful information, however—for instance, on how fast a drug that has reached toxic levels is being removed from the body during treatment of an overdose. A second limitation on the usefulness of blood levels is that they should be used as a guideline, not a commandment.[6] Patients vary. In one patient, a blood level "in the therapeutic range" may be too much and cause toxic side effects. That patient may respond clinically to a lower dose that is not toxic *in that patient*. In principle, a particular patient might benefit from a higher than recommended blood level of a medication. However, prescribing that much of a medicine is risky, both for the patient and for the prescriber. The easier and safer explanation of why a drug is not effective even though it is present at a therapeutic blood level is that it is the wrong drug. These limitations on using blood levels as an individualized guide to dosage reflect considerations of both pharmacokinetics and pharmacodynamics.

Pharmacodynamics deals with the actions of the drug on the body. Those actions that are the desired effects of the treatment are by definition *therapeutic effects*. Those actions of a drug that are not desired are by definition *side effects*. Several factors influence the ratio of therapeutic effects to side effects. One is the inherent properties of the drug. For some drugs, the therapeutic effects occur at much, much lower doses than do side effects. This is true, for instance, of penicillin in people who do not have penicillin allergies. For other drugs, doses that provide a clinical benefit can be perilously close to toxic doses. Prime examples are *digitalis* alkaloids.[6] The term *therapeutic window* refers to the range between the therapeutic dose and the toxic dose. Penicillin has a large therapeutic window, digitalis a small one. The term *therapeutic index* summarizes that information in another form. It refers to the ratio of the dose at which 50% of patients develop significant side effects to the dose at which 50% of people receive significant therapeutic benefits. Drugs with a large therapeutic window and a high therapeutic index are easier for clinicians to use because they are safer for patients, that is, less likely to lead to side effects in normal clinical practice. As discussed above, side effects have a tendency to impair compliance. However, drugs with small therapeutic windows and low therapeutic indexes are sometimes the most effective and sometimes the only medications available to treat an illness effectively.

The pharmacodynamic mechanisms of medications that act on the nervous system vary markedly. Antibiotics typically inhibit specific enzymes or other metabolic processes in bacteria. General anesthetics typically alter the properties of membranes. Many drugs that act on the nervous system, and particularly in psychiatric illnesses, do so via their actions on neurotransmitter systems. In this monograph, the mechanisms by which specific drugs act are discussed with the commentary on the use of those medications for clinical indications. Excellent reviews of the pharmacodynamics of different classes of drugs and of individual drugs are available in the recent literature.[1]

Actions on neurotransmitter systems are of course actions on the major mechanisms by which nerve cells communicate with each other. Until the beginning of the twentieth century, neuroscientists in general assumed that the brain was a *syncytium* in which nerve cells communicated with each other through direct contacts. The work of Sir Henry Dale on acetylcholine established that excitable nerve cells (neurons) communicate with each other via chemical signals, that is, neurotransmitters. Recent work has shown that nerve cells also have direct contacts with each other. However, little is known about the functional importance of these direct contacts, and there is essentially no neuropharmacology related to them. In contrast, a mountain of data exists on neurotransmission and the neuropharmacology of neurotransmission. For most neurotransmitters, agents are available that can modify their manufacture (synthesis), their release into the synaptic cleft between neurons, their removal from those points of communication by uptake into cells (sequestration) or by breakdown, and their action on the "downstream" *postsynaptic* nerve cell (neuron). The actions on postsynaptic nerve cells are typically mediated through the action of a neurotransmitter on a receptor in that neuron. Agents that block the action of a neurotransmitter on its receptor are called *neurotransmitter antagonists.* Chemicals that directly mimic or otherwise increase the action of a neurotransmitter are known as *neurotransmitter agonists.* Other classes of agents can also modify the responses of specific receptors to specific neurotransmitters. Often drugs have effects on receptors in the nerve ending of the neuron that secretes the neurotransmitter of interest (the presynaptic nerve ending). Often neurotransmitters and medications that act on them have multiple actions. There are obviously many possibilities for individualized treatment based on the intricacies of these mechanisms. Knowledge of the relevant mechanisms constitutes the specialized field of clinical neuropharmacology.

As the dose of a drug is increased, new effects become prominent and sometimes overwhelming. This is summarized in the pharmacologist's saying that, "Different doses are different drugs." For instance, small doses of morphine relieve pain in most people. Large doses of morphine depress respiration in most people. In pharmacological terms, the lower doses act on the endorphin system to reduce pain perception, while the larger doses depress the brainstem respiratory center. When present, the clinical manifestations of the second effect dominate over the first, particularly if the patient stops breathing and dies. The need to consider dose effects adds yet another layer of complexity to neuropharmacology.

DRUG ACTION AND HUMAN VARIATION

The rapid advances in knowledge of human genetics have documented effects of specific gene variations on responses to specific medications. Genetic variations in components of the CYP system that metabolizes many drugs are well known to influence appropriate dosages of those drugs. Recent reviews describe the *pharmacogenetics* of drugs for psychoses.[7] Many human geneticists hope that it will be possible to collect genetic information rapidly and accurately enough within the clinical setting to allow practitioners to predict responses of specific patients to specific medications. Bringing that hope to fruition will require technical advances. It will also require improved understanding of interactions among different human genes involved in drug metabolism.[8]

No two human beings are identical. That is a critically important principle in treating patients and specifically those with disease of the nervous system. Each of us who is not an identical twin differs genetically from every other human being. Even for identical twins, environmental influences can create differences between them even in utero—for instance, a more severe intrauterine illness in one of the fetuses. Many studies document that even twins experience important environmental differences once they are born. Among the effects of environmental experiences are changes in DNA (deoxyribonucleic acid)—experience sculpts genes (epigenesis).[9] As life goes on, the effects of environmental variations accumulate. A cliché in geriatrics and gerontology is that old people tend to differ from each other even more than young people do, biologically as well as culturally. That is largely because of the different things that have happened to them during their long lives, including the effects of intercurrent illnesses. Because DNA is subject to damage that can be cell specific and by its nature "random," and because of technical limitations in studying it, it is impossible to know the genome of any adult individual at the level of individual bases in single living cells in that individual. (When we talk about "knowing the whole genome," we are stating an approximation.[10])

Environmental influences on an individual are relatively "random." Both genetic variation and environmental variation are formally "chaotic" in the sense of chaos theory. In other words, apparently minor events can have major consequences. (Consider, for instance, cancers caused by the impact of cosmic rays on DNA.)

Clinical studies accepted as highly informative are getting larger and larger, as computers and computer programs allow the efficient handling of more and more information and an increasingly wealthy society can afford to accumulate the necessary data. In principle, medical investigators continue to recognize that each human being differs from every other human being. In practice, clinical studies that lead to clinical guidelines now require making generalizations from larger and larger groups of people. Individual case reports are considered anecdotes, and studies of relatively small groups of individuals are not considered good guides to clinical practice. The high standards of epidemiology of the Cochrane database analyses are a good example. There are many advantages of using large studies in terms. Perhaps most important, they tend to limit potentially misleading conclusions that arise from random variations among small samples, that is, from statistical drift. But large studies can also have important disadvantages. Effects in significant subgroups can be lost—"washed out"—if the subgroups are unwittingly submerged in larger groups from whom they differ meaningfully. The larger the group being studied, the larger the groups whose variation from the average is easily lost unless appropriate statistical precautions are taken.

Clinical skill requires the ability to treat each patient as an individual, different from everyone else biologically as well as in terms of other aspects of humanity that are harder to define. That includes individualizing pharmacological therapy so that it is optimal for the individual being treated. In actual practice, recommended doses and medications provide a starting point for good care. If the patient responds to standard doses of standard medications, well and good. If not, or if side effects are unacceptable, the skilled clinician can modify doses or medications in the attempt to take better care of the patient. Sometimes doing so helps; sometimes it doesn't. None of us can help everyone, and there are some patients whom none of us can help. Medicolegal considerations are making it harder and harder—and riskier and riskier—to vary from textbook standards, that is, from "standard clinical practice in your area, doctor." But taking the best care we can of those who come to us for help requires individualization of care, often beyond the constraints of textbook teaching. We are taking care of our fellow human beings, not laboratory rats or other experimental animals. The results in one rat that differs from the other eleven in an experiment can be disregarded, and there are rigorous statistical tests to allow legitimately discarding such "aberrant" observations. With human beings, each individual matters, even those who respond differently than most other patients who have been placed in the same diagnostic category. The patient who suffers a side effect suffers, even if theoretical formulations and the pronouncements of pharmaceutical companies proclaim that side effect to be aberrant.

TALK THERAPY AND DRUG THERAPY

Although this volume focuses on treatment of the nervous system with medicines—that is, on clinical neuropharmacology—nothing written here is meant to disparage the importance of nonpharmacological *talk therapies*. Counseling is a vital part of the management of any chronic or recurrent disease. That is at least as true for diseases of the nervous system as for diseases of other organ systems like the heart or lungs or liver.

The following example illustrates such a nonpharmacological therapy.

> A young woman was brought to the hospital after taking a life-threatening overdose of a sedative in a well-thought-through suicide attempt. Her breathing was supported mechanically, and her blood pressure was maintained in a healthy range with intravenous pressors. After a few days, the drug in her system had been metabolized down to a level that allowed her to wake up and maintain her own physiological functions unaided. She then explained that she had taken the overdose because her boyfriend had left her. On closer questioning, it turned out that a major reason he had left her was that he had become sleep deprived. She had been waking up in the middle of the night nearly every night, and keeping him awake with her weeping and pacing. She had also become unattractively thin, and her sex drive had dwindled to nearly nothing. The young woman was treated successfully with an antidepressant to which she responded, first as an inpatient and then as an outpatient. However, even when the biological imbalance in her brain had been well treated, she still faced difficult problems. Her boyfriend was now engaged to marry another woman. At work, she had been moved off the "fast-track" because she had performed so poorly on her job during her depression. Many of the people who had been her good friends were now much more distant, in part because of the things she had said and done while depressed. The woman needed support and counseling while getting her life back in order. She needed follow-up to monitor her continued compliance with her medication, including the maintenance doses she went on after the severe depression had cleared. She also needed follow-up because of the risk of another suicide attempt, since one of the main risk factors for successful suicide is a previous unsuccessful suicide attempt.
>
> This young woman initially needed intensive medical treatment to maintain key physiological functions so that she did not die as a result of her overdose. She then needed neuropharmacological treatment—specifically, antidepressant medicine—to correct the chemical imbalance in her brain that had led to her pathological sadness. But then, as a human being, she needed counseling, not only to maintain herself on the regimen necessary for her health but also to help her put her life back together.

There are aberrations of behavior that neither need nor benefit from treatment with medicine. These include aberrations of behavior that were primarily learned, often at a young age. Medication is seldom an appropriate way to treat existential angst or guilt about one's normal sexuality induced by an excessively rigid home. Those kinds of problems are better dealt with by talk therapies, including psychotherapy and psychoanalysis. A number of controlled studies support the effectiveness of psychotherapy based on current concepts in experimental psychology, namely, *cognitive-behavioral therapy* (CBT). Talk therapy is often valuable for a suffering person. It is not, however, the subject of this monograph. This book is about neuropharmacology. However, nothing written here is meant to demean the importance of counseling for people with brain disease, particularly disease with prominent psychiatric manifestations. A wide and excellent literature discusses the broader issues of nonpharmacological approaches to psychiatric diseases.

REFERENCES

1. A classic monograph is Cooper JR, Bloom F, Roth RH. *The Biochemical Basis of Neuropharmacology*. NY, Oxford, 7th ed, Oxford University Press, 1996. This book, which is suitable for medical and graduate students as well as clinicians in practice, provides an informative, accurate, and relatively concise discussion of how drugs work on the nervous system at the neurobiological level.

   For more complete discussions of the neurobiology, an impressively perceptive but older reference is Kandel ER, Schwartz JH, Jessel TM. *Principles of Neural Science*. 3d ed, Elsevier, New York, 1991. A new edition is reportedly in preparation.

   A recent, useful compendium of psychiatric medications is Sadock BJ, Sadock VA. *Pocket Handbook of Psychiatric Drug Treatment*. 3d ed, New York, Lippincott Williams & Wilkins, 2001. This relatively short monograph is oriented around medications rather than disease entities. It is rich in useful tables, including tables of drug interactions and side effects. An encyclopedic volume (1296 large pages) is Shatzberg AF, Cole JD, DeBattista C, *Textbook of Psychopharmacology*, 3d ed, American Psychiatric Publishing, 2004.

   Detailed discussions of the pharmacology of agents of interest can be found in Hardman JG, Limbird LE. *Goodman and Gilman's The Pharmacological Basis of Therapeutics*. This book remains a classic American text on pharmacology. It includes first rate, erudite discussions of medications that act on the nervous system.

2. When I was a second-year medical student, we were taught that the properties of halothane were close to those of the ideal anesthetic. When I came back after a year's research fellowship, we were taught that halothane should be used only under special circumstances because it could induce acute and sometimes fatal liver failure. This was an important lesson in my medical education, and not because I was ever in a position to give a patient halothane. This experience taught me that medical knowledge is always provisional. That generalization applies emphatically to what is written in this monograph.

   Guidelines arrived at in *consensus conferences* are also inherently provisional. Consensus conferences have been referred to as *Delphic conferences*. That terminology is appropriate, since the oracles at Delphi were typically misunderstood. (Oedipus was not the only one who got it wrong.)
3. About 25 years ago, there was great interest in genes that were expressed only in the nervous system. This interest was sparked by reports of mRNAs (messenger ribonucleic acids) in brain extracts that were not found in extracts of other tissues. At that time, "brain-specific gene expression" was considered a potential explanation of unique properties of the nervous system. However, these "unique" messages are present in low concentrations if at all. Direct demonstrations of their biological significance are lacking, and interest in them has waned.
4. Loss of bowel control can be a major issue for both the patient and caregivers. Anecdotally, it has been a reason for placement in a nursing home. Bowel incontinence can be a potentially fatal complication, if it leads to calling in the "mercy squad" because of "quality-of-life" issues (i.e., to deciding it is time to stop effective medical care because the patient's life has become so unpleasant). Nausea and vomiting, potentially leading to aspiration, are obviously dangerous. They call for stopping a medicine, unless that medicine is necessary to maintain life or reasonable health.
5. Physician's Desk Reference: Descriptions of medications in the PDR are the same as those in package inserts.
6. The same considerations are true for other biological rather than clinical indicators of when a patient has received enough of a medicine. During my residency in internal medicine in the 1960s, we were taught that a patient was not "fully digitalized" until a *digitalis* effect was evident on the ECG (electrocardiogram). In other words, standard practice was to induce mild *digitalis* toxicity. That may be one of the reasons we ended up treating so much serious *digitalis* toxicity. Happily for patients in atrial fibrillation whose heart rate was being controlled with *digitalis*, the clinical benefit was accepted as a therapeutic end point even without a "dig effect" by ECG. In these patients, even at that time we adjusted the dose of medicine according to clinical effect rather than to physiological theories.
7. Malhotra AK, Murphy GM Jr, Kennedy JL. Pharmacogenetics of psychotropic drug response. *Am J Psychiatry.* 2004;161:780–796.

8. Basile VS, Masellis M, Potkin SG, Kennedy JL. Pharmacogenetics in schizophrenia: the quest for individualized therapy. *Hum Mol Genet.* 2002; 11:2517–2530.
9. Fraga MF, Ballestar E, Paz MF, et al. Epigenetic differences arise during the lifetime of monozygotic twins. *Proc Natl Acad Sci USA.* 2005;102: 10604–10609.
   Martin GM. Epigenetic drift in aging identical twins. *Proc Natl Acad Sci USA.* 2005;102:10413–10414.
10. Of course, describing that approximation enthusiastically plays well in both the lay and the scientific media. The limitations on genetic data are now receiving wider attention by the public.

CHAPTER THREE

Mood Disorders: Depression and Mania

There are many reasons for people to be miserably unhappy and many reasons for them to be wildly elated. When troubled mood results from biological abnormalities of the brain, physicians have special skills to offer. We are trained in human biology, and our medical licenses allow us to prescribe drugs. Unless the neurobiological abnormalities are treated effectively in the affected people, the damage to their brains prevents them from incorporating even the wisest counsel into their lives. Physicians may also, by dint of special training or native ability, be effective at counseling troubled people. Clinical psychologists, clergy, or other appropriately trained nonmedical personnel can also be useful as counselors. A specific type of psychotherapy, *cognitive-behavioral therapy*, has been reported to be as beneficial as medications in treating mild depression. Nonmedical counselors are not, however, as effective as physicians at helping people who require not only *talk therapy* but also medical treatment for the chemical imbalances in their brains. The need for talk therapy to accompany drug therapy is emphasized both in the body of the text below and in the stories of the individual patients used as examples. This discussion assumes that physicians will be complete doctors and treat the whole patient. However, this monograph focuses on treatment with medications.

It is important for general clinicians to recognize mood disorders in their patients and to institute prompt and appropriate treatment. Precise diagnosis and choice of treatment is best done by or in consultation with a psychiatrist. Mood disorders can be life-threatening. Textbook teaching is that left to themselves these diseases get worse, particularly *manic-depressive disease*. Not treating mood disorders is analogous to not treating heart failure. The damaged organ is likely to deteriorate more rapidly without treatment than with proper management.

The words *mania* and *manic* are usually used in a more or less restricted medical sense, but the word *depression* has a confusing variety of meanings in ordinary language. In common parlance, it can mean anything from culturally adaptive *Weltschmerz* to a life-threatening form of madness. General clinicians should be aware that depression fills more hospital beds than do many common "real medical illnesses." Both depression and manic-depressive disease can lead to suicide, and patients who kill themselves end up just as dead as if they had died of cancer or of heart disease.

DEPRESSION

Depression is one of the most common diseases of the nervous system seen by general clinicians in their patients. Treatment with antidepressant medications helps people with so many superficially different clinical syndromes that discussion of the neuropharmacology of depression and antidepressants is appropriate in the beginning of this monograph.

The word *depression* in this monograph refers to negative alterations in mood that have as a major component a biological and functionally significant abnormality in the modulation of mood (*affect*) by the brain. As noted earlier, treatment with medication and sometimes with even more drastic biological interventions is typically necessary for people with these neurobiological abnormalities, in addition to counseling.

The characteristic complex of signs and symptoms that characterizes medical depression appears to reflect functional deficiency of the neurotransmitters serotonin and often also norepinephrine. The diagnosis is, however, clinical. There is no laboratory test for depression or mania.

Classification and Diagnosis

The current American classification of types of depression and the diagnostic terms it uses are defined clinically, not biologically. The classification was developed by consensus committees. There is no reason to think that the behaviorally defined syndromes it describes represent discrete biological entities. Indeed, there is good reason to think that they do not. Drugs that work on the same biological mechanisms are effective in different behaviorally defined types of depression. The widely cited example for depression is medication that increases the efficiency of a specific neurotransmitter—*serotonin*. These drugs are helpful not only in the various subtypes of depression but also in a number of other psychiatric syndromes, including anxiety disorders and obsessive-compulsive behavior. Years ago, all these syndromes were thought of as variant behavioral expressions of the same underlying disease. The term used for them was *depressive equivalents*. That terminology has been dropped in favor of a more detailed classification of psychiatric disorders (Table 3-1).

TABLE 3–1

Classifications of mood disorders in DSM IV

Mood episodes
Major depressive episode
Manic episode
Mixed episode
Hypomanic episode
Depressive disorders
Major depressive disorder (296.xx)
Dysthymic disorder (300.40)
Depressive disorder not otherwise specified (311.00)
Bipolar disorders
Bipolar I disorder (296.xx)
Bipolar II disorder (296.89)
Cyclothymic disorder (301.13)
Bipolar disorder not otherwise specified (296.80)
Other mood disorders
Mood disorder due to (*indicate the general medical condition.*) (293.83)
Substance-induced mood disorder (29x.xx)
Mood disorder not otherwise specified (296.90)

The numbers in parentheses are the numerical codes used for the specific conditions. DSM-IV provides detailed lists of the abnormalities necessary and sufficient to distinguish these different categories of mood disorder from each other. These have been carefully worked out by consensus committees.

It is instructive to compare the classifications of depressions in the first and in more recent versions of the Diagnostic and Statistical Manual of the American Psychiatric Association (DSM). In *DSM I* in 1952, five types of depression were listed. Four were classified under *Psychotic Disorders*. They were:

manic-depressive reaction, manic type

manic-depressive reaction, depressive type

manic-depressive reaction, other types

psychotic depression

The fifth type, depressive reaction, was listed under Psychoneurotic Disorders. In DSM IV, in 1994, the list was three times as long (Table 3-1).

The general clinician can be confident of seeing patients who need treatment with a medicine that ameliorates depression. Brain disorders that lead to this symptom complex and benefit from medication occur in something between 10% and 15% of the population, depending on the population and the definitions used. The conventional numbers for the one-year prevalence of serious depression in the United States are 4–8%, again depending on definition. Many individuals seek medical help for what turns out to be a depressive illness. Often their complaints are somatic rather than psychiatric. Such somatic complaints may be vague, but can be misleadingly precise, particularly in medically sophisticated individuals. A classic example of "masked depression of the high achiever"[1] is *pseudo angina* in a physician with an underlying depressive disorder. Abnormalities in sexual functioning typically accompany depression and can be the presenting problem. Anger rather than overt sadness can be the most obvious clinical abnormality of a depression. The anger can be focused on a spouse and precipitate divorce. Depression associated with menopause (*involutional psychosis*) can lead to divorce in what had previously appeared to be a stable marriage. *Involutional melancholia* can also lead to suicide in a woman who was medically and psychiatrically well before the hormonal storms of menopause, and would have been well after they had subsided had she survived.

Neurobiology of Depression

Both hereditary and environmental factors play a role in causing depression, as they do in most complex groups of illnesses. Sometimes one and sometimes the other appear to be more important in a particular patient.

Previous classifications of types of depression reflected those differences. *Psychotic depression* was depression where endogenous, probably genetic factors played the major role, and only limited environmental stress was needed to precipitate an acute attack. *Depressive reaction* was a bout of depression precipitated by a stress in the environment, although the person presumably had an inherent genetic predisposition to that reaction. As the molecular genetics of depression becomes clearer, those descriptive terms have been recognized as carrying little biological information. An analogy is the way the terms *infectious hepatitis* and *serum hepatitis* dropped from clinical use once the relevant viruses became known and readily identifiable in clinical practice. Psychiatrists in the United States no longer use the term *reactive depression.*

Gene-Environment Interactions: Modern molecular genetics has demonstrated specific gene-environment interactions in causing depression. A clear example has recently been demonstrated at the Institute of Psychiatry of the University of London (UK).[2] It involves a gene that encodes a component of the transporter for serotonin. More precisely, it involves a genetic variation in the region of that gene that influences the rate at which the gene is transcribed, that is, in the *promoter* region. Depressive symptoms and full-blown and often suicidal depression are more likely to develop after stressful life events in people with the short form of this gene than in those with the long form. This genetic variation is a clear example of a *susceptibility gene* for depression. Other molecular genetic data implicate other susceptibility gene loci as biological predispositions to becoming depressed. Those data are too extensive to discuss in any detail here. They provide molecular evidence at the DNA (deoxyribonucleic acid) level that supports the long-standing clinical impression that certain people suffer from a susceptibility to depression, that is, a *depressive diathesis.* In any individual patient, the clinical (i.e., behavioral) expression of such a genetic predisposition will depend on a number of factors, including the individual's other genes (*genetic background*) and life experiences. The latter will include how the patient has been taught to respond to stress, particularly what he or she was taught as a child. In some individuals, a genetic variation alone seems to be adequate to cause depressions, even in the absence of unusually stressful life events.

Other genes associated with depression are also being identified. There is a relatively weak association with the gene coding for a protein necessary for the synthesis of serotonin in the brain, namely, tryptophan hydroxylase 2 (*TPH2*).[3] Patients with this genetic abnormality, which interferes with the synthesis of serotonin, appear to be relatively unlikely to benefit from medications that spare serotonin, such as the SSRIs discussed later. Abnormalities in genes encoded on the DNA in mitochondria (mtDNA) have also been suggested to be associated with depression in general, and variation in a gene coding for a stress response (*CRH1*, encoding the corticotrophin releasing hormone receptor) with prominent anxiety in depressed people (anxious depression).

Other investigators have identified genes that are copied (*transcribed*) in abnormal amounts in the brains of patients with depression. For technical reasons, they have had to select which genes to study. (The *gene chip* methods they use only allow looking at perhaps 1/10 of human genes at a time [i.e., 10% of the human genome]). Understandably, they have generally chosen genes implicated as "reasonable candidates" by the major current theories of depression. Their studies confirm the importance in depression of the mechanisms they chose to study (i.e., genes involved in monoamine neurotransmission). More detailed examination of the whole human genome will be necessary to determine the abnormalities of gene expression that are most prominent in depression. Changes in the extent to which a gene is expressed (transcribed) can reflect reactions to, rather than causes of, the disease process. It would not be surprising if that included relatively wide panoply of genes. The fragments of data available suggest other genes may also be important in mood disorders.

The Bioamine Model: The major neurobiological mechanism by which the genetic and environmental causes of depression express themselves involves a specific subset of the chemicals by which nerve cells communicate with each other. These are the *monoamine neurotransmitters serotonin* (*5-hydroxytryptamine* [5-HT]) and *norepinephrine* (*noradrenalin*). This *bioamine hypothesis* is a particularly relevant model for clinical neuropharmacology.[4] To simplify greatly, this hypothesis states that the biological basis of depression is a functional deficiency in the brain of serotonin (5-HT) or of *norepinephrine* (NE) or of both. Extensive neurochemical and genetic data support this hypothesis. For instance, the gene mentioned in the previous paragraph that predisposes to depression affects serotonin metabolism. Neuropharmacological support for this hypothesis comes from the observation that medicines that relieve depression typically act on neurotransmitter systems involving serotonin and often NE. Selective serotonin reuptake inhibitors (SSRIs) and other newer antidepressants appear to have much more effect on serotonin than on NE systems. However, some of the other newer antidepressants such as *bupropion* (Wellbutrin, Zyban) appear to act primarily on NE pathways and to a lesser extent on *dopamine* synapses. The older tricyclic antidepressants act on both serotonin and NE systems and sometimes on other neurotransmitter systems—for instance, that involving *acetylcholine*. Inhibitors of the enzyme *monoamine oxidase* (MAO inhibitors) are an effective if clinically risky group of antidepressants that act on both serotonin and NE and also on dopamine. The relation between deficiency of serotonin and deficiency of noradrenalin in depression is complex and unsettled. The *somatic signs* of depression tend to reflect functional deficiency of serotonin more than that of epinephrine. For instance, depression is associated with sleep disorders rather than with low blood pressure. Even antidepressants that appear to act primarily on NE mechanisms tend to clear up the somatic manifestations of *central serotonergic deficiency* listed below. The pharmacological rationale for this observation is not certain.

Recently, a flurry of interest has arisen about the role of another signal compound in depression, namely, the neurotransmitter *y-aminobutyric acid* (GABA). Functional deficiency of GABA is associated with anxiety disorders. (See Chap. 6, Anxiety.) It is therefore tempting to speculate that depressed patients with GABA deficiencies are likely to be anxious as well (i.e., have *anxious depressions*). Some animal data support that idea, but whether it is true for humans remains uncertain.

The structure and metabolism of a specific part of the brain, the *orbitofrontal cortex*, may be abnormal in a significant proportion of depressed patients, according to studies with modern imaging techniques. Those observations are compatible with the chemical and pharmacological mechanisms, in terms of the known connections among nerve cells (*neural circuitry*) and the signal compounds (*neurotransmitters*) involved.

Structural damage to the brain can lead to disorders of mood if it affects parts of the brain that mediate the modulation of mood. Typically, such damage involves the parts that contain cells using the neurotransmitters discussed in the last paragraph. (The principle is known as gangsters' neurochemistry: "Dead cells make no neurotransmitters.") The most common mood disorder resulting from brain damage is depression. Brain damage causing a mood disorder can arise from a variety of sources. Among these are unusual manifestations of infections of the brain, including later effects of syphilis. (This disease is known historically as "the great imitator.") Patients with new onset depression deserve a blood test for syphilis, even though the diagnostic yield of untreated disease is likely to be very low. In areas where *Lyme disease* is endemic, they deserve a blood test for that disorder as well.

In older people, two common causes of depression are vascular disease (stroke) and degenerative diseases (e.g., Alzheimer disease, Parkinson disease, Lewy body disease, and so on.) At least two types of *depressive syndrome* can be distinguished in the elderly. One is recurrent depression in people who have suffered from depressions on and off throughout their life. These individuals often have a family history of depression, as would be suggested by the gene-environment interactions. In them, the mechanisms leading to the mood disorder are likely to be the same as they were in younger people: indeed, in themselves when they were younger. In other elderly people, the first episode of clinically relevant depression occurs when they are older and often in conjunction with a brain injury. Depression frequently follows stroke, perhaps more often strokes involving the left (*dominant*) side of the brain than the right. Depression is also often associated with brain damage due to a degenerative disease. Marshall Folstein and his colleagues suggested, on the basis of autopsy studies, that depression in Alzheimer disease (AD) tends to be more associated with damage to the noradrenergic *locus ceruleus* than with the serotonergic *raphe nuclei*. Nevertheless, elderly patients with depression including depression in AD characteristically respond to medications that act primarily on the serotonin system (such as the SSRIs).

Thus, from the viewpoint of clinical neuropharmacology, the question of whether or not to treat with an antidepressant comes down to whether or not there is clinical evidence that there is likely to be a functional deficiency of a biogenic amine transmitter in the brain. The more important of these neurotransmitters is probably serotonin, even though experimental studies indicate that a number of effective antidepressant work more on NE-mediated synapses than on serotonergic systems. The question of whether or not to prescribe modern "antidepressant" medication for a specific patient can therefore be rephrased in more biological terms. Is the patient likely to have a functional deficiency of a biogenic amine in the brain—and specifically of serotonin?

Recognition of Central Biogenic Amine Deficiency

Unfortunately, clinically convenient biological tests for central serotonergic deficiency are not yet available. Metabolic studies in patients with severe depression tend to show decreased function in dominant (left-sided) prefrontal structures, that is, reduced blood flow or reduced utilization of glucose and oxygen. This observation has not reached the level of diagnostic usefulness. Measurements of serotonin or its major metabolite (*5-hydroxyindoleacetic acid*) in spinal fluid or in urine[5] are also inconvenient and have not been adopted into ordinary clinical practice. One can hope that clinically applicable techniques to diagnose central serotonergic deficiency will come out of the development of specific molecular probes combined with modern brain imaging technology (MRI [*magnetic resonance imaging*], PET [*positron emission tomography*], and SPECT [*single-photon emission computerized tomography*]). Perhaps molecular genetics will help. At the time of this writing, however, those pious hopes were irrelevant to clinical practice, except perhaps in a few specialized research centers. Therefore, when diagnosing central bioamine (serotonin) deficiency in patients who are pathologically sad or have other manifestations consistent with depression, the clinician must look for *clinical* clues implicating central serotonergic dysfunction.

The clinician can do so by looking at several physiological functions modulated in part by serotonin. One is sleep. Application of serotonin to the *suprachiasmatic nucleus* (*preoptic area*) induces slow-wave sleep in animals. Treatment of animals with an inhibitor of the conversion of tryptophan to serotonin impairs sleep. Clinically, ingestion of the serotonin precursor *tryptophan* can induce sleep. Another effect of serotonin is on appetite. It can enhance appetite even in invertebrates. Its actions on feeding behavior in mammals including our species may be mediated via a specific part of the brain, namely, the *hypothalamus* and particularly the *paraventricular nucleus* and the *lateral hypothalamic area.* Serotonin also effects human sexuality. It is a transmitter for the sexually *dimorphic nucleus* of the thalamus in experimental animals and presumably in humans as well. Still another effect of serotonin is on bowel movement. This is believed to be mediated by serotonin in specific cells of the bowel (the *enterochromaffin cells*). Many patients who respond to treatment with serotonergic medication with improvement of mood also tend to normalize their bowel movements. Therefore, evidence of serotonergic dysfunction in depression is not limited to the central nervous system but occurs in cells in the bowel as well.

The apparent defect in serotonin in cells in the gut has interesting theoretical implications for the etiology of serotonergic dysfunction in depression. It is hard to see how *psychogenic stressors* would induce serotonergic deficiency in the large bowel, in cells that are not in direct contact with the nervous system. If that is true for cells of the gut, it is likely to be true as well for cells of the brain. That view agrees with the molecular genetic data.[2]

As the discussion earlier indicates, serotonergic deficiency can lead to the characteristic "somatic signs of depression," namely:

- sleep abnormalities (often sleeplessness and particularly early morning wakefulness; sometimes excessive sleep [*hypersomnolence*])
- eating difficulties (often weight loss, sometimes weight gain)
- decreased sex drive
- constipation in younger people (Constipation is not a reliable sign of depression in older people, because they often complain of constipation anyway.)

The presence of this constellation of somatic signs should increase a clinician's index of suspicion of a neurobiologically based depressive syndrome even in a patient who has somatic complaints or "free-floating anger" but denies a depressed mood.

Part of the workup for patients with weight problems, including obesity, is to check for an underlying mood disorder. People with mood disorders tend to have weight problems. Many lose weight, often to the point of malnutrition and even starvation. Some gain weight to the point of malignant obesity. People can try to eat their way out of sadness. Manic patients can gain weight because they carry eating, like their other activities, to excess. Further, some of the medications used to treat depression can also lead to weight gain. Patients with mood disorders are at risk not only for malnutrition but also for medical complications of obesity including the *metabolic syndrome*.

Excessive amounts of serotonin can cause disease as striking as that caused by relative deficiency. *Carcinoid syndrome* is a relatively clean example of serotonin poisoning in humans. Serotonin excess can cause apparently psychotic behavior, sometimes including mania. A number of toxins that can induce psychotic manifestations have structures that resemble serotonin. A classic example is LSD (*d-lysergic acid diethylamide*). Chapter 4 (Thought Disorders) discusses these issues, as does Chap. 14 (Disorders of Conduct.) Thus, both too much and too little serotonin is harmful, as expected for a living system that depends on balance (*homeostasis*). Of interest, serotonin receptors have been identified that both reduce the symptoms of depression and anxiety ($5HT_{1A}$) and increase those symptoms ($5HT_{2A}$). The antidepressant nefazodone is believed to stimulate the former and antagonize the latter.

Clinical Course of Depression

Episodes of depressions tend to be recurrent but self-limited (unless the patient commits suicide). The tendency of depressions to recur is in accord with the gene-environment interactions. The genetic predisposition (*diathesis*) is permanent, and disappointments and other stressful life events are part of normal life. Losses are hard to avoid, particularly as one gets older and one's contemporaries get older and sicker and die. Some clinicians think of depression as a chronic disease with episodes of *flares* and periods of remission, rather like *gout* or *lupus*. Bouts of mania typically recur in manic-depressive disease. The tendency to recur raises the question of how long medication should be given in the treatment of mood disorders. This is discussed under medications for these disorders.

MANIA

Clinically, mania is often described as the "mirror image" of depression. Instead of being inappropriately sad, patients are inappropriately elated. They tend to need little sleep. Their appetites are good, often excessive. Their sex drive is usually increased. Instead of being hopeless, they are typically full of plans—often grandiose and unrealistic plans. Instead of feeling helpless, they typically describe being powerful and become irritable if people disagree with them. When severely manic (*hypermanic*), their irritation can trigger violent incidents. As they get more and more manic, they can become so angry at having their power and their decisions questioned that they act paranoid. Severe mania is often associated with frank hallucinations and delusions. It then merges into a syndrome hard to distinguish from a primary thought disorder, that is, from a form of *schizophrenia*. (See Chap. 4, Thought Disorders.) One of the physical types associated with recurrent episodes of mania is the loud, pushy, "oversexed" man with a charming manner who is often strikingly attractive to women, at least transiently. Women who suffer from mania can be strikingly attractive to men, for similar reasons. The relation between mania and *hypersexuality* is also discussed in Chap. 14 (Disorders of Conduct).

However, it is simplistic to think of manic patients as "happy." First, despite the often-infectious elation and "manic humor" of these patients, they tend to come across as more pressured than happy. The observer may get the impression that their mania is a way to try to hold off depression.[6] Second, the victims of this condition can often be strikingly successful, at least in the short run, if the mania does not become debilitating. Thus, *hypomania* tends to be associated with worldly success if not with stable relationships. That is particularly true in certain professions that put a premium on charisma, such as the theater and related media. A classic example is the "manic clown." Another is the theatrical producer who is hated by the cast but puts on shows that are smashes. Physicians who are proud that they enjoy working through the night without sleep may want to be careful about how loosely they use the terms manic or mildly manic (*hypomanic*).[7]

Neurobiologically, less is known confidently about the causes and mechanisms in mania than in depression. Genetic factors have been studied more intensively in relation to manic-depressive disease than to "pure" mania. The efficacy of *lithium* in treating mania has led to investigations of *phospholipid metabolism* in mania. Robust, compelling findings are unfortunately lacking. In a few percent of patients, treatment with drugs that increases central serotonergic activity leads to episodes of mania. It would be attractive if there was convincing evidence for a "serotonin hypothesis of mood," that is, too little serotonin ⇒ depression; too much serotonin ⇒ mania. Unfortunately, a clear and robust relationship between mania and any specific neurotransmitter(s) or intracellular messenger(s) has not yet been identified.[8]

Patients who experience bouts of mania without any bouts of depression are rare. The depressive episodes may be short and well-hidden, but it is when they crash that patients who have come through bouts of mania are at the highest risk of killing themselves. In the rest of this monograph, mania is discussed in the context of manic-depressive disease—in modern terminology, *bipolar disease*.

MANIC-DEPRESSIVE DISEASE

Clinically, as noted in the preceding paragraph, if one looks closely enough, most patients who appear to have only episodes of mania also have at least subtle manifestations of depression between manic attacks. Of course, even "normal" people are sometimes happier and sometimes sadder, often in reaction to the pleasures and pains inherent in the human condition.[9] They may sometimes benefit from counseling—for instance, during grief after a loved one has died. They do not need drug therapy. Pathological variations from an average state of contentedness (*euthymia*) do, however, typically benefit from treatment with medications.

Classification and Diagnosis

The term *Bipolar I* refers to a form of manic-depressive disease in which mania predominates clinically; and *Bipolar II* to a form of manic-depressive disease in which depression predominates. Bipolar II disorder is easy to confuse with pure depression unless a detailed and accurate history can be obtained. This distinction is important for choosing the right medication. The distinction between manic-depressive disease and *schizophrenia* or *schizoaffective disorder* can also be difficult to make clinically, particularly in people who are crazy. Fortunately, the treatment of the acute psychotic phase of both of these clinical entities can be the same. In fact, the distinctions among these syndromes serve mostly as statistical guides to counseling the patient and family and to deciding which medication to prescribe first. The aim is to find a medication regimen that works for the individual patient. Overlaps are so large that individualization of treatment should be guided by empirical experience in the particular patient being treated. Syndromic distinctions do not clearly separate, for instance, lithium-responsive mental disease from SSRI-responsive mental disease or neuroleptic requiring mental disease. Objective studies of primary care physicians indicate that they frequently mistake patients with manic-depressive disease (bipolar disease) for patients with depression alone (unipolar depression). Since treatment with antidepressants alone can precipitate mania in a patient with bipolar disease, this clinical diagnostic distinction is important. Detailed questioning about states of excessive elation and energy may be difficult with depressed patients, but family and other informants may provide the critical information to guide the choice of treatment.

As discussed, both manic and depressive episodes tend to be recurrent, although frequently self-limited. Maintenance treatment as well as treatment for acute episodes are usually indicated. There are unfortunate people who cycle rapidly between mania and depression, sometimes even within a few days. Such "rapid cyclers" need specialist treatment by a qualified psychiatrist.

The term *cyclothymia* refers to the condition in which the ups and downs of mood are prominent but are not severe enough to reach criteria for mania or depression. Cyclothymic people can be strikingly successful if often difficult to live with. Judging when to treat mood swings without interfering with a person's productivity can be a difficult and necessarily subjective decision.

Neurobiology

Genetics: Strong and increasing data support a genetic predisposition to manic-depressive disease.[10,11] For instance, having a first degree relative with bipolar disease increased risk for this condition, over tenfold, in a population-based study in Denmark.[11] Some of the genetic loci that have been implicated for a predisposition to manic-depressive (bipolar) disease have also been associated with other kinds of psychoses, including schizophrenia. (See Chap. 1, Introduction, section on Classification and Diagnosis, and Chap. 4, Thought Disorders, section on Neurobiology.) Other loci appear more specific for bipolar disorders. Anatomic abnormalities of the brain have also been reported in some patients with bipolar disorder—specifically, increase in the ratio of gray-to-white matter in specific regions.

SUICIDE

Clinicians are obligated to worry about the possibility of suicide in patients with mood disorders. That is true even though suicide is actually almost as common in *psychoses* such as schizophrenia as in disorders of mood such as depression or bipolar disease.[12] Suicide, of course, kills a person just as dead as do "medical" conditions such as cancer or heart attack or stroke. In theory, suicide is always a preventable death. In practice, no way is known to prevent all suicides. In retrospect, however, family and physicians frequently convince themselves that the suicide of the person they were trying to help could have been prevented, if only they had been smart enough or loving enough. Despite all efforts, suicide remains a major cause of death among young people, even though the demographic group most likely to commit successful suicide is older white men.

Risk factors for suicide have been an area of intensive study (Table 3-2). The most powerful single predictor is a previous suicide attempt. Even patients whose previous suicide attempts have been "just gestures" have to come closer to completion in subsequent "suicide attempts" in order to get the people whose attention they want to keep worrying about their suicidality. One of these increasingly serious attempts may actually kill the person, even if the person who committed suicide actually only wanted to make another gesture. Suicide rates peak in older people, and

TABLE 3–2
Major risk factors for suicide

Risk factor	Specifics
Previous suicide attempt	Often associated with mood disorder
Age	Elderly > adolescents > others
Sex	Men > women
Race	White > Black
Religion	Protestant, Jewish, or secular > Roman Catholic
Marital status	Single > married
Socioeconomic status	High and low status > average status
Method used	Violent, irreversible > overdoses
Physical illnesses	Particularly fatal, painful illnesses and those causing psychiatric problems
Psychiatric illness	Particularly mood disorders

are higher in adolescents than in adults or children. That is particularly true for men, who have a higher rate of completed suicide than women. White people have consistently committed suicide more than Black people, although that may be changing. Suicide in inner cities is not rare. Whether some of the violence in inner cities results from suicidal behavior is not clear. The Roman Catholic Church teaches that suicide is a sin, and at least in the United States, Roman Catholics are less likely to kill themselves than are people of other religious traditions, including secular people who deny having any religion. Married people are less likely to commit suicide than single people. Perhaps that is in part because they have better support systems and also because they are more immediately aware of the effect their suicide would have on those who love them. Both high socioeconomic status and low socioeconomic status are associated with successful suicide. Doctors and other medical personnel have been considered to be at particularly high risk. Controlled studies indicate that belief to be incorrect for the United States but perhaps correct in Great Britain and Scandinavia. Even in the United States, the suicide rate for female doctors is higher than that for other women. The more violent and irreversible the method of suicide chosen, the less likely is survival.

Putting a gun to one's head and pulling the trigger allows fewer second thoughts than taking pills, which take hours to be effective. People who are physically ill are at increased risk of suicide, particularly if their illness is incurable and painful, for instance, late stage cancer. Suicide is also a risk in physical illnesses, which can induce disease of the brain. An example is a person with *Cushing's disease* (*adrenal steroid excess*) who becomes physiologically depressed.

A common teaching is that suicides are almost always planned. That statement can, however, be misleading. Most people who commit suicide have thought about doing so for some time before the event. Not rarely, have they obsessed about suicide. Usually they signal their suicidal thoughts, although the signals are sometimes subtle enough to be missed by the unwary or by family members who cannot bear the thought of their loved one killing himself or herself. Such signs can be as subtle as putting one's possessions in order or an inexplicable calm in a person who has been upset. At the moment of committing the act, when one must pull the trigger or take the pills, there is always a last instant when one must decide to go through with it or not. Going through with a planned suicide is thus in some sense always an impulsive act. The literature documents that many people who survive serious suicide attempts then say, "I regretted it as soon as I had done it." There are, however, people who survive an attempted suicide and are disappointed that they are still alive.

In treating a person with a mood disorder, the physician should not be shy about asking directly about suicide. While treatment must always be adapted to the individual patient and his or her social environment, it is often useful to ask the patient directly, "Do you want to die?" or "Do you think about committing suicide?" An offhanded denial of suicidal intentions need not be accepted as convincing. The worried clinician can go on to ask the patient, "If you were to commit suicide, how would you do it?" When patients give detailed descriptions of what they would not do to kill themselves, a red flag should go up. Those patients have clearly been thinking about suicide even if they deny any intention of carrying it out. Similarly, it pays to ask patients who wake up in the early morning what they think about when they are lying awake. If they brood about "bad things," it pays to ask again if they consider suicide during those sleepless times.[14] Again, if the patient lies awake brooding about suicide but denies being "serious" about it, a red flag goes up. Recent studies suggest that focusing on the suicidal behavior itself can help to prevent suicides, particularly by using "*cognitive-behavioral*" techniques.

The maximum risk of suicide in a person with a mood disorder is generally accepted not to occur in the depths of depression or at the height of manic elation. Rather, risk is greatest when the patient is on the slope back toward a more normal mood. Patients in the depths of depression are often too dispirited to get themselves together enough even to kill themselves – at least to kill themselves actively.[15] When they have been improving, they have more of the necessary energy to undertake goal-directed activities. They may be particularly vulnerable to suicide if they feel that they are slipping back toward unbearable despair, a condition they never want to be in again. As discussed below, there is an ongoing argument about whether or not treatment with specific SSRIs increases the risk of suicide, particularly in young people. Patients with manic-depressive disease are at relatively higher risk of suicide when they are sliding from mania toward depression, that is, when they are "crashing." To use psychoanalytic jargon, suicide risk in bipolar patients is often maximal when their mania is no longer an adequate defense to hold off their despair. Physicians who care for patients being treated for depression or mania need to be aware that the same medications that ameliorate the signs and symptoms of depression or mania may transiently increase the risk of suicide in patients in the early stages of recovery. That is certainly true if the patients stop taking the medication, for whatever reason, and start slipping back into madness. Suicide risk can increase because of an intercurrent life stressor to which a patient is vulnerable. And the acting out of suicidal ideation can occur with little or no warning, certainly with no obvious change in an apparently recovering patient's ideation or behavior.

The risk of suicide is one of the major reasons that medication for mood disorders is best provided in consultation with a psychiatrist. If a general clinician thinks the patient is an active suicide risk, emergency psychiatric consultation is mandatory, in part because emergency admission to a psychiatric facility may prove advisable. Even if no active suicide risk is detected, specialized psychiatric consultation provides an extra level of assurance that the outpatient treatment being given is appropriate. Psychiatric consultation will not prevent all suicides nor will psychiatric admission. "Suicide precautions" in a mental hospital involve extreme invasion of privacy. A patient may decide that suicide is preferable to undergoing a second such admission. But at least the general clinicians can tell their own consciences and the grieving family and can demonstrate in court that they did their best to protect the patient. Some suicidal patients refuse to see a psychiatrist. That may reflect the same self-destructive urges that make them suicidal. If suicidal patients refuse referral, the general clinician then has no choice except to treat them or to abandon them. The latter choice is dangerous not only for the patient but also, medicolegally, for the physician. Also, few of us went to medical school in order to abandon sick people. If a suicidal patient refuses referral, the physician's own self-protection requires careful documentation in the patient's chart of the attempts to treat and prevent suicide.

Whether or not there is such a thing as "rational suicide" is a sociological question that is beyond the scope of this monograph. In medical school in New York and residency in Boston, I was taught that suicide is always irrational. In postgraduate training in England, I was taught that rational suicide does exist. In the Netherlands, physicians are allowed to assist patients to commit suicide—typically, patients already dying from a hopeless, painful disease. A hundred years ago, European society assumed there were circumstances where a "gentleman" was obligated to blow his brains out. One of my wife's ancestors was in that position but continued to live because he so loved life. In northern Europe at that time, his failure to kill himself was considered a sign of weakness rather than of mental health. Analogies to medieval Japan and the code of Bushido come to mind.

TREATMENT FOR DEPRESSION

Prescriptions for depression can be divided into those for acute illness and those for maintenance therapy. In current practice, doses for the latter purpose are generally similar to those for the former. There is a bewildering variety of *antidepressants*. The rules of medication use in general clinical medicine discussed in Chap. 2 (General Principles) apply to depressive disorders as well. Compliance with medication is a major problem in general clinical medicine, certainly in psychiatric diseases, and very much in mood disorders.

One of the most important things that a general clinician can do in caring for patients with depression is to encourage them to continue taking their medication. Many clinicians including the author have noticed that patients with affective disorders are particularly likely to stop medication even if it is helping them. A patient and family can become obsessed about a possible side effect listed in the package insert, even if that side effect is much less dangerous than the risk of suicide from the mood disorder. Why the rejection of these necessary medications? The answer is uncertain. Side effects can be one reason. A woman who is no longer depressed may well long for the orgasms that her SSRI prevents her from having. Another reason may be that previously depressed patients slip into mild mania, and develop the conviction that they are too strong and healthy to need the medicine. But another reason may be that having a mood disorder heightens emotions even as it makes them less pleasant. Perhaps an analogy is the difference between van Gogh's sunflowers and a pleasant watercolor of a lakeside vacation retreat. Life without the mood disorder, and specifically without mania, may feel passionless compared to life with it. Whatever the reason, depression appears to interfere frequently with its own treatment, by altering the function of the parts of the brain that are required to motivate the patient to comply with treatment.[13]

As discussed, in patients in the depressive phase of manic-depressive disease, antidepressant therapy often has untoward effects such as induction of rapid cycling. Current psychiatric opinion generally holds that a clear distinction exists between patients who suffer only from depression—unipolar illness—or from mania as well as depression—bipolar illness. (As noted, bipolar illness is divided into Bipolar I and Bipolar II, depending on the intensity of the manic manifestations.) As mentioned earlier, before starting an antidepressant, the physician should be reasonably confident that the patient has *unipolar* rather than *bipolar* depressive illness. The patient may be too depressed to give an accurate history, and that information may need to be obtained from the family or other people who know the patient. However, the value of obtaining a good psychiatric history should not preclude timely pharmaceutical treatment of the depression. Depression not only makes a person miserable but also threatens his or her life.

If the diagnosis of (unipolar) depression is made, then treatment should be active and last at least 3 months. A short treatment trial of an antidepressant "to see if it helps" is not good medical practice. All depressed patients do not respond to all antidepressants. A treatment trial may fail simply because the wrong antidepressant was used. Many psychiatrists have reported that it takes 3 months for a depressed patient to show an impressive response to treatment. It is common for consultants to treat depression successfully in patients who have "already had a trial of antidepressant," simply by giving an adequate dose of antidepressant for an adequate length of time. The resulting "therapeutic successes" may result from nothing more than the effect of taking an antidepressant for long enough. What matters, of course, is that the patient gets better.

Selective Serotonin Reuptake Inhibitors (SSRIs)

Selective serotonin reuptake inhibitors (SSRIs) are now widely used as the first line medication for depression. Table 3-3 lists SSRIs widely used in the United States in the beginning of 2005.[16] The mechanism of action of these agents is to reduce the rate at which specific uptake mechanisms inactivate serotonin. They thereby prolong the time serotonin molecules stay in the synaptic cleft and thus favor serotonergic transmission. In general, the medications listed in Table 3-3 are selective for serotonergic uptake mechanisms. However, fluoxetine weakly inhibits the uptake (inactivation) of norepinephrine, sertraline weakly inhibits reuptake (inactivation) of NE and dopamine, and paroxetine has weak anticholinergic effects that may become noticeable at higher doses.

Choice of which SSRI to prescribe, depends on many factors. If a patient has previously responded well to one of these agents without important side effects, then that is clearly the medicine to use again in that patient. If a patient reports significant side effects with the first SSRI tried, it generally pays to switch to another. Susceptibility to side effects to particular SSRIs does differ among patients. Even if the "side effects" are not due to identifiable physiological mechanisms, switching to please the patient will often improve compliance and convince the patient that the treating physician "listens." Formal studies of relatively large series of patients with depression

TABLE 3-3
Selective serotonin reuptake inhibitors (SSRIs)

Medication	Trade name	Time to steady state	Dosage (mg/day)	Major side effects
Fluoxetine	Prozac	1 month	20-40	↓ sexuality, anxiety (early), headache
Sertraline	Zoloft	1 week	25-50	↓ sexuality, GI, insomnia
Paroxetine	Paxil	1 week	20	↓ sexuality, dizziness; odd dreams
Citalopram	Celexa	1 week	20-40	↓ sexuality, GI, somnolence
Escitalopram	Lexapro	1 week	10-20	↓ sexuality

have not shown major differences in clinical effectiveness among the SSRIs. Other careful studies indicate that it is impossible to tell whether or not a patient will respond to a specific SSRI (or other antidepressant) until the patient has actually taken adequate doses of that medication for 3 months. However, a number of experienced clinicians have convinced themselves that patients often respond to one SSRI better than they do to others. Sometimes a patient appears to respond to only one of the SSRIs and not at all to the others. My own experience tends to agree, perhaps in part because when patients do not appear to be responding to an SSRI after a month, I have typically switched them to another SSRI. The "effective" SSRI tended to be the last one used, that is, the one that they took after the longest exposure to SSRIs (and were therefore taking after 3 months). In general, SSRIs tend to improve somatic signs of depression such as difficulties with eating and sleeping before the patient describes improvements in his or her mood.

Absorption of these medications by the oral route is usually good. The rate of removal tends to be slow, being slowest for fluoxetine (Table 3-3). Therefore, these medications tend to build up in the body. When safe, persisting with a lower dose is more likely to lead to therapeutic levels without side effects than moving quickly up the dosage scale. Controlled investigations have demonstrated that older people with more severe depression require doses of SSRIs as high as younger people. However, my own experience indicates that lower doses than those given in Table 3-3 often provide a fully satisfactory therapeutic effect in individual patients, particularly in older people with dementia or other evidence of brain damage. Some of my patients over 75 have responded gratifyingly to as little as 25 mg of Zoloft a day, with no further improvement when the dosage was increased or other SSRIs tried. On the other hand, a major reason for failure of treatment with an antidepressant is not taking enough for long enough. As always, doses need to be individualized and clinical judgment exercised.

Inactivation of the SSRIs is largely by oxidation in the CYP system (*cytochrome P450 system*) in the liver. Somewhere around a half of the medications in common use are metabolized by or at least interact with this system. Therefore, clinically significant drug interactions between SSRIs and other drugs metabolized by this system can occur.

Side Effects: Certain side effects tend to be characteristic of the group of SSRIs as a whole, although some are more common with one of these medications than with the others.

Impaired sexual functions are now said to occur in a majority of patients taking these drugs. The general effect is reduction in libido and increased length of time to orgasm. The latter effect has led to the use of SSRIs to treat premature ejaculation. This side effect can be pleasing to a man and to the woman he is sleeping with. That is notably true if the man has been worried about his performance, which may have been impaired by his depression. On the other hand, requiring more stimulation to reach orgasm can be distressing to a woman who has had difficulty finding a man who lasts long enough to satisfy her sexually. Central serotonergic deficiencies themselves characteristically reduce sex drive and performance, complicating any discussion of the effects on sexual function of treating these disorders. The complicated social role sexuality plays in any human society also makes that discussion more difficult. (See the discussion of sexuality in Chap. 14, Disorders of Conduct.) In the United States, in the beginning of this millennium, there is a great emphasis on the technical aspects of copulation to the point where it can replace concern with tenderness and togetherness. In common usage in the United States in this new millenium, the word *sex* refers to copulation rather than to cuddling. In this environment, sexual performance can become a kind of competitive athletic contest.[17] "Decreased libido" and fewer orgasms than a patient wants to achieve, or remembers having had, can be threatening, particularly to a fragile person recovering from a mood disorder. There are medical ways to deal with this problem. One is concomitant treatment with both SSRIs and the antidepressant *bupropion*. The latter does not appear to act primarily on serotonergic mechanisms, does not have sexual side effects, does appear to act synergistically with SSRIs in the treatment of depression, and appears to counteract the sexual side effects of SSRIs. Another medical approach to the sexual side effects of SSRIs is concomitant use of *sildenafil* (Viagra) to help men achieve "satisfactory" erections. And, of course, one can discontinue the SSRI and go on to another class of antidepressant, such as bupropion.

Gastrointestinal symptoms are also relatively common side effects of SSRIs. These include loss of appetite, dyspepsia, diarrhea, nausea, and sometimes vomiting. They tend to clear with continued dosage. However, weight should be monitored in patients on SSRIs, as in all patients with depression.

Headaches are more common with fluoxetine (Prozac) than with other SSRIs. Often they clear with continued use. In other patients, they require switching to another SSRI or antidepressant. Headaches can also be a "*depressive equivalent*," that is, a somatic consequence of central serotonergic deficiency. In some patients, SSRIs including Prozac can be an effective treatment of chronic headache. As always, clinical judgment and close observation of the patient are necessary.

Suicide: There has been controversy over whether SSRIs and specifically fluoxetine can precipitate suicide in depressed people. When these medications were first introduced, anecdotal reports fueled a marked concern about giving this medication and by implication other SSRIs to people at high risk of suicide—as so many depressed people are. That was a particular concern for depressed adolescents. Later, controlled studies did not confirm the earlier clinical impression that patients on Prozac or other SSRIs are at greater risk of suicide, during the early stages of treatment, than are patients being treated with other antidepressants. More recently, the controversy has again been raised in the literature. The newest publications fall on both sides of this debate. Suicide is a risk in all patients with mood disorders, particularly in the early stages of treatment. A reasonable proposal is that all such patients be monitored as carefully as possible, whatever antidepressant they are on.

Overdoses: Committing suicide by taking an overdose of an SSRI is difficult. The amount of SSRI that needs to be taken is enormous. Of course, committing suicide by overdosing on other pills or by some other means unfortunately remains as possible in patients on SSRIs as in patients on any other treatment.

Other Newer Antidepressants

Newer antidepressants are being introduced into clinical practice with gratifying frequency (Table 3-4). The steady introduction of a variety of medicines for depression increases the likelihood that an agent can be found that is effective in any particular patient, even a patient who did not respond to "standard antidepressants." For the time being, conservative practice is for these medications to be prescribed by psychiatrists rather than by general clinicians, except in unusual circumstances. The medications discussed in this section are all taken orally.

Buproprion (Wellbutrin, Zyban*)* is a newer but relatively widely used antidepressant. How bupropion acts pharmacologically is still not clear. However, it is now thought to act primarily on systems using signaling compounds (neurotransmitters) other than serotonin. Specifically, it is believed

TABLE 3–4
Other newer antidepressants

Medication	Trade name	Dosage (mg/day)	Major side effects
Bupropion	Wellbutrin, Zyban	100–300	Seizures (rare), euphoria with overdose
Venlafaxine	Effexor	50 (or more)	Agitation (mania), sleep disorders
Nefazodone	Serzone	300–600	Headache, dry mouth, somnolence, nausea, dizziness
Mirtazapine	Remeron	15	Agranulocytosis, sleepiness, cognitive problems, weight loss
Trazodone	Desyrel	50–600	Sleepiness,* priapism, migraine, anxiety, weight loss

*This "side effect" is utilized therapeutically when trazodone is prescribed for sleep, that is, as a hypnotic.

to act primarily on NE-mediated and somewhat on dopamine-mediated systems. The chemical structure of bupropion resembles that of *amphetamine*, which is known to act on specific dopamine receptors, but pharmacological studies do not support a primary action of this medication on dopamine synapses. As discussed elsewhere, this antidepressant is also marketed as an aid to stopping smoking, under the trade name Zyban. (See Chap. 14, Disorders of Conduct; discussion on substance abuse.)

Dosage of bupropion should be increased gradually. The starting dose is 100 mg/day. Doses increase by 100 mg/day every 4 days until a stable dose of 300 mg/day (100 mg 3id[15]or 150 mg of sustained release form 2id[15]) is reached. Of course, full clinical response without side effects is a satisfactory end point even at lower doses.

Bupropion's reported side effects include headache, insomnia, nausea, restlessness and irritability, and weight loss. A slight increase in the risk of seizures occurs at full doses. Hallucinations or other psychotic manifestations mentioned in the literature are very rare. Bupropion does not appear to impair sexual function. At high doses, as in drug overdoses, it can induce euphoria. Fatal overdoses are about as hard to achieve with this medication alone as with SSRIs alone.

Venlaflaxine (Effexor) inhibits reuptake of both serotonin and NE and to a lesser extent dopamine. Its chemical structure differs from that of other antidepressants. One might therefore hope that it might be effective in patients who do not respond to other antidepressants because genetic variation has caused the structures of their relevant "responding" molecules (receptors) to be different from those molecules in most other people.

The usual starting dose of venlafaxine is 37.5 mg/day. This should be slowly increased to 150 mg/day (in divided doses) and in people who need it to 375 mg/day. Increases in dosage, particularly to these high levels, should be done *incrementally*, at intervals of no less than several days. This medicine is metabolized primarily in the liver and excreted primarily in the urine. Dosage needs to be monitored carefully in patients with significant liver or kidney disease.

Side effects are similar to those with other antidepressants. Excess agitation verging on mania occurs in some patients at higher doses. Sleep disturbances have also been reported but are, as always, hard to evaluate in a disease characterized by disturbances of sleep. Loss of appetite and nausea occur in perhaps 10% of patients. Sexual side effects have also been reported in a somewhat lower percentage of patients than for SSRIs. Few overdoses have been reported, none fatal.

Mirtazapine (Remeron) appears to be effective in the treatment of major depressions but also has side effects that militate against its widespread use. This medication acts on both serotonin- and NE-mediated systems in the brain. It is metabolized largely in the liver by CYP systems and excreted largely in the urine. The half-life is usually 1–2 days. Elderly people metabolize this drug more slowly, as do people with liver and kidney disease.

The standard starting dose is 15 mg/day, by mouth, initially usually at bedtime. The dose should be increased at intervals, no shorter than 1 week, to up to 45 mg/day. As noted earlier, doses should be kept low in older people or those with liver and kidney problems.

Side effects can be prominent. Central nervous system side effects include sleepiness in over half the patients, impairment of cognition that may be linked to decreased attention, dizziness, and increased appetite often associated with weight gain. The most feared complication is wiping out the bone marrow (*agranulocytosis*). This potentially fatal side effect argues that mirtazapine should be prescribed only when less dangerous antidepressants have proven ineffective, that is, by a psychiatrist who is following the patient closely in collaboration with a generalist clinician. Successful suicide by taking mirtazapine alone has not been recorded. A fatal overdose did occur in a patient who also took an overdose of tricyclic antidepressants.

Nefazadone (Serzone) is rarely used because of the risk of liver damage. A "black box" warning about liver toxicity has led to virtual abandonment of this antidepressant.

Reboxatine (Vestra) is an antidepressant described in the literature that was not approved for use in the United States because of lack of efficacy.

Trazodone (Desyrel) is an effective medication for sleep, a nonaddicting *tranquilizer*, and a weak antidepressant even when used at high doses. Its hypnotic effect can be particularly useful in patients in whom sleep disturbances are important and debilitating. That includes patients in whom depression complicates conditions such as AD. Trazodone is often used as a hypnotic in conjunction with another antidepressant rather than for its antidepressant activity alone. It can be used with an SSRI, when sleeplessness persists or is exacerbated by SSRI treatment. Synergism between the effects of SSRIs and trazodone has not been documented objectively. However, a number of clinicians who have prescribed both medicines simultaneously have been impressed with the benefit of these drugs together compared to the sum of their individual actions. In practice, trazodone is now used mainly as a nonaddictive tranquilizer. Trazodone has been used successfully to treat erectile dysfunction in men, although that problem is now treated more often with sildenafil (Viagra). The mechanism of action of trazodone on erections appears to be more specific than simply relieving depression-related impairment of sexuality, since this medication can induce painful and excessively prolonged erections (*priapism*).

Trazodone appears to act primarily by blocking the serotonin receptors whose activation is associated with the symptoms of depression ($5HT_{2A}$ and $5HT_{2C}$). It is well-absorbed orally. It should not be used together with monoamine oxidase (MAO) inhibitors. Trazodone should be "washed out" of the system of patients before they undergo electric shock therapy (i.e., *electroconvulsive therapy*, ECT).

Doses of trazodone can vary over a large range. The starting dose is 50 mg/day, usually given at bedtime (i.e., 50 mg hs) Doses up to 600 mg a day in divided doses may be necessary to achieve a satisfactory action against depression. On the other hand, doses as low as 25 mg at bedtime have been reported by families to be useful in helping patients with AD to sleep.

Trazodone has definite side effects that can limit its use. It can cause sleepiness that the patient and caregivers regard as a disability. Even at low doses, it can induce prolonged erections (priapism) that requires prompt treatment. It can cause transient drops in blood pressure when people stand up (*orthostatic hypotension*). That side effect tends to be less marked if the medicine is taken with food. A metabolite of trazodone stimulates a group of receptors ($5HT_{2C}$) whose actions are associated with migraine headaches. This metabolite has also been associated with anxiety and weight loss. Since headaches, anxiety, and weight loss are also typical manifestations of depression itself, the clinician can be hard-pressed to tell whether these clinical manifestations reflect failure of drug action or side effects of the drug. The obvious solution in this case is to go to another antidepressant when feasible.

Tricyclic and Tetracyclic Antidepressants (TCAs)

These medicines were the main drugs used to treat depression until the introduction of the SSRIs and other newer antidepressants. More side effects are known for the tricyclics and tetracyclics, which have been widely used for many years, than for the newer antidepressants. The TCAs are now usually second- or third-line drugs, used only after treatment with SSRIs or other newer antidepressants has been unsuccessful. However, many psychiatrists do try treatment with a TCA if treatment with one of the newer antidepressants fails. Table 3-5 lists TCAs commonly available in the United States in 2005. The TCA antidepressants that continue in relatively wide use are nortriptyline and less so desipramine. These two are significantly safer than the others. Both of these medications cause relatively little sedation compared to the other TCAs. Neither of these drugs are prominent blockers of systems using acetylcholine as a neurotransmitter (i.e., they are relatively weak *anticholinergics*). As a result, they are less likely to induce delirium, including delirium in older people with minimal or mild dementia. (See Chap. 5, Cognitive Disorders.) Nortriptyline alone among TCA antidepressants is not a significant cause of transient drops in blood pressure on standing (orthostatic hypertension). It therefore does not increase risk of hip fractures and other dangerous complications of falls in the elderly.

The mechanisms of action of the TCAs generally involve inhibition of reuptake of serotonin and norepinephrine, which is a major mechanism for inactivating these neurotransmitters. As a group, the TCAs also tend to block some actions of acetylcholine (at *muscarinic* receptors) as well as

TABLE 3–5
Tricyclic antidepressants

Medication	Trade name	Blood levels available	Dosage (mg/day)	Specific side effects
More commonly prescribed at the present time				
Nortriptyline	Pamelor, Aventyl	yes	75–150	sedation
Desipramine	Norpramin, Pertofrane	yes	150–300	–
More rarely prescribed at the present time				
Trimipramine	Surmontil	yes	150–300	H_2 blocker, useful for allergies and stomach ulcer
Doxepin	Sinequan, Triadapin	yes	100–300	like trimipramine, an H_2 (histamine) receptor blocker
Amitriptyline	Elavil	yes	150–300	sedation
Imipramine	Tofranil	yes	150–300	–
Protriptyline	Vivactil	yes	15–60	–
Amoxapine	Asendin	yes	150–600	antipsychotic (neuroleptic)
Maprotiline	Ludiomil	yes	150–230	seizures
Clomipramine	Anafranil	yes	130–250	seizures

blocking some actions of histamine (at H_1 receptors) and adrenaline (at α_1 and α_2 receptors), that is, the TCAs frequently have anticholinergic effects. As expected, different TCAs vary in their properties. Nortriptyline and desipramine have the most attractive side effect profiles. Like them, maprotiline tends to have less anticholinergic activity than other TCAs. A metabolite of amoxapine blocks dopamine receptors. That can lead to beneficial antipsychotic effects and deleterious hormonal effects. Doxepin and also trimipramine have antihistaminic effects that can be useful in patients with gastritis or stomach ulcers or in some patients with allergies.

Since depression is so common and the TCAs were the best antidepressants available for decades, many general clinicians have significant experience in the use of these drugs in clinical settings. However, these medications should probably now be prescribed only by a psychiatrist or in consultation with a psychiatrist. Certainly, only psychiatrists should initiate treatment with TCA antidepressants other than nortriptyline and perhaps desipramine. In fact, psychiatrists are unlikely to use those drugs any more. With the development of newer antidepressants, there is little justification now to fall back on the more dangerous TCAs in patients who do not respond to nortriptyline or desipramine.

One of the great advantages of the TCAs is the relatively wide availability of techniques to measure the blood levels of many of them. This is important not only to avoid overdose but also to monitor compliance. In prescribing a TCA for an actively suicidal patient, it is wise to choose a medicine for which blood levels are available. TCAs are effective drugs for committing suicide, particularly if a patient saves them for that purpose. The patient doing so may very well lie to a physician about his or her compliance. A low or absent blood level of a TCA in a patient who claims to be taking the medicine regularly amounts to two red flags: (1) the treatment is not successful, and (2) the patient is in danger. The therapeutic blood levels for nortriptyline (60–150 μg/ml) and for desipramine (>115 μg/ml) in the elderly are the same as for young adults. However, older people can often achieve these levels with lower daily doses.

The TCAs are well-absorbed orally and metabolized slowly. Their half-lives vary from 10 hours to 70 hours or more. They are therefore "blood level medications." They are inactivated primarily in the liver, by the CYP system, and therefore have the expected interactions with other medications metabolized by that system. The clinical benefits of TCAs become evident relatively slowly. Full benefit is typically not seen in less than 3 months. Clinically significant improvement cannot be expected in the first 2 weeks of treatment. That lag time appears to be a characteristic of neurobiologically based depressive disease, even depression treated with the newer antidepressants.

The *side effects* of TCAs are well-known and can be dangerous.

- Mania. All antidepressants can induce mania, but TCAs are thought to be more likely than the newer antidepressants to do so.
- Sedation. This can be useful in patients with sleep problems but can also be an unpleasant and even dangerous side effect. The most sedating TCAs are amitriptyline, trimipramine, and doxepin; the least sedating are desipramine and protriptyline. Others are intermediate.

- Weight gain. This common side effect of TCA treatment does not always respond to degrees of dietary restriction that are practical in human beings not on a metabolic ward or in prison.
- Sexual side effects. These can include impotence, problems with ejaculation, and failure to reach orgasm. These are particularly prominent with amoxapine.
- Anticholinergic actions. The anticholinergic side effects of the TCAs as a group include dry mouth (which sounds minor but can be extremely unpleasant), urine retention, constipation, and blurred vision. The TCAs with the most prominent anticholinergic side effects are amitriptyline (Elavil), imipramine, trimipramine, and doxepin; the least anticholinergic in most patients is desipramine. Anticholinergic actions can also contribute to the cardiac side effects of the TCAs, including rapid heartbeat (*tachycardia*).
- Delirium. At higher doses, the TCAs can induce delirium including psychotic manifestations. Risk of delirium increases as the anticholinergic side effects of the TCA increases. This makes sense because drugs which interfere with acetylcholine-mediated systems in the brain are typical causes of delirium. (See Chap. 5, Cognitive Disorders.)
- Heart damage. Even at standard doses, the TCAs tend to affect the heart. They can lead not only to palpitations but also an excessively rapid heartbeat that can last for months and require discontinuing the medicine. On ECGs (electrocardiograms), TCAs can cause ST- and T-wave abnormalities, including depressed ST segments and flattened T waves. They can prolong the QT interval and are contraindicated in people with a QT interval of 450 milliseconds. TCAs must not be given to people with *bundle branch blocks*, because 10% of these patients would then develop *second-degree block*. Imipramine (which is now rarely used) has a quinidine-like action on the heart. It can reduce the number of premature ventricular contractions but can also depress cardiac function. Overdoses of TCAs can lead to fatal irregularities of the heartbeat (*arrhythmias*).

  Depression itself puts a strain on the heart. When the TCAs were the best antidepressants available, it was often hard to decide clinically whether the risk to a depressed patient with heart disease would be increased or decreased if a TCA were given. With the availability of the newer antidepressants that have relatively little toxicity for the heart, the decision to treat depression accompanying heart disease has become relatively straightforward.
- Orthostatic hypotension. Transient episodes of low blood pressure on standing can occur in people taking TCAs. As noted, nortriptyline

seldom if ever causes this side effect. The drops in blood pressure, although transient, can lead to serious effects such as falls and fractured hips in older people. Treatment includes lowering the dose of TCA and increased intake of fluids, particularly coffee. Appropriate low doses of salt-retaining steroids such as *fludrocortisone* (Florinef) have been used, but should be prescribed cautiously, particularly in older patients and in patients with hypertension or cardiac disease.

- High blood pressure. TCAs can also cause high blood pressure (*hypertension*). For this reason, they should be discontinued for several days before elective surgery.
- Sweating. Apparently, TCAs mediate this unpleasant effect through the autonomic nervous system.
- Seizures (fits). Although these are not a common side effect of TCAs, clomipramine and amoxapine can lower seizure threshold and maprotiline can cause seizures. (See Chap. 10, Disorders of Awareness.)
- Motor effects. (See Chap. 11, Disorders of Motility.) Amoxapine is metabolized in part to a dopamine antagonist that can cause parkinsonism and even *akathisia*. Other motor effects of TCAs can include *myoclonic* twitching, tremors of the tongue and arms and/or hands, and rarely *ataxia*, *paresthesias*, and *peroneal nerve* weakness with foot drop.
- Rashes. These are seen particularly with maprotiline.
- Agranulocytosis. This decrease in the number of white blood cells is a rare complication of TCA treatment, but it is obviously serious and potentially life threatening. High white cell count (*leukocytosis*), low white cell count (*leucopenia*), and excess eosinophilic cells (*eosinophilia*) are also rare results of treatment with TCAs.
- Hormonal side effects. These can include inappropriate production of breast milk (*galactorrhea*), breast enlargement in men (*gynecomastia*), and menstrual irregularities in women.
- Drug interactions. Interactions with other medicines are well-documented for the TCAs. They should, for instance, never be taken within 2 weeks of taking a MAO inhibitor Taking a TCA with a sympathomimetic, such as certain weight-loss preparations, can lead to serious cardiac arrhythmias. Newer antidepressants should be used cautiously with TCAs. For instance, fluoxetine or paroxetine can increase blood levels of TCAs sixfold even though the dosage of the TCA has not been changed. That effect is due to by interactions at the level of drug inactivation mechanisms in the liver. (Specifically, the CYP system; see Chap. 2, General Principles). Other drugs that should be used cautiously in combination with TCAs include antihypertensives including *thiazides*, medicines affecting cardiac

rhythm, drugs that mimic the action of the neurotransmitter dopamine (*dopamine receptor agonists*); CNS depressants; oral contraceptives; and even aspirin. This list is not exhaustive. Careful prescription of TCAs requires looking up their interaction with other medications a patient is on. When putting a patient who is taking a TCA for depression on some other drug for some other indication, the potential interactions of that drug with the TCA being used should be checked.

- Suicide risk. The TCAs are effective drugs with which to commit suicide. Overdoses have dangerous effects on the heart as well as on other organs. Unlike committing suicide with an SSRI, which is relatively difficult, committing suicide effectively with a TCA is tragically easy. It is particularly easy in the presence of underlying and even asymptomatic heart disease. In patients who are recognized to be active suicidal risks, good clinical practice requires prescribing no more than a week's supply of TCA with no refills. Such patients should, of course, be seen at least at weekly intervals, when the prescriptions can be renewed and blood levels tested.

Dosages of TCAs are outlined in Table 3-5. Most of the medications listed in this table are seldom prescribed nowadays. Before starting any TCA, including nortriptyline or desipramine, medical history and physical examination, complete blood count and liver chemistries, and ECG should be done. The medications should be started at low doses and increased relatively gradually. The doses listed in Table 3-5 are for medically healthy younger adults. As with all medications, doses should be adjusted for the individual patient. The correct dose is "enough but not too much," that is, that which gives maximum benefit with minimum significant side effects. Blood levels are a good guide. The importance of allowing for interactions with other medications has been stressed earlier. Doses should be lowered for patients with liver or kidney disease. The elderly typically respond to much lower doses than those listed; the average for older people is about 1.2 mg/kg body weight. The author has never found it necessary to give a person above 70 years old more than 150 mg of a TCA in order to get a full therapeutic result. Current practice strongly discourages the use of TCAs to treat the symptoms of depression in people with AD; when they were used surprisingly small doses were sometimes effective. On the other hand, a major reason for failure of antidepressant treatment is inadequate dosage, either because too little is prescribed or because the patient does not take it or take it for long enough. Compliance is a problem in all patients with mood disorders, but the often prominent and unpleasant side effects of the TCAs can make it even more of a problem with them than with the newer antidepressants.

MAO Inhibitors

MAO inhibitors were among the first medications used to treat major depressions successfully. They remain effective but, unfortunately, they can be dangerous particularly in potentially suicidal people (as most depressives are). MAO inhibitors increase the activity of the neurotransmitters serotonin, norepinephrine, dopamine, and a number of related metabolites by reducing the inactivation of these *biogenic monoamines*. The double negative (reduce inactivation) results in a positive (increase activity). Two major enzymes are responsible for inactivating these neurotransmitters by oxidizing them. Their names are, reasonably enough, monoamine oxidase A and monoamine oxidase B. These enzymes, and particularly monoamine oxidase A, also act on constituents of the normal diet that can cause high blood pressure if not inactivated promptly. If patients taking MAO inhibitors eat foods or take other drugs they have been warned against, their blood pressures can rise to levels that cause fatal bleeding into their brains. The recommended diet excludes many appetizing foods including, for instance, many cheeses. The diet is difficult enough to stick to that it can be unclear whether patients on MAO inhibitors who bled into their heads were careless, tempted, suicidal, or any combination of those three. A retrospective explanation is not much help once the cerebrovascular accident has occurred.

Selective inhibitors of monamine oxidase B are available and are less likely to cause hypertensive crises than nonselective inhibitors of both forms of the enzyme. One is the drug *selegiline*. However, the high doses of selegiline that treat depression effectively also inhibit monoamine oxidase A. The use of MAO inhibitors to treat depression is best left to psychiatrists, who will often restrict their use of these effective but dangerous drugs to inpatient settings where the patient's diet and exposure to other drugs can be relatively well-controlled.

Antiepileptics

The relation between madness and aberrant electrophysiology is discussed in Chap. 10, Disorders of Awareness in relation to seizures. Clinical experience, as well as controlled studies, indicates that disordered moods are common in people with epilepsy. The general rule is to treat the seizures first, with standard antiseizure (*anticonvulsant*) medications. Sometimes effective anticonvulsant treatment also treats the mood disorder effectively. Anticonvulsants are so effective in treating manic-depressive disease (bipolar disorder) that two of these medications, valproate and carbamazepine, are among the mainline treatments for bipolar disease. These and other anticonvulsants are not conventionally used to treat depression alone. On occasion temporal lobe epilepsy can present clinically like classic episodes of mania or depression in a manic-depressive disorder. This differential diagnosis can be difficult, unless a clear history of seizures is elicited or the patient is kind enough to have a seizure in front of the examiner. Some physicians use a trial of treatment with an antiepileptic medication as a "last resort" in medical therapy of a psychosis, including bipolar disease before moving on to more interventive approaches such as ECT. Successful treatment with an antiseizure medication of a patient who failed to respond to a series of other medicines is a pleasing resolution of a difficult problem, for the physician who prescribed the antiepileptic as well as for the patient and the patient's family.

Antiseizure medications are discussed primarily in the discussion of epilepsy in Chap. 10 (Disorders of Awareness). Their use in mental illnesses is discussed at greater length in the chapter on psychoses (Chap. 4, Thought Disorders).

Lithium

This medication can reduce the incidence of attacks of depression as well as of attacks of mania, particularly in patients with manic-depressive (bipolar) illness. It is discussed later with the treatment of manic-depressive disease.

St. John's Wort and Other "Natural" Products

St. John's Wort is a herbal extract (*Hypericum*) used in Europe and particularly in the German-speaking world to treat depression. Double-blind studies in Europe have generally confirmed its efficacy; these studies used European preparations where the amount of the active ingredient per dose is standardized.[18] Double-blind studies in the United States have not found it useful, and this material is not widely recommended by

U.S. psychiatrists or neurologists. However, if a patient who has been taking it is doing well on it and swears that it helps him or her, there is no reason to stop it, unless signs of depression or mania develop and a more universally proven medication is needed. It is important to know if a patient is taking St. John's Wort on his or her own, since the active principle does alter the metabolism of a number of other medications, including specifically medications metabolized by the CYP 3A4 system.[19] A number of other "harmless herbal preparations" that a troubled person may decide to take without telling his or her physician can also alter drug metabolism. As always, it is important to know accurately what a patient is actually taking.

Methylphenidate and Other Psychostimulants

"Liaison (consulting) psychiatrists" often prescribe *methylphenidate* (Ritalin) or other stimulants for severely ill patients who have clinically significant loss of energy (*anergia*) and will (*abulia*). Ritalin acts rapidly. It can be useful in relatively emergency situations where patients are too sick to be treated with ECT, for instance, where a medically ill patient becomes suicidal. Ritalin earned a bad reputation when it was overused some decades ago, but as currently prescribed by psychiatrists it can be a useful and even life-saving medicine.

The dosages to be used in severely ill people follow the adage "start low, go slow." Methylphenidate is available in tablets of 5 mg and 10 mg, and patients should be started on one tablet a day. Doses can be increased while watching for side effects, that is, doses can be titrated up. The maximum according to textbooks is 90 mg/day, but this is likely to be too much for a sick person—particularly an old, sick person. Treatment with this drug for more than a month is generally unwise. Tolerance develops rapidly, so that the beneficial effects of the treatment are lost. Increasing or prolonging dosage can lead to side effects that include loss of appetite, irritability and agitation, and difficulty sleeping with nightmares.

Maintenance Therapy

Depression tends to be a more or less chronic disease with recurrent exacerbations. U.S. practice has tended to shift toward maintenance antidepressant therapy rather than only treating the exacerbations. Generally, current guidelines for maintenance therapy recommend using the same medicines in the same doses that helped the particular patient in an acute phase. That can be assumed to be the medicine to which the particular patient's unique body chemistry responds well. Of course, apparent response to a medication may have been accidental in a patient who was improving anyway. Common sense and close attention to the response of the patient being treated are always necessary. Benefit to the patient is as always more important than theory.

Recovery from depression can induce strains into the life of a person who has been chronically depressed and has adjusted the circumstances of his or her life to that depression. For instance, family members may have developed habits of interaction with the patient that are no longer suitable when the patient is no longer "always down." As emphasized previously, counseling is usually a necessary part of the successful treatment of depression as of most other illnesses—not just psychiatric illness. Counseling is also important in maintaining patient compliance with the prescribed treatment regimen, even when the patient "feels fine."

How long to continue maintenance therapy is an unsolved issue. Patients tend not to like to think of themselves as chronically mentally ill. After months or a year or two with no exacerbation, they may decide to go off their medicine. Probably it is better to go along with that urge, unless the patient suffers from bipolar illness. The patient is likely to do what he or she wants despite the MD's advice (certainly in our catchment area in New York). It is vital that the physician knows what medications the patient is actually ingesting rather than wrongly assuming that an illness "broke through" despite adequate doses of a medication that the patient was not actually taking. Scolding the patient can just lead to the patient lying. Of course, patients who have gone off maintenance treatment for a mood disorder must be monitored reasonably closely and treated promptly if signs and symptoms of an exacerbation appear.

TREATMENT OF MANIA AND MANIC-DEPRESSIVE ILLNESS

The chronic treatment of manic-depressive disorders is best left to specialists. These disorders are difficult to treat well. For instance, prescribing an antidepressant to a patient in the depressive phase of a bipolar illness can lead to mania or to rapid cycling between mania and depression. Manic-depressive patients are at high risk of suicide or other violent expressions of their disease. As discussed earlier, most patients with mania sooner or later develop some degree of depression as well, so it is safe to assume that the same precautions must be exercised in patients with "isolated" mania as with manic-depressive disease.

General clinicians have two major roles in the treatment of mania/manic-depression. They may have to care for patients with acute mania who need prompt treatment even if psychiatric referral cannot be arranged with the requisite speed. Also, lithium and other medicines used to treat chronic mania have potential medical side effects to which the general clinician should be sensitive, as part of the general medical care of these dangerously ill patients.

Lithium

Salts of the metal Lithium are the first choice drug for treatment of both the manic and depressive phases of manic-depressive disease. It is useful chronically and for maintenance therapy to reduce the incidence of attacks. Since its onset of effective action requires 1–3 weeks, it is not effective in rapidly "cooling down" acute mania. However, lithium treatment is typically part of the initial treatment of mania because of its benefits in maintenance therapy of what is typically a chronic disease with exacerbations and remissions. Lithium is generally a better treatment for the depressive phases of manic-depressive disease than a conventional antidepressant. Conventional antidepressants can induce mania or rapid cycling in these patients. Therefore, in initiating treatment for depression, the skilled clinician must first find out whether the patient also suffers from manic episodes. That may require interviewing family or others familiar with the patient. The patient may be too depressed or otherwise too crazy to give a reliable history. If the patient is in the depressive phase of a bipolar illness, both lithium therapy and consultation with a psychiatrist are indicated. Simply giving a patient who presents with depression an antidepressant "to see what happens" is not optimal medical care. Sometimes addition of lithium dramatically increases the efficacy of other antidepressant treatments in a patient who has not previously responded. It is tempting to speculate that such patients may have a manic-depressive illness in which the episodes of mania have been too mild to call attention to themselves clinically. The brain disease in such patients is best treated by a psychiatrist familiar with the complexities of the pharmacology.

The mechanism of action of lithium is not known. Chemically, it is the lightest of the group of elements in the Periodic Table that also includes sodium and potassium. Some data suggest that the effect of lithium on phospholipids is important in its therapeutic actions.

Maintenance therapy with lithium is generally indicated after even one episode of mania. Longitudinal studies indicate that such treatment can lower the rate of recurrence by 20- to 30-fold and prevent the deterioration that is often characteristic of untreated manic-depressive illness. Therefore, the general clinician is likely to see people who are taking lithium chronically. Lithium doses in older people and adolescents are similar to those in adults.

The *side effects* of lithium are many, potentially serious, and can affect many organ systems. Patients who require lithium maintenance therapy need reasonably close medical monitoring. The physician doing that needs a good background in internal medicine. Collaboration between general clinicians and psychiatrists in the care of these patients is often a wise course and safer for the patients, although some psychiatrists have strong enough medical training and knowledge to monitor these effects themselves. Having two doctors monitoring patient compliance can be an advantage in itself. Patients requiring lithium maintenance are, by definition, at least intermittently crazy and typically suffer from episodes of mania. They are at high risk of stopping the medicine because they come to feel that they are too healthy and strong to need it or become too depressed to continue it. Perhaps even more dangerous, the patients may take a manic excess of medication if they break through maintenance therapy and fall into another attack of frank mania.

General physicians need to be familiar with the side effects of lithium, since they are likely to provide general medical care to patients in their practice who are on maintenance lithium. The following side effects are relatively common.

Birth Defects: Lithium should not be taken by women in the first trimester of pregnancy since it can cause significant birth defects. Therefore, its use in women who are likely to get pregnant is worrisome. Patients who need lithium are by definition at risk of unpredictable behavior, and the decision to make love is often impulsive (blessedly so). Physicians taking care of potentially fertile women who require lithium maintenance need to be sensitive—and, where necessary, sensitize the patients—to these issues. Lithium is excellent for maintenance treatment of manic-depressive disease, but other treatments are also available for women who are likely to become pregnant. Unfortunately, anticonvulsants that are effective treatment for bipolar disease can also cause birth defects. The safest medication from the point of view of the fetus may be calcium channel blockers. If those are not effective, another possible choice is antipsychotics despite their many potential side effects. (See Chap. 4, Thought Disorders.)

Excessive urination and a compensatory increase in fluid intake occur in perhaps a third of people on lithium. The apparent cause is lithium antagonism of the action of *antidiuretic hormone* on its receptor. This side effect can be managed by standard medical procedures, for example, drinking more fluids (*fluid replacement*). Drinking enough fluids is particularly important in hot weather, since patients on lithium can become dehydrated relatively easily. Giving the lithium in a single daily dose often helps avoid problems with fluid (and *electrolyte*) balance. Rarer kidney complications are *nephrotic syndrome*, *renal tubular acidosis*, and an interstitial renal *fibrosis* in chronic lithium users that can even lead to kidney failure.

Thyroid hormone levels in blood alter in perhaps half of patients on lithium maintenance. Perhaps 5% of lithium-treated patients develop clinically significant thyroid disease. Whether or not to treat elevations of *thyroid-stimulating hormone* (TSH) with thyroid replacement in a patient on lithium who has no clinically significant thyroid dysfunction (i.e., is *euthyroid*) is a clinical decision. Sometimes thyroid replacements lead to remissions in patients in an apparently drug-unresponsive depressive phase of manic-depressive illness.

Heart problems are an uncommon but serious side effect of lithium treatment. These are problems with the conduction of the heartbeat. Sometimes these are benign ECG alterations resembling those of *hypokalemia* (low potassium), since lithium can replace potassium within cells. More serious abnormalities arise from lithium-related depression of the pacemaking activities of the *sinus node*. Lithium should not be prescribed to patients who already have a "*sick sinus*." Occasional patients on lithium develop potentially life-threatening *ventricular arrhythmias*. Heart failure has also been reported.

Skin conditions including acne can result from treatment with lithium. Treatment of the acne with tetracycline must be done with attention to lithium levels since tetracycline can increase the retention of lithium in the body. Acne (and weight gain) may be particularly bothersome in adolescents who are subject to acne anyway. Other skin conditions more rarely associated with lithium therapy include leg ulcers, exacerbation of *psoriasis*, and occasionally hair loss.

Neurological side effects of lithium include tremor. Typically this is *postural tremor*, incoordination (shaking) that develops when muscle groups are activated. It can be detected by asking a patient to hold their hands outstretched while standing up. Another side effect of lithium treatment is mental blunting that can mimic depression or a cognitive disorder. Rare side effects include peripheral nerve problems, increased susceptibility to seizures, and mild parkinsonian signs and symptoms. Ataxia, including impaired speech, is a sign of lithium toxicity but can also occur with blood levels in the putatively therapeutic range. (See Chap. 11, Disorders of Motility, for a fuller discussion of these motor disorders.)

Blood Levels and Toxicity: Lithium toxicity can occur, particularly in its milder forms, even in patients with appropriate blood levels. The standard rule applies—treat the patient, not the laboratory values. However, one must remember that manic-depressive episodes are themselves life threatening. As so often in medicine, the clinician must use judgment to balance conflicting considerations—the seriousness of the underlying disease versus the seriousness of the side effects.

The prominence of different groups of side effects of lithium tends to vary with the degree of toxicity. Even mild lithium toxicity can cause behavioral changes that can mimic either depression (e.g., lethargy) or mania (e.g., excessive excitement). Associated signs and symptoms that can provide clinical clues to excessive lithium levels are gastrointestinal distress (vomiting, abdominal pain), ataxia (staggering gait, dizziness, slurred speech, *nystagmus*), and muscle weakness. Moderate lithium toxicity leads to more striking manifestations of dysfunction of the same organ systems. Behavioral changes can extend to frank delirium, stupor, or coma with abnormalities detectable on EEG (electroencephalogram). Gastrointestinal distress can extend to loss of appetite and persistent nausea and vomiting. Neurological signs can include seizures, abnormal movements (*choreoathetosis*), and overactive reflexes. Lowered blood pressure and cardiac conduction abnormalities and arrhythmias can lead to failure of circulation. Severe lithium toxicity is associated with convulsions and compromised kidney function. It can cause renal failure and kill the patient.

The blood levels of lithium associated with mild toxicity are 1.5–2.0 mEq/L, with moderate toxicity 2.0–2.5 mEq/L, and with severe toxicity >2.5 mEq/L. However, clinical findings are as always more important than the results of laboratory tests. The recommended laboratory values (0.5–1.5 mEq/L) are the averages for relatively large groups of patients. People vary in their response to lithium as to other medications. Some patients become toxic with therapeutic blood levels. Occasional patients do best with blood levels slightly above the normal therapeutic range.

Clinical Laboratory Values: Lithium treatment can alter a number of commonly determined clinical laboratory values. It tends to increase values for glucose, magnesium, and white cells, and decrease levels of potassium, uric acid, and thyroxin.

Drug interactions occur between lithium and often medically necessary medications. Most *nonsteroidal anti-inflammatory* medications, with the fortunate exception of aspirin, increase lithium levels and can do so to the point of clinical toxicity. Many diuretics including *thiazides* increase blood lithium levels. So can ACE (*angiotensin converting enzyme*) inhibitors, although not *angiotensin II receptor blockers*. The antibiotic *metronidazole* increases lithium blood levels too. Osmotic and loop diuretics reduce lithium levels, as do acetazolamide and other carbonic anhydrase inhibitors and sodium bicarbonate. Even caffeine can reduce lithium levels. Patients who pour strong coffee into themselves with manic intensity can increase their excitement by this effect on lithium levels as well as by the stimulant effects of the coffee itself. Calcium channel blockers are *contraindicated* in patients on lithium since this combination can cause fatal neurotoxicity.

Anticonvulsants can be useful in patients who require lithium but can also increase blood levels of lithium. Antiseizure medicines that do so include *carbamazepine* (Tegretol), *valproate* (Depakote), and *clonazepam* (Klonopin).

The use of antipsychotics together with lithium has been associated with increased toxicity of both lithium and the antipsychotic drugs. The latter include *parkinsonian* and other *extrapyramidal* signs and life-threatening *neuroleptic malignant syndrome*. (See Chap. 4, Thought Disorders, for a fuller discussion of side effects of antipsychotic drugs, and Chap. 11, Disorders of Motility, for discussion of these abnormalities of motor function) Antidepressants can lead to rapid cycling of mania and depression in patients who require lithium. Serotonin agonists in patients on lithium occasionally lead to a *hyperserotonin* syndrome resembling manifestations of *carcinoid* syndrome.

Dosages of lithium need to be adjusted carefully for each patient. Patients should have a general medical examination if possible before and if necessary as soon as possible after initiation of lithium therapy. Specific attention should be paid to kidney function, including electrolytes, to thyroid function, to heart function, including baseline ECG, and to baseline blood count. Pregnancy testing should be done in women of child-bearing potential. Prescribing lithium to women who are likely to get pregnant creates a serious risk to the children they bear while on the drug. Patients also need to be warned that sharp alterations in diet including fad diets can play havoc with their lithium therapy and can lead to serious toxicity. Of course, no one should have exaggerated expectations that such warnings will be heeded in patients who have manic breaks.

The standard starting dose for patients who have not had lithium before is 300 mg 3id, orally. Dosage is increased over weeks to a total of 900–1200 mg/day in the maintenance phase and to as much as 1200–1800 mg/day in treatment of acute mania. Doses are lower in patients with compromised kidney function. The use of divided doses tends to minimize stomach upsets from this medicine. Published guidelines suggest that blood levels of 1.0–1.5 mEq/L are optimal in most patients for treatment of the acute illness and of 0.4–0.8 mEq/L in the maintenance phase. Conventionally, lithium levels are determined 12 hours after the last dose of lithium in a patient who has been on a stable dose for at least 5 days, generally dosing several times a day. Blood for lithium determination should obviously not be collected in a tube containing lithium heparin anticoagulant.

When patients on lithium maintenance come to elective surgery, it has been common practice to stop the lithium while the patient is not taking anything by mouth and restart as soon as he or she is allowed to drink and take pills. The decision on whether to stop lithium for this interval should be taken jointly by the surgeon and the treating psychiatrist. No one wants a manic break in a patient in the recovery room or with a fresh wound and intravenous or other tubes in place.

In summary, lithium is a valuable drug for the treatment of both acute exacerbations and maintenance in manic-depressive patients, and is also effective preventive therapy in this disabling, frequently life-shortening, and potentially life-threatening disease. However, lithium comes with a serious set of medical and neurological side effects. In manic-depressive patients, the dosage of lithium and if needed other psychotropic medications are best left to the psychiatrist. However, the general clinician caring for these patients also has to be knowledgeable about and sensitive to the side effects and interactions with other common medicines.

Anticonvulsants

Antiepileptic medications have proven useful in treating mania and manic-depressive disorder. They can be used together with lithium, with care that lithium levels remain in a nontoxic range. The properties of the anticonvulsants are discussed in more detail in Chap. 10, Disorders of Awareness (in the discussion on seizures).

Valproate (Depakote; Depakene) is effective in about 60–70% of people with mania. Response has been claimed to be relatively rapid, within a week, but can take much longer. Rapid dosing regimens are available to reach the therapeutic levels of 50–100 (g/mL within a few days. Valproate is less effective in treating the depressive symptoms of this disease. It can be used for maintenance therapy.

Carbamazepine (Tegretol) is usually effective for the treatment of both acute mania and for prophylactic maintenance treatment of manic-depressive disease. It is as effective in the acute phase as lithium or antipsychotics. It appears less effective than lithium or valproate in maintenance therapy to reduce recurrences. Sometimes people respond to this medication although they do not respond to lithium or valproate. (The reverse can, not surprisingly, also occur.) It can be more effective than valproate in treating depressions. Unfortunately, tolerance to the anti-manic effects of carbamazepine can develop in people in whom this medicine was previously effective. As discussed in Chap. 10 (Disorders of Awareness, in the discussion of seizure disorders), life-threatening bone marrow suppression is a rare (<1/100,000) but dangerous side effect of Tegretol. That risk is much lower than the risk of suicide in manic or manic-depressive patients.

Other anticonvulsants are sometimes prescribed for manic-depressive disease when first-line medicines (lithium, valproate, carbamazepine) have failed. The use of these second-line anticonvulsants to treat bipolar disease should be restricted to psychiatrists. Both *gabapentin* (Neurontin) and *lamotrigine* (Lamictal) are sometimes beneficial for depression but seldom if at all for mania. *Topiramate* has been little studied for these indications.

Calcium Channel Blockers

The calcium channel blockers nimodipine and verapamil have been reported to be anti-manic, although less effective than the first-line medications. These drugs may be particularly useful in patients who cycle rapidly. They can also be used with relative safety in patients who are or might be pregnant. Calcium channel blockers should *not* be given to patients who are also taking lithium.

Antipsychotics

Some of the same medicines that are used to treat thought disorders are also widely used in the treatment of acute mania, in part because they have a more rapid onset of action than lithium and anticonvulsants. Their use in prophylactic maintenance therapy is controversial, in part because of less-reliable effectiveness and in part because of a relatively high incidence of serious side effects. Antipsychotic medications are discussed at greater length in Chap. 4 (Thought Disorders).

In general, both older antipsychotic medications (*haloperidol* [Haldol], *chlorpromazine* [Thorazine], and *thiothixene* [Navane]), and newer antipsychotics (*risperidone* [Risperdal], *olanzapine* [Zyprexa], *quetiapine* [Seroquel], *clozapine* [Clozaril], and *ziprasidone* [Zeldox]) appear to be equally effective in cooling down mania. There have been reports of risperidone and olanzapine inducing mania. That effect might conceivably relate to their action in blocking serotonin receptors.

An appropriate starting dose of haloperidol in acute mania is 5–10 mg by mouth or 5 mg parenterally. In older people, doses of 1–2 mg are more appropriate. Repeated doses every hour until symptoms are controlled is often a wiser practice than fewer but larger doses. The acute toxicity of these antipsychotic medications is low, although their chronic side effects are significant. (See Chap. 4.) Acute mania can be associated with violence to the patient or to others. Furthermore, severe mood disorder and particularly severe mania can put a strain on the heart and other organs. As always, the optimal dose is that which benefits the patient without inducing untoward side effects. In treating acute psychoses, including acute mania, risking giving a little more medicine than is necessary may be safer than risking giving too little.

Benzodiazepines

The *benzodiazepines*, which are widely used as calming agents, are useful adjuncts in the treatment of acute mania. They improve and calm agitation and anxiety. When used together with antipsychotic medications, benzodiazepines tend to "cool" symptoms faster and lead to lower doses of antipsychotic drugs. The favored benzodiazepines for this purpose are *lorazepam* (Ativan) and *clonazepam* (Klonopin). Lorazepam can be given intravenously and intramuscularly as well as orally. It is relatively short acting, with a half-life of 8–30 hours and is therefore relatively safe even when given by injection (parenterally). The benzodiazepines are discussed at greater length in Chap. 6 (Anxiety).

TREATMENT OF ACUTE PSYCHOSIS BY THE GENERAL CLINICIAN

Even experts can have trouble telling whether a patient with severe mania suffers primarily from a disorder of mood or primarily a disorder of thought, that is, manic, schizophrenic, or schizoaffective. Even Bleuler, the expert clinician who invented the distinction between thought and mood disorders, found this differential difficult. When a general clinician needs to treat a patient in an acute break, which may be *manic* but might be *schizophrenic*, a safe course is to use treatment that is suitable for both. This would be a classic antipsychotic and a benzodiazepine. A reasonable combination is Haldol (10 mg by mouth or 5 mg intramuscularly) and lorazepam (2 mg by mouth or intramuscularly), repeated as necessary at intervals of not less than 1 hour. The patient should then be transferred to the care of a psychiatrist or neurologist. These patients typically require hospitalization until consultation is available. If at all possible, the consultant should decide on the longer-term therapy including the appropriate drugs.

Acutely manic or otherwise, psychotic patients can present as medical-surgical emergencies. An example is a patient who castrates himself in what he believes is a religious vision, and is bleeding rapidly from the penile arteries. In these patients, the need for simultaneous medical-surgical and psychiatric treatment is obvious. Acute psychosis is a life-threatening condition. Appropriate treatment of these often difficult patients requires mobilization of medical resources comparable to that done for life-threatening illnesses of other organs.

Not rarely, the only way to be confident that acutely psychotic patients will not hurt themselves or other people is to put them into a mental hospital or a psychiatric ward of a general hospital. Assuming the facility is appropriately run, the patient will then receive skilled supervision and medication until the danger is reduced to a more acceptable level. Admission can be necessary not only for patients who are a risk to themselves but also for patients who are a risk to the people around them. That includes some manic patients, especially manic patients who are also paranoid. Emergency admission can also be necessary for patients so underweight from their depression as to be in danger of a fatal medical complication of starvation. Patients with combined psychiatric and medical problems often benefit from combined care by both psychiatrists and general clinicians. Often this can be best given in a general hospital setting, either on the psychiatric service of the general hospital or, if that is not available, in a private room with special nursing focused on that patient.

When admission is medically (psychiatrically) indicated, then the patient should be admitted. To the author's knowledge, there is nowhere in the United States that does not have appropriate specialized facilities in general hospitals or specialized psychiatric hospitals, including state psychiatric institutions. Appropriate transport is also generally available.

Voluntary (self) admission is desirable but not always attainable. When patients need to be hospitalized, then they should be hospitalized even if they or their families disagree. Being one of the two doctors necessary for such an admission can be embarrassing and can strain a relationship with a patient and a family. But the embarrassment and the strain are better than a person killing himself or herself, and sometimes killing other people as well. Death of a patient or of someone killed by the patient is permanent—even if the death is "inadvertent" or classified as "accidental." Under current U.S. law in almost all jurisdictions, courts review involuntary admissions within a few days. Relatively verbal and well-behaved but still suicidal or otherwise violent patients can too often convince a judge that they are undergoing a form of extralegal incarceration. In my view, that is unfortunate. Medical decisions should be made by doctors, not by courts and not by professional civil libertarians.[20] That is as true for diseases of the brain as it is for diseases of other organ systems where there are more, and more reliable, laboratory tests to document a diagnosis. Physicians can be biased, incompetent, or venal. Unfortunately, so can lawyers, judges, and lay people.

NONPHARMACOLOGICAL TREATMENTS

More interventive, nonpharmacological treatments fall outside the scope of this monograph. However, when pharmacological treatment fails in a patient suffering from a severe disorder of mood, such treatments need to be considered. That is particularly true in a patient who is suicidal—actively or passively. It is also true in a patient who is suffering so severely and is so disabled that the risks and side effects of highly interventive therapies seem worth accepting.

An almost risk-free treatment is light therapy. This is often effective for mood disorder that comes on regularly at a particular time of year (i.e., *seasonal affective disorder*). For the subgroup of patients who benefit from light therapy, it can increase the effectiveness of antidepressant medications and sometimes make those medications unnecessary. Light therapy is unlikely to harm patients, except perhaps for a somewhat increased risk of skin cancers and other skin lesions.

A more interventive treatment is electric shock therapy (ECT). This can be done with relatively little trauma and small risk of significant permanent memory impairment. ECT can be beneficial in acute mania, where it is almost a specific. It can also be the optimal way to treat the depressive phase of a manic-depressive illness.

Psychosurgery is highly interventive. It may be indicated particularly in patients in whom the psychiatric disorder is associated with a discrete lesion in the brain, including a discrete epileptic focus. More general, risky psychosurgical procedures such as *frontal lobotomy* are seldom done at the present time, now that so many effective psychotropic drugs are available.

A recently introduced method for *treatment-resistant depression* is stimulation of the *vagus* nerve.[21] Experience with this form of treatment is as yet limited.

REFERENCES

1. High achievers may have committed themselves so much to emotional strength and to self-control that they will not admit to being depressed, to others or even to themselves. In caring for a patient who is obviously depressed but denies depression, Prof Lars Gustafson in Sweden sometimes resorts to declaring energetically, "Yes, you are depressed! You are depressed!" To quote Prof Gustafson, "That often releases the patient's tears and allows effective treatment to begin." In my own experience in the United States, a typical encouraging response from the patient is, "Doctor, you'd be depressed too if you were in my situation." Then the real discussion can begin.
2. Caspi A, Sugden K, Moffitt TE, et al. Influence of life stress on depression: moderation by a polymorphism in the 5HTT gene. *Science.* 2003;301: 291–293.
3. Zhang X, Gainetdinov RR, Beaulieu JM, et al. Loss-of-function mutation in tryptophan hydroxylase-2 identified in unipolar major depression. *Neuron.* 2005;45:11–16.
4. Standard textbooks discuss the various theoretical models for depression and provide lead references for further reading. Standard current American textbooks of psychiatry include Hales RE, Yudofsky SC . *Textbook of General Psychiatry*, 4th ed, American Psychiatric Publishing, Washington, DC, 2005; and Sadock J, Sadock VA, Kaplan HI. *Kaplan and Sadock's*

Comprehensive Textbook of Psychiatry, 7th ed, Lippincott Williams & Wilkins, Philadelphia, PA, 2002. A briefer version of the latter is Sadock BJ, Sadock VA, Synopsis of Psychiatry, 9th ed, Lippincott Williams & Wilkins, Philadelphia, PA, 2003. In addition, a large variety of books on specialized psychiatric approaches and techniques including psychotherapy are available. Some of the inevitable cultural biases in American psychiatry can become clear from reading a foreign text as well as a U.S. textbook. The foreign texts typically display a different set of cultural and sometimes of biological biases. A standard current British text is Gelder MG, Lopez-Ibor JJ, Andreasen N eds. *New Oxford Textbook of Psychiatry*. Oxford University Press, Oxford, London UK, 2003. A British textbook by Meyer-Gross, Slater, and Roth published in 1960 is now out-of-date technically but still stimulating in the way it analyzes psychiatric phenomena.
A thoughtful discussion of modern classification of mood disorders, specifically in the elderly, is Alexopolous GS, Schultz SK, Lebowitz B. Late-life depression: a model for medical classification. *Biol Psych.* 2005;58:283–289.

5. For the urine measurements to be interpretable, the patient must be on probenecid to prevent reuptake of the relevant compounds.
6. As in an old joke: A passenger hears a Pullman car porter singing at work and says, “You’re happy!” The porter responds, “No, sir. I’m just trying to get happy.”
7. The comment has been made that “the best physician is a well-compensated, hypomanic, obsessive-compulsive.” That is not necessarily true, but it is not entirely wrong, either.
8. Of interest, K.L. Davis and M. Murphy and their coworkers in the 1970s found that intravenous doses of acetylcholine agonists could reduce and even reverse manifestations of mania.
9. A relevant quote is “most people live lives of quiet desperation.” My Italian American neighbors taught me to try to enjoy life even when life is miserable: “You work hard and then you die. Anything better is gravy.”
10. Green E, Elvidge G, Jacobsen N, et al. Localization of bipolar susceptibility locus by molecular genetic analysis of the chromosome 12q23-q24 region in two pedigrees with bipolar disorder and Darter’s disease. *Am J Psychiatry.* 2005;162:35–42.
11. Mortensen PB, Pedersen CB, Melbye M, et al. Individual and familial risk factors for bipolar affective disorders in Denmark. *Arch Gen Psychiatry.* 2003;60:1209–1215.
12. A clinical anecdote describing a rather typical suicide attempt associated with central serotonergic deficiency is presented in the chapter on general principles. Depression can sometimes alter cognition so much that the depressed person feels irreversibly cut off from the more normal life that he or she knew before the depressive episode. A number of gifted artists have described that state, including the poet Verlaine:

"My God, my God, life is there,
Simple and tranquil."
["Mon dieu, mon Dieu, la vie est là
Simple et tranquile."]

The distortions of thinking that sometimes accompany mood disorders can make getting through to these patients difficult. In a play about her illness by a playwright who committed suicide not long after finishing it, the psychiatrist is a half-seen figure behind a semi-opaque screen. (The play, *4.48 Psychose*, by the Englishwoman Sarah Kane, was originally written in French.) The quality of suicide associated with thought disorders can be different from that in mood disorders, although the result is just as deadly. A teaching joke illustrates this point. Two psychotics are standing on the information deck of a tall building that is a tourist site. One says to the other, "Hey, man, I'm flying," jumps off the observation deck, and falls to his death many stories below. A tourist turns to the other psychotic and says, "Why didn't you stop?" The second one answers, "Hey, man, I thought he could make it."

13. A somewhat forced analogy can be drawn with AIDS, in which the virus attacks parts of the immune system necessary to mobilize a response to viral infection.
14. A period of distressed sleeplessness in the early hours of the morning has been referred to in Scandinavian languages as "the hour of the wolf." Ingmar Bergman made a movie with that title.
15. Whether eating so little that one dies or failing to take necessary medications to maintain health count as "passive suicide" is largely a matter of definition, i.e. of "therapeutic viewpoint." What does one say about the skilled internist with mild emphysema who does not stop smoking after a heart attack? Or, for that matter, an internist who frequently patronizes prostitutes, refuses to wear a condom, and dies of AIDS?
16. In this monograph, the notation "2id" for twice a day is used rather than "bid" and "3id" for three times a day rather than "tid."
17. With bonus points given for mutual orgasm, as compared to two individual orgasms separated in time.
18. Szegedi A, Kohnen R, Dienel A, et al. Acute treatment of moderate to severe depression with hypericum extract WS 5570 (St John's wort). *Brit Med J.* 2005;330:503–507.
19. Markowitz JS, Donovan JL, DeVane CL, et al. Effect of St John's wort on drug metabolism by induction of cytochrome P450 3A4 enzyme. *JAMA.* 2003;290:1500–1504.
20. There is little independent evidence to support the claim that transferring patient rights from the medical to the legal system actually benefits most people, even though most lawyers and judges accept that as axiomatic.
21. Rush AJ, Sackheim HA, Marangel LB, et al. Effects of 12 months of vagus nerve stimulation in treatment-resistant depression: a naturalistic study. *Biol Psych.* 2005;58:355–363.

CHAPTER FOUR

Thought Disorders: Including Schizophrenias and Related Psychoses

For the last century, it has been conventional to separate primary disorders of mood from primary disorders of thought, that is, *mania* and *depression* from *schizophrenias*. This distinction has been maintained even though the clinical syndromes can overlap. Patients with depression and particularly with manic-depression can think in weird ways. Patients with schizophrenia can have major problems with mood, to the point where they are classified as having a *schizoaffective disorder*. More important, many patients with a *mood disorder* benefit from treatment with an antipsychotic medication, and many patients with a *thought disorder* benefit from treatment with an antidepressant. Often patients in both categories benefit from simultaneous treatment with both types of medication. The categories of mood disorder and thought disorder should not be looked on as mutually exclusive—biologically, clinically, or pharmacologically.[1] However, the distinction between mood disorders and thought disorders is well-established in the literature and is convenient for clinicians in deciding what medicines to prescribe first. It is a useful clinical approximation so long as it is regarded as an approximation rather than a limitation—a guideline for what treatment to try first rather than a rigid rule.[1,2] Empiricism trumps theory, and patient welfare is the ace of trumps.

In general, most psychotic people try to use the undamaged parts of their brains to enable themselves to live as best they can, despite the aberrations in perception and thought arising from the damaged parts of their brains. To use a computer analogy, they try to run what software they can with the undamaged part of their hardware. The results are often garbled—sometimes analogous to what comes out of a computer that is contaminated with a virus. Erik Kandel, who was trained in psychiatry before embarking on his extraordinarily productive career in the laboratory, has proposed a reductionist neurobiological basis for the attempt to use the parts of the brain that are working well to compensate for the dysfunction of the parts that are not.

> The functions localized to discrete regions in the brain are not complex faculties of mind, but *elementary operations* [italics in original]. More elaborate faculties are constructed from the serial and parallel (distributed) interconnections of several brain regions. As a result, damage to a single area need not lead to the disappearance of a specific mental function as Flourens, Lashley, and many later neurologists had predicted. Even if the function does disappear, it may partially return because the undamaged parts of the brain can reorganize to some extent to perform lost functions. Thus, interrelated local brain functions do not represent a series of links in a single chain, for in such an arrangement all related functions stop when one link is disrupted. Rather, interrelated functions are processed by many neural pathways distributed in parallel. The interruption of a single link within a pathway disrupts only the one pathway, but this need not interfere permanently with the performance of the system as a whole. The remaining parts of the system can modify their performance following the breakage of a link.[3]

Here Kandel is referring to higher functions of the brain. Removing the optic chiasm or the striate cortex leads to complete blindness with no prospect of recovery. If one includes simple as well as complex activities, then some of the functions of the brain are organized in series and some in parallel.

Kandel's formulation does, however, provide a clear basis for variations in complex behavior as a result of a disease. For instance, people who hear voices can have various attitudes to what they hear. One of my patients recognized the voices she heard as a sign of her brain disease (schizophrenia) and was able to disregard them. She was a successful businesswoman, perhaps a bit brassy, but well within accepted standards of behavior in the tolerant city in which she lived. The voices in the head of another patient in the same city led this other woman to write a bitter letter to the dean of a university medical school. She claimed that the electrophysiological equipment in the laboratory of a handsome young associate professor was putting the awful thoughts into her head that led her do "awful things" with many different men.[4] The responses to the core phenomena of schizophrenia can be as varied as the people who experience them.

The ability of people who are quite mad to compensate partially for their madness can lead to an "in and out" kind of behavior that is epitomized in certain teaching jokes. For instance

> A young psychiatrist is walking around a state mental hospital and sees a patient fishing in a toilet bowl. The psychiatrist asks, "What are you fishing for?" The patient answers, "Whales." The psychiatrist asks, "Catch any?" The patient responds, "What, are you crazy? In a toilet bowl?"

Or

> A man goes to see a psychiatrist to get help for his brother. The man says, "You know, Doctor, my brother is really crazy. He keeps goats in the house." The psychiatrist responds, "That is certainly strange behavior." The man says, "And with all the windows closed, the smell is terrible." The psychiatrist asks, "Why don't you at least open the windows?" The man replies indignantly, "What, are you crazy? And let out all my pigeons?"

The point of teaching anecdotes of this type is that even crazy people need not act totally crazy all the time. The clinician has to be sensitive to which statements by a patient are valid and are justifications for insane thoughts. For instance, a patient who comes in wearing a bizarre bracelet might, when complimented on her bracelet, explain that she wears it to protect herself "against them—you know, the Martians."[5] Of course, the bracelet might also have a rational explanation, for instance, a badly chosen gift to her by her husband. The skilled clinician has to be sensitive, to avoid being judgmental or otherwise inhibiting the patient's willingness to communicate, and to check the accuracy of the patient's statements with relatives or other caregivers.[6] Recognition and differential diagnosis of insanity are sometimes easy and sometimes hard. Diagnostic errors can be as dangerous as for other life-threatening illnesses.

CLASSIFICATION AND DIAGNOSIS

As with mood disorders, the classification of psychoses has changed during the iterations of DSM (Diagnostic and Statistical Manual of the American Psychiatric Association) from *DSM-I* to *DSM-IV-TR* (Table 4-1). Although the classifications have changed, there is no reason to think that the patients have. The current system avoids some of the more egregious problems of the past. When I was in medical school half a century ago, *pseudoneurotic schizophrenia* was a commonly used diagnostic term. The

TABLE 4–1
Classification of psychoses

DSM-I	DSM-IV
Affective reactions Psychotic depressive reaction	Schizophrenia
Schizophrenic reactions Simple type	Schizophreniform disorder
Hebephrenic type Catatonic type	Schizoaffective disorder
Paranoid type Acute undifferentiated type	Delusional disorder
Chronic undifferentiated type Schizoaffective type	Brief psychotic disorder
Childhood type Residual type	Shared psychotic disorder
Paranoid reactions Paranoia Paranoid state	Psychotic disorder due to a general medical condition
Psychotic reaction without clearly defined structural change	Substance-induced psychotic disorder Psychotic disorder not otherwise specified

definition of that condition taught to me in medical school was, "the diagnosis for a patient who does not respond to psychotherapy whom the psychiatrist does not like." The professor of psychiatry who used that phrasing was fully conversant with the scholarly, textbook definitions of pseudoneurotic schizophrenia, but he was also a realist who knew what that diagnostic category meant in actual clinical practice.

The diagnostic classifications presented in Table 4-1 are those used in DSM-IV. According to this schema, *schizophrenia* is a clinically significant disturbance of behavior that lasts at least 6 months if untreated and is characterized by at least two of the following abnormalities: hallucinations, delusions, disorganized speech, grossly disorganized behavior (including *catatonia*[7]), and negative symptoms such as flattening of *affect* (emotion), reduced speaking, and/or lack of persistence in activities. Function typically declines over time in untreated schizophrenics. Schizophrenia remains a diagnosis of exclusion. The insanity must occur without another identifiable cause such as substance abuse or a recognized anatomic lesion of the brain. Schizophreniform disorder resembles schizophrenia but lasts less than 6 months, typically 1–6 months. Delusional disorder requires at least 1 month of nonbizarre delusions without the accompanying symptoms of schizophrenia. Brief psychotic disorder has manifestations like schizophrenia but lasts more than 1 day and less than 1 month. Shared psychotic disorder is a mental disturbance in a person who shares the same delusions with another person. Shared psychosis has been referred to by a French term—*folie à deux*. Psychotic disorder due to a general medical condition is a psychotic reflection of delirium, that is, *agitated delirium*. In this monograph, agitated delirium is discussed with delirium in Chap. 5, Cognitive Disorders. Substance-induced psychotic disorder can be attributed to a toxic reaction to a drug of abuse, a medication, an environmental toxin, or some other toxic exposure. It, too, is a form of delirium. (See also Chap. 14, Disorders of Conduct.) Psychotic disorder not otherwise specified is the necessary grab-bag category for people who cannot be fit into the other categories.[8] Sometimes that failure to meet criteria for other types of psychoses reflects lack of data. Sometimes it reflects variations in real patients that are not reflected in the available diagnostic categories.

Recognizing that a patient is insane is the first and most critical decision that a general clinician must make in dealing with these conditions. That can be easy or difficult. Some of these patients are raving mad, but others present in a more controlled state. As a medical student in the

1960s, I was taught that "If you spend an hour interviewing a patient and at the end of the hour neither one of you know what the other was talking about, at least one of you is probably psychotic." While sounding flip, that is actually a useful way to recognize a thought disorder (presumably in the patient). This idea has been put more pithily, if more crudely, in the maxim, "Crazy people are nuts. If they thought straight, they would not be crazy." J.K.Wing at the Maudsley proposed that the central phenomenon of the schizophrenias is "thought broadcasting."[9] That term describes the feeling that someone or something else is putting thoughts into one's brain ("thought insertion"). In other words, someone else is controlling one's brain. The patient sometimes recognizes the "broadcast" thoughts as inappropriate and sometimes does not. Other investigators have put forward other ideas about the psychological phenomena in schizophrenia and other thought disorders.[10,11] It is beyond the aims of this monograph to review the extensive studies of the different types of aberrant thinking that have been observed in patients with thought disorders or the attempts to classify the bizarre thought patterns that result.

Once the existence of a thought disorder is recognized, the next critical decision is whether the psychosis is the result of a medical illness, including exposure to a recreational drug or other toxin, or has no recognized organic cause. In jargon, the diagnostic question is whether the psychosis is "exogenous" or "endogenous". In the former case, it is usefully thought of as a form of delirium or perhaps dementia, and is discussed in Chap. 5 (Cognitive Disorders). As noted there, even if an organic cause is identified, the psychosis usually needs to be treated, in addition to the underlying illness. The subject of the current chapter is psychoses for which no organic cause is identified, that is, endogenous psychoses. Of course, an endogenous psychosis does not protect a person against developing an organic illness. Patients are at risk of having taken toxic recreational drugs or other materials, sometimes as misguided forms of self-medication. Mixed exogenous/endogenous psychoses are discussed in Chaps. 5 and 14.

For the general clinician, history is often the best guide as to whether a psychosis is the result of a recognizable medical illness or is endogenous. Patients with endogenous psychoses tend to have a history of odd behavior before they go frankly mad, although such a history is neither always present nor always obtainable. Nor does a history of progressive psychological disability rule out the presence of an organic disorder. Common examples of disorders that lead to people acting progressively crazier include accumulating toxicity from recreational drug abuse or slowly developing *hypothyroidism*. As discussed in Chaps. 5 and . 14, the differential diagnosis between endogenous and exogenous psychosis is sometimes relatively easy but can often be difficult.

The Hippocratic physicians or ancient Greek physicians did not make a clear distinction between endogenous and exogenous insanity. Modern advances in understanding the neurobiology of psychiatric diseases may yet lead us to use their concepts again.

NEUROBIOLOGY

The subject of this chapter is thought disorders for which no organic cause can be identified. If an organic cause can be identified, the condition is discussed in Chap. 5 (Cognitive Disorders), as a form of delirium or dementia. Therefore, by definition, the biology of the thought disorders discussed in this chapter is poorly understood. Even the meager information available has, however, led to wide acceptance of some aspects of their origins and mechanisms.

First, and perhaps most important in clinical practice, schizophrenia itself is not now thought to be a single disorder biologically. To quote a standard textbook.

> Schizophrenia is discussed as if it is a single disease, but the diagnostic category includes a group of disorders, probably with heterogeneous causes, but with somewhat similar behavioral symptoms.[11]

In the rest of this discussion, the plural term *schizophrenias* is used for this group of disorders.

The schizophrenias and other thought disorders are rarely purely psychogenic in origin. In the large majority of cases, they reflect brain disease. They can be the major and sometimes the only manifestation of a brain disease. The causes of the brain diseases that lead to these clinical disorders are usually a mixture of genetic and environmental factors.

Genetic predispositions have been identified in schizophrenia. Twin studies are revealing. In identical (monozygotic) twins, the chance of one twin developing schizophrenia is roughly 50% if the other twin has it, compared to about 1% in the general population. For nonidentical twins, the chance is about 12%, the same as the odds if one parent has schizophrenia. Adopted twins reared separately have almost the same genetic risks as twins reared together. These robust, well-documented findings indicate that genetic load is a major factor in the development of schizophrenia. On the other hand, genes are clearly not the only factor. If they were, the concordance between identical twins would approach 100%. The extent to which genetic and environmental factors are responsible for the clinical disabilities presumably varies among patients, even within the same family (kindred).

Whether or not genes that lead to thought disorders have been identified or not is partly a matter of definition. Attempts to identify genetic abnormalities common to many or most schizophrenics have had mixed results.[12,13] A number of loci have been proposed (Table 4-2). A gene that appears to be reproducibly associated with schizophrenia syndromes is *DISC1* (Disrupted in Schizophrenia 1). This gene encodes a multifunctional protein that appears to be involved in a number of aspects of nerve cell (neuron) function. The protein appears to be associated with a specific substructure in the cell, namely the *centrosome*. *DISC2* is a related gene that appears to encode a message that inactivates the product of *DISC1*. *DISC2* appears to specify a nontranscribed RNA (ribonucleic acid) message that is antisense to *DISC1,* that is, inactivates the *DISC1* message. Variations in the amount of *DISC2,* relative to that of *DISC1,* provide a way to regulate the formation (*translation*) of the *DISC1* protein. (Regulation by a *missense* mRNA (*messenger ribonucleic acid*) is not a rare mechanism in genetics.)

In addition to the genes listed in Table 4-2, a number of genes causing *inborn errors* can sometimes lead to syndromes clinically indistinguishable from classic forms of schizophrenia. The abnormalities in these genes have been well characterized at the DNA (*deoxyribonucleic acid*) level. Examples include *Tay-Sachs disease* (GM_2 gangliosidosis) and *metachromatic leukodystrophy* (*sulfatide lipidosis*). Of course, not all patients who have the mutation (in the *HEXA* gene) that leads to Tay-Sachs disease present clinically as psychotic. The best-known form of this illness is severe psychomotor degeneration in infants, often Ashkenazi Jewish infants with an exaggerated startle reflex. However, mutations in this gene can lead to at least seven clinically distinct syndromes, and schizophrenia can be one of those syndromes. Metachromatic leukodystrophy can also present clinically as a number of different syndromes, one of which is schizophreniform insanity. A number of investigators, including my coworkers and me, have suggested that anomalies in "housekeeping" genes such as those for energy metabolism may lead to schizophrenias, if the damage they cause is not severe enough to lead to

TABLE 4-2
Proposed genes for schizophrenia

Gene	Reference
DISC1	Millar, et al. *Hum Mol Genet.* 2000;9:1415-1423. Morris, et al. *Hum Mol Genet.* 2003;12:1591-1608. Hannah, et al. *Hum Mol Genet.* 2003;12:3151–3159. Callicott, et al. *Proc Natl Acad Sci U.S.A* 2005;102: 8627-8632.
DISC2	Devon, et al. *Psychiatr Genet.* 2001;11:71-78.
CAG repeats	Morris, et al. *Hum Mol Genet.* 1995;4:1957-1961.
C1q32-q42	Ekelund, et al. *Hum Mol Genet.* 2001;10:1611-1617.
C2q locus	Paunio, et al. *Hum Mol Genet.* 2001;10:3037-3048.
C5q locus	Paunio, et al. *Hum Mol Genet.* 2001;10:3037-3048.
C7q22 locus	Ekelund, et al, *Hum Mol Genet.* 2000;9:1049-1057.
DTNB1	Numakawa, et al. *Hum Mol Genet.* 2004;13:2699-2708.
G72/G30	Maiet, et al. *Eur Arch Psychiat Clin Neurosci.* 2005;255:159-166.*
MLC1	Verma, et al. *Biol Psychiatry.* 2005;58:16-22.
NRG1	Green, et al. *Arch Gen Psychiatry.* 2005;62:642-648.*
PRODH	Jaquet, et al. *Hum Mol Genet.* 2002;11:2243-2249.
RGS4	Chowdri, et al. *Hum Mol Genet.* 2003;12:1371-1380.*†
ZFHHC8	Hum Mol Genet 2004;13:2991-2995 .

This list does not include genes for inborn errors sometimes associated with insanity. See the text for discussion of some of those genes.

*Also reportedly associated with bipolar disease. (See Chap. 3, Mood Disorders).

† Erratum appears in Hum Mol Genet. 2003;12:1781.

severe psychomotor retardation in early life. My colleagues and I have proposed that such defects can lead to relatively subtle developmental abnormalities that present clinically as thought disorders—schizophrenias—that develop during the changes in brain function that accompany puberty. This suggestion is in line with observations that a variety of genetic abnormalities can predispose to the development of psychosis in early childhood, that is, to autism.[14]

The difficulty in discovering genes that predispose to thought disorders including schizophrenias may lie in large part with the conceptual requirements that such a gene is still required to fulfill in order to be convincing to the biomedical community. A *schizophrenia gene* is expected to contribute significantly to the development of schizophrenia and only schizophrenia and to do so in a significantly large proportion of the individuals who receive this diagnosis. However, data on the genetics of schizophrenia and bipolar disease suggest that some genetic loci are associated with both conditions (Table 4-2).[15–17] The failure of specific genetic abnormalities to correlate with specific behaviorally defined syndromes is not surprising if one considers the details of the biology involved. For instance, the *NRG1* gene that predisposes to schizophrenias and manic-depressive disease encodes a protein, neuregulin, involved in signaling between nerve cells (*synaptic transmission*). It is not surprising that abnormalities in this protein can not only scramble thinking but can also affect connections among nerve cells involved in regulating mood. Nor is it surprising that sometimes the latter change is more prominent clinically than the former.

The available evidence thus makes it unlikely that the genes that predispose to thought disorders will always lead only to thought disorders. Kandel's comments quoted earlier on how the brain is organized suggest that different people with different brains and different environments may well respond differently to the same genetic impairment of a primitive brain system. The "one gene, one clinical syndrome" hypothesis has broken down for a large number of well-understood genetic diseases including classical inborn errors like Tay-Sachs disease. There is no reason to think it will not break down for such heterogeneous conditions as the schizophrenias. In other words, the difficulty in identifying genes that predispose to schizophrenia may lie less in the multiplicity of genes involved than in the multiplicity of syndromes these genes can cause. If the same gene can be a risk factor for a number of syndromes, how does an investigator decide who should be classified as controls—and specifically disease controls—in the appropriate genetic studies? These considerations are inconvenient. They militate against some time-honored medical traditions including ways of classifying psychiatric diseases. But physicians have to deal with human biology as it is, not as we would find it convenient if it were. Claude Bernard pointed out that the physician does not command behavior but obeys her. (Actually, he quoted a Latin maxim: *medicus naturae non imperat nisi parendo*.)

Environmental factors typically interact with genes in causing thought disorders, as they do in other diseases including diseases affecting organ systems other than the brain. The studies of twins cited earlier suggest that what are inherited in the psychoses are usually biological risk factors. The extent to which genetic or environmental factors are important varies from patient to patient and family to family over a wide spectrum. In some families, genetic factors seem dominant. In other people, environmental factors seem to be primarily responsible. Epidemiological studies suggest that among the important environmental factors are infections, while the nervous system is still developing, in the unborn fetus or in infancy. Madness can also follow encephalitis or other brain damage in later life.[18] *Tertiary syphilis* can lead to madness, and patients with psychoses need to be tested for syphilis and, in areas where it is endemic, *Lyme disease*. Chronic *amphetamine* abuse can lead to a syndrome closely resembling schizophrenia, and that syndrome can be irreversible. The roles of other toxins are less clear. Psychological theories such as the "cold, schizophrenogenic mother" have been discarded by almost all people who now treat psychotics.[19]

The *brain damage* in schizophrenics is now widely thought to have been developmental in many and perhaps most patients. Several lines of evidence support that view. The genetic data including twin studies are discussed earlier. Epidemiological studies suggest that obstetric complications, malnutrition during pregnancy, and pregnancy during periods when minor maternal illnesses are common, appear to predispose to the development of thought disorders in the offspring. Neuropathologists have described developmental anomalies in the organization of the brains of some schizophrenics.[20] MRI (magnetic resonance imaging) during life has provided evidence for subtle differences between the anatomy of schizophrenic and normal brains. Regions reported to be affected in schizophrenia include, among others, the frontal lobes and thalamus. Neurophysiologic abnormalities have been described that are explicable as flaws in integration of brain activity. Neuropsychological studies have identified abnormalities that precede the development of frank thought disorder. Some of these anomalies occur in the first few years of life of the unfortunate individuals who go on to develop thought disorders.

Recent studies of the composition of the brains of patients with schizophrenias have found that the chemistry of their brains differ from those of normal individuals in many ways. Some of these studies use new techniques for looking at the level at which a large number of genes are expressed (i.e., gene chip technology to measure the levels of specific mRNAs).[21] Cellular mechanisms implicated by these studies include the breakdown of proteins (*proteosome* and *ubiquitin* pathways) and energy production and signaling mechanisms (in *mitochondria*). These abnormalities can be predicted to have widespread, if sometimes subtle, effects on nerve cell function. Other abnormalities continue to be described, for instance, in proteins that participate in enriching the connections between nerve cells.

Neurotransmitter abnormalities in schizophrenias and other thought disorders are of particular interest for treatment. Abnormalities in these signals by which nerve cells talk to each other are intuitively easy to link to disorders of the organization of the brain's higher functions. The neurotransmitter most implicated in the schizophrenias is *dopamine*. Classical antipsychotics are dopamine receptor blockers—specifically D_2 blockers. The simple hypothesis that schizophrenia results from functionally excessive dopamine activity is, however, no longer widely accepted. Davis and coworkers[22] suggested over a decade ago that schizophrenia may be associated with functional overactivity of dopamine in the mesolimbic cortex and functional underactivity in the prefrontal cortex. That revision of the dopamine hypothesis is consistent with the anatomical, pathological, and neurophysiological findings discussed in the previous paragraphs. As mentioned earlier, abuse of amphetamine, which acts on dopamine receptors, can cause a syndrome clinically almost indistinguishable from schizophrenias. Aberrations in other neurotransmitter systems also appear involved in the schizophrenias, however, including serotonin. Some of the newer atypical antipsychotics act on both dopamine and serotonin, including a few that act primarily on serotonin systems. Historically, a *serotonin hypothesis* of schizophrenia preceded the currently more popular *dopamine hypothesis*.

TREATMENT

In the United States today, psychiatrists rather than general clinicians are usually responsible for treating endogenous psychoses. The behavior of psychotic patients, including their compliance with treatment, is unpredictable. If their behavior made sense, they wouldn't be crazy. The behavioral abnormalities in these people are frequently life-threatening. Their diseases can lead to suicide and to inappropriate behavior involving others. Psychotic people are far more likely to be victims of crime than to perpetrate crimes; statistically they are at least four times more likely to be victims of violence and over ten times more likely to be victims of other crimes. Sometimes, however, insane people become violent, occasionally even murderous. Statistically, psychotics are not significantly more likely to commit murder than are other people, but when they do the crime may be senseless and therefore unpredictable.

The drugs used to treat psychoses have powerful and sometimes irreversible side effects. A significant proportion of psychotic patients do not benefit from any treatment. Depending on the population studied, that includes anything from 10–50% of schizophrenics. Also, psychoses can "break through" even in patients who appear to have stabilized on a drug and even if they have in fact been taking their medicine as prescribed. In other words, medication that previously seemed effective can become ineffective as a disease process progresses. (That is of course a general principle in medicine, in cardiology and infectious disease at least as much as in psychiatry or neurology.) Furthermore, some psychotic patients become better without treatment. Given these complexities, the general clinician who chooses to treat a patient for his or her psychosis not only puts the patient at risk of suboptimal care but also puts himself or herself at risk medicolegally. Collaborating with a psychiatrist who consults regularly about a psychotic patient's care can reduce the risk of less than optimal care as well as the risk of doing something that a court will decide did not meet standards of care.

There are, however, situations where treatment of a thought disorder by a general clinician is appropriate. One is "cooling down" an acute psychotic state, if a psychiatrist is not available in a timely manner. That is particularly important for a patient who is an immediate threat to himself or herself or to others. The acute treatment of psychosis was discussed in Chap. 3 (Mood Disorders). General physicians may also have to treat psychoses in those patients who will comply more or less with medication or other interventions prescribed by a "real doctor" but not by a psychiatrist. Such patients and/or their families may insist that the patient is not crazy.[23] In that case, however, regular consultations with a psychiatrist are very much the better part of valor for the general clinician forced to do the prescribing.

Providing good general medical care to psychotic people is challenging.[24] Their behavior is unpredictable (crazy), and they are by definition unreliable historians. Some specialists in treatment of diseases of the nervous system have enough training and interest in internal medicine that they can effectively monitor patients for diseases of organ systems other than the brain. However, knowledge is advancing too fast for it to be easy to keep up with more than one medical specialty. The medicines used to treat psychoses can have serious systemic side effects. A major role of the general clinician in caring for psychotic patients is recognizing and dealing appropriately with side effects of antipsychotic medications, even if those medications are prescribed by a psychiatrist. In the care of psychotic people, close collaboration between a psychiatrist treating the patient's psychosis and a general clinician monitoring the patient's general health is typically the optimal arrangement. Such collaboration requires that the psychiatrist and the general clinician talk to each other regularly. The information the patient and family provide about what the other doctor said is inherently unreliable, even when the patient and family are trying to tell the truth.[23]

The side effects of antipsychotic medications tend to vary with the class of medication used. These medicines can be divided into three broad categories: (i) typical antipsychotics, that is, *dopamine receptor antagonists*; (ii) atypical antipsychotics, that is, *dopamine-serotonin receptor antagonists*; and (iii) other drugs with antipsychotic activities. Among the dopamine receptor antagonists, high-potency medications tend to have neurological side effects and low-potency medications to have systemic side effects (Table 4-3). The latter can include serious cardiac arrhythmias.

Typical Antipsychotics

The use of the terms *typical*, *traditional*, or *conventional* to describe this group of antipsychotic agents will become increasingly out-of-date, as younger physicians come into practice who are as familiar with newer medications as with these older drugs. The following discussion therefore

TABLE 4–3

High and low potency dopamine receptor antagonists

High potency	Low potency
Haloperidol (Haldol)	Chlorpromazine (Thorazine)
Fluphenazine (Prolixin)	Mesoridazine (Serentil)
Trifluoperazine (Stelazine)	Thioridazine (Mellaril)
Thiothixene (Navane)	—
Pimozide (Orap)	—

Chemically, the low-potency agents are phenothiazines and the high-potency agents are piperazines, a butyrophenone, and a thioxanthene.

uses a pharmacological term that is less likely to become outdated, namely *dopamine receptor antagonists*. These medications are widely regarded as having more side effects and being less effective than the newer *atypical antipsychotics,* which are combined dopamine-serotonin antagonists.[25] The latter are more desirable for chronic use but in general do not have as rapid an onset of action in the acute situation as the older drugs do.

Table 4-4 lists the dopamine receptor antagonists now in reasonably common clinical use.[26] Haloperidol is listed first because its use is so widespread. The large number of agents in Table 4-4 indicates both that the market for antipsychotics is lucrative and that an ideal antipsychotic with negligible side effects has not been found.

The mechanism of action of these medications is blockage of dopamine receptors, primarily D_2 receptors. Different parts of the brain are believed to be involved in the beneficial effects and the side effects:

TABLE 4-4
Typical antipsychotics

Generic name	Trade name	Oral dose*	I.M. dose*
Haloperidol	Haldol	6-20	2-6
Thioridazine	Mellaril	200-700	NA
Mesoridazine	Serentil	75-300	25
Thiothixene	Navane	6-30	2-4
Chlorpromazine	Thorazine	300-800	25-50
Triflupromazine	Vesprin	100-150	20-60
Promazine	Sarine	40-800	50-150
Prochlorperazine	Compazine	40-150	10-20
Perphenazine	Trilafon	8-40	5-10
Trifluoperazine	Stelazine	6-20	1-2
Fluphenazine	Prolixin, Permitil	1-20	2-5
Pimozide	Orap	1-10	NA

This is an incomplete list of antipsychotic medications that have a primary action against dopamine receptors. They belong to a number of chemical classes. For details and more extensive discussion, see reference 11.

*Doses are usual adult doses in mg. Doses for older subjects are often lower.

NA = Not Applicable.

antipsychotic effects primarily via actions on *mesolimbic* systems; parkinsonian and related side effects by actions on the *nigrostriatal* system; and endocrine side effects by actions on the *tuberoinfundibular* tract. Dopamine receptor antagonists tend to be more effective against positive symptoms of schizophrenia such as delusions and hallucinations than on negative symptoms such as apathy. Indeed, these drugs can sometimes exacerbate negative symptoms.

Choice of which antipsychotic to use is best left to a psychiatrist who has training in psychopharmacology. In general, a patient who has discontinued an antipsychotic medication to which he or she has responded well will usually respond well to reinstitution of the same medication. In making this determination, one must remember the rule that "crazy people are nuts." There are many reasons for such patients to give even more inaccurate medication histories than do putatively sane patients. Psychiatric patients may or may not have been taking or not taking pills in accord with what the (broadcast) voices in their heads have been telling them. In other words, they may listen to their hallucinations more than to their doctors. Their insanity may keep them from knowing what they took. If a patient truly breaks through a medication that he or she has in fact been taking regularly in the prescribed doses, consultation with a specialist is indicated. Choice of an antipsychotic in an acute situation is discussed later.

Doses of antipsychotics including dopamine receptor antagonists vary greatly from patient to patient. The numbers given in Table 4-4 are only guidelines. In general, older people or people with significant other illnesses may require smaller doses. However, it should be remembered that extreme excitement could strain the heart or raise blood pressure. In highly agitated patients, doses of an antipsychotic that are relatively not toxic to the heart ("noncardiotoxic") but adequate to calm the psychotic excitement can protect the heart.

The dopamine receptor antagonists are absorbed orally and continue to remain in active forms for relatively long times in the body (i.e., have relatively long half-lives). Daily dosing is usually adequate. Blood levels can increase over time, eventually requiring reductions in the daily dose.

Side effects of these medications are common and potentially serious. **Neurological side effects** of antipsychotics can unfortunately be common, disabling, and sometimes irreversible.

<u>Tardive Dyskinesia:</u> This serious complication of longer-term treatment with a dopamine receptor antagonist consists of involuntary, "wormy" (choreoathetoid) movements of the head, arms and legs, or trunk. Abnormal

movements of the mouth are typical. Tardive dyskinesia must be distinguished from abnormal movements that are part of the patient's psychotic behavior as well as from other conditions that can cause abnormal writhing movements (e.g., Huntington disease or toxicity from other drugs). Tardive dyskinesia usually appears after relatively prolonged therapy. It affects up to 15–20% of people in treatment for more than a year. Women are said to be more susceptible to it than men. The onset can be gradual but is often sudden. The abnormal movements can be mild or disabling. Fortunately, in contradiction to earlier ideas, it is now clear that tardive dyskinesia tends to remit when the offending drug is stopped and sometimes even when it is not. Over half of mild cases remit, and from 5% to 50% of more established cases do. (Of course, that means that from 50% to 95% of established cases do not remit.) Clinicians need to be sensitive to the early signs of tardive dyskinesia. Common practice when it develops is to switch the patient to one of the newer atypical antipsychotics that appear to be less likely to cause this condition. Unfortunately, reducing the dose or discontinuing the medicine sometimes makes the symptoms transiently worse. No medication is known to be robustly effective against tardive dyskinesia. Treatment is best left to a specialist, either a psychiatrist or a neurologist.

Dystonia: Abnormal movements that occur hours or days after initiating therapy with a dopamine receptor blocker usually represent drug-induced dystonia. These movements result from a relatively slow muscular contraction or spasm that eventually leads to an abnormal movement. They often involve the neck, jaw, and/or tongue. Sometimes they involve the whole body (*opisthotonos*). Involvement of the glossopharyngeal muscles of the mouth and throat can lead to difficulty swallowing or even breathing. Involvement of the eyes, which can occur suddenly even after prolonged use of one of these drugs, can lead to spasm of the lids (*blepharospasm*) or to unwilled movements of the eyes (*oculogyric crisis*). Dystonia is seen most often in young men who have been given intramuscular injections of high-potency dopamine receptor antagonists, but it is not limited to this group of patients. Injections of *anticholinergic agents* or of *diphenhydramine* usually relieve the symptoms. A number of other interventions have also been reported to do so, including hypnosis. This side effect typically leads the prescribing psychiatrist to change to one of the newer atypical antipsychotics.

Parkinsonism: Perhaps 15% of adults treated with dopamine receptor antagonists develop parkinsonism.[27] (See Chap. 11, Disorders of Motility, for a description of the signs of parkinsonism.) The incidence tends to be higher in older people. Aging itself is associated with a progressive decrease in the number of cells containing the neurotransmitter dopamine (*dopaminergic neurons*) in the relevant region of the brain (the *pars compacta* of the *substantia nigra*). People who have lost dopaminergic cells are likely to be more sensitive to the effects of dopamine antagonists. Parkinsonism resembles classical Parkinson disease. The symptoms usually improve with withdrawal of the offending medication. Treatment with an anticholinergic drug such as *amantidine* can help. Continuation of such treatment may benefit patients in whom the parkinsonism does not go away. Unfortunately, L-DOPA tends not to be effective in patients with drug-induced parkinsonism and can exacerbate their psychosis.

Akathisia: This term refers to a sense of discomfort associated with restlessness. The preferred treatment of *akathisia* is to use another antipsychotic or, if that is not practical, to reduce the dose to the lowest level consistent with adequate control of psychotic symptoms. Sometimes akathisia responds to treatment with the *β-adrenergic blocker propranolol* (30–120 mg a day) or with *benzodiazepines*. Sometimes it does not appear to respond to anything. Vague discomfort and restlessness are, of course, often manifestations of an underlying brain disease that also manifests itself as a psychosis. They typically occur in Alzheimer disease, where evidence of organic brain damage is well characterized. (Many high achievers are driven by restlessness and internal discomfort, but it is not conventional to label them as having mild akathisia or even well-compensated hypomania.)

Seizures: Dopamine receptor antagonists can predispose to epileptic fits (*seizures*). These drugs tend to lower seizure thresholds, perhaps because they tend to slow and synchronize the EEG (electroencephalogram). Low-potency dopamine receptor antagonists are more likely to lead to this side effect than the high-potency drugs. This consideration can be important in prescribing for a patient who has already had seizures.

Sedation: The calming effects of the dopamine receptor antagonists can extend to making people sleepy, that is, to sedative side effects. A simple way to deal with this complication is for the patient to take the medication before going to sleep. Chlorpromazine and, to a somewhat lesser extent, thioridazine are particularly sedating, and may be useful in patients in whom sleep is a problem. The high-potency antipsychotics tend not to be sedating. If sleepiness is a problem, patients should avoid driving a car or operating machinery. That may be impractical, however. Not being able to drive a car has become a major disability in much of the United States and, indeed, in other developed countries. Similarly, someone whose job involves using machinery should not be forced to choose between making a living and staying reasonably sane. If the doses of an antipsychotic necessary for satisfactory symptom control are also sedating, then changing to another antipsychotic may be the best option. Fortunately, this side effect often diminishes with time.

Confusion and Other Central Anticholinergic Effects: The dopamine receptor antagonists can lead to delirium, stupor, and coma. (See Chap. 5, Cognitive Disorders.) These effects appear to be due to their antagonism of the neurotransmitter acetylcholine (i.e., their *anticholinergic* effects). Pharmacological treatment is sometimes necessary, for instance in a patient who has received depot injections of the responsible drug. The accepted treatment is with a medication that increases the amount of acetylcholine (a *cholinergic agonist*), namely *physostigmine* (*eserine*). This drug blocks the breakdown of acetylcholine—in other words, it is a cholinesterase inhibitor. The therapeutic window for physostigmine is small, and overdose also needs treatment, usually with atropine (an anticholinergic). Obviously, the treating physician wants to avoid using the patient as a titration vessel in which more drugs are given to block the effects of having given too much of a drug or drugs.

Nonneurological side effects of dopamine receptor antagonists are of particular concern to general physicians.

Neuroleptic Malignant Syndrome: Neuroleptic malignant syndrome is a dangerous complication of treatment with dopamine receptor antagonists.[28] Death rates can be 30% or more when the reaction is to a depot injection of an antipsychotic. Men are affected more often than women. Fortunately, this condition is uncommon, but when it does occur this medical emergency must be promptly recognized and equally promptly treated.

The syndrome can develop rapidly, over 1–3 days or even more rapidly, and can last up to 2 weeks. It can occur at any time in the course of treatment with a dopamine receptor antagonist. The earliest manifestations often include agitation or withdrawal that can easily be mistaken for increased psychosis. The motor signs, which include rigidity and involuntary muscle contractions (dystonia), agitation or lack of movement, lack of speech, or clouded consciousness, can also be mistaken for worsening psychosis (e.g., catatonia). However, the dramatic medical manifestations of the syndrome tend to make themselves noticed. Temperature can rise very high (e.g., 107°F/41.7°C). An older name for the syndrome was malignant hyperpyrexia. Accompanying autonomic symptoms are, not surprisingly, sweating, hypertension, and rapid heart beat (*tachycardia*).

Treatment is supportive, that is, to take care of the manifestations of the syndrome while the body gets rid of the offending medication. Obviously, the drug must be discontinued, although it is difficult to remove a depot injection. The patient needs to be cooled to and kept at a physiological temperature. Electrolyte status, fluid balance, and fluid intake and output need to be monitored. If rigidity is excessive, antiparkinsonian medications may help. (See Chap. 11, Disorders of Motility). A muscle relaxant such as *dantrolene* may also help. (Dosage: IM dantrolene at 0.8–2.5 mg/kg per day, not to exceed 10 mg per day; or oral dantrolene at 100–200 mg/day). Treatment of neuroleptic malignant syndrome obviously needs to continue until the patient is stable and out of danger, usually 5–10 days.

Bone Marrow/Blood: Transient, mild drop in white cell count is common and unimportant. Unfortunately, all of these drugs can depress the bone marrow, with frank *agranulocytosis* occurring in perhaps 0.05% of patients. Blood counts are not routinely done in patients treated with these drugs, but the clinician should be sensitive to early signs of bone marrow depression including susceptibility to infection, bruising, or anemia. As usual, serious bone marrow depression requires serious medical attention by the appropriately qualified clinicians. Fortunately, there is now such panoply of antipsychotic medications that treatment of the psychosis can be continued with a drug of a completely different chemical structure.

Heart and Circulation: The dopamine receptor blockers can lead to drops in blood pressure on rising (*orthostatic hypotension*). Chlorpromazine and thioridazine are particular offenders in this regard. The mechanism appears to be partial blockade of receptors for the transmitter noradrenalin (i.e., *adrenergic receptors*). Fortunately, this side effect usually clears after the first few days of therapy. Blood pressure should if possible be tested before administering these drugs, and the usual precautions taken for patients with orthostatic hypotension. Teaching the patients not to get up too quickly and to hold onto something until they stop feeling light-headed is good in principle, but may well not work for people who are psychotic. Occasionally support stockings or *pressor* agents are necessary, even though it is undesirable to give potentially toxic medications to people who are potentially suicidal.

The association of sudden death with treatment with dopamine receptor antagonists is controversial. One complication is that these patients are typically mad, and one cannot be sure what else they have ingested or what other damage they have done to themselves. Thioridazine at higher doses can cause dangerous irregularities of the heartbeat (*malignant arrhythmias*). It must be used cautiously in people who have or are at high risk for heart disease. ECG (electrocardiogram) changes associated with chlorpromazine include prolonged QT and PR intervals, ST-segment depression, and blunted T waves.

Weight Gain: Weight gain is a common side effect of dopamine receptor antagonists. It can interfere with compliance and in some people lead to medical complications associated with obesity. The treatment of choice is to change the medication.

Pregnancy: Pregnancy is obviously not a complication of treatment with these medicines, but it does complicate their use. Preferable clinical practice is to avoid these medications in women who are pregnant, particularly in the first trimester, or who are nursing. However, doing so may not be realistic. As always, judgment must be used. If a woman who has been relatively stable on these medicines is abruptly taken off them, her recrudescent psychosis may increase the risk of her damaging herself and/or her fetus much more than the low risk of fetal abnormalities from these drugs. Also, women who need antipsychotic medications can no more be presumed to restrain their sexual urges or use contraceptives consistently than can nonpsychotic women. Women being treated for psychoses may take a dopamine receptor antagonist well into the first trimester without being aware that they are pregnant.

Endocrine/Sexual: These types of side effects are unfortunately common. These medications can lead to breast enlargement, inappropriate lactation, and loss of menses. Reduction or loss of sex drive and orgasms can occur in both men and women treated with these drugs. Perhaps 50% of men on these medications claim to have problems with erection and/or ejaculation. Some become frankly impotent. Prolonged and often painful erections (*priapism*) are rarer but do occur.

In treating these side effects, it is important to remember that sexual functions are needed for reproduction but not to maintain life. Many societies over many years have admired chastity and celibacy. Some still do. In modern America, sexual performance is often important to a man's or a woman's sense of self. Diminished performance can lead to a fear that a cherished relationship is threatened, and sometimes it is. Few people want to have less ability to enjoy the pleasures of sex and orgasm. These considerations can affect people with psychoses just as they can those of us who are supposed to be sane. However, it is important for the treating physician to remember that sexual side effects of medication are in general not life-threatening, except for the lives of children who might otherwise have been conceived. (See the discussion of sexual disorders in Chap. 14, Disorders of Conduct.)

Skin: Dopamine receptor antagonists, like most other drugs, can cause allergic skin reactions. These usually appear within weeks after the medication is started. Sensitivity to the sun (*photosensitivity*) can occur, particularly in patients taking chlorpromazine. That drug is sometimes associated with skin discoloration—blue, gray, or gold.

Eyes: Thioridazine can damage the retina. It can induce a form of *retinitis pigmentosa* that can progress to blindness, sometimes even if the medication is stopped. Chlorpromazine can induce a relatively asymptomatic discoloration of the retina after the cumulative lifetime dose exceeds 3 kg or more.

Liver: Cholestatic jaundice is a rare but well-documented complication of treatment with dopamine receptor antagonists. It is an indication for immediately stopping the offending medication, and if necessary replacing it with another antipsychotic.

Atypical Antipsychotics

These agents are typically more effective symptomatically than the older "typical" antipsychotics, and most of them have much more attractive side effect profiles. Their attractive characteristics are supported by many, though not all, studies.[25] These medications are antagonists not only at dopamine receptors but also at serotonin receptors. Many act on other neurotransmitter receptors as well, depending on the specific medication. These medicines are referred to as dopamine-serotonin receptor antagonists.

Table 4-5 lists these drugs and typical doses during maintenance therapy. Again, the doses given in the table are only guidelines. These medications, like the dopamine receptor antagonists, belong to several chemical classes. Patients who become allergic to one of these medications may not be allergic to others of different chemical structures (i.e., to other *haptenes* with the same pharmacological but different immunochemical profiles). In

TABLE 4–5
Atypical antipsychotics

Generic name	Trade name	Oral dose*	I.M. dose
Risperidone	Risperdal	2-6	NA
Olanzapine	Zyprexa	10	NA
Quetiapine	Seroquel	300-400	NA
Ziprasidone	Zeldox	80-160	10 mg; ≤40 mg/day
Clozapine	Clozaril	300	NA

This is an incomplete list of antipsychotic medications that antagonize both serotonin and dopamine receptors. They belong to a number of chemical classes. For details and more extensive discussion, see reference 11

*Doses are usual adult doses in mg. Doses for older subjects are often lower.

NA = Not Applicable.

general, the side effects of these agents are the same as but milder and less frequent than for the pure dopamine antagonists (typical antipsychotics).

Risperidone (Risperdal) is probably the medication in this group that is most widely prescribed by nonpsychiatrists. It is often used where haloperidol (Haldol) was used previously, in part because of its attractive side effect profile. It is readily absorbed after oral dosing, and has a half-life of about 20 hours. Only one dose a day is necessary. Risperidone has been reported to cause a much lower incidence of motor side effects than Haldol does, even though it has just as high an affinity for dopamine receptors. The most common reasons for discontinuing risperidone are extrapyramidal or other movements, seen primarily after doses in excess of 6 mg/day. Other relatively common side effects are dizziness, sleepiness, and nausea.

Risperidone, like haloperidol, is available in solution as well as in pills. The oral solution contains 1 mg/ml of risperidone, that is, 50 μg per drop. The solution form therefore allows convenient administration of very low doses. As discussed in Chap. 5, surprisingly low doses of risperidone or Haldol—perhaps 0.05–0.1 mg—have in my experience often been effective in controlling symptoms in geriatric patients with psychotic symptoms as complications of Alzheimer disease or other dementia. Whether the results are pharmacological or just "placebo effects" matters less than that the patient and family perceive themselves to be benefiting. Even if such small "homeopathic" doses act only by empowering the caregiver, they can stabilize a care situation.

Olanzapine (Zyprexa) is also prescribed relatively frequently. This medication often has useful antidepressant effects. Psychosis complicated by depression (or depression complicated by psychosis) is often difficult to treat and life-threatening because of the risk of suicide. Chronic care of such patients is best left to experts. That is strikingly true of adolescent onset schizoaffective disorder. Olanzapine is more likely than risperidone to lead to weight gain and diabetes. Patients on olanzapine can develop *transaminase* elevations that require stopping the drug. Monitoring these blood values is appropriate in patients taking this drug.

Ziprasidone (Zeldox) has also been reported to have antidepressant actions. If the low incidence of side effects that have been reported for this medication holds up with more extensive use, this may become a popular dopamine receptor antagonist.

Clozapine (Clozaril) and quetiapine (Seroquel) reportedly do not have extrapyramidal side effects, perhaps because they are less-effective dopamine receptor blockers than the other medications. Treatment with clozapine, like that with olanzapine, has been reported to lead to weight gain and diabetes.

Lithium

This medication can help to reduce psychotic symptoms in as many as half the patients who receive the diagnosis of schizophrenia, even if it is more commonly thought of as a drug for manic-depressive disease. As discussed in Chap. 3 (Mood Disorders), the clinical manifestations of schizophrenia and manic-depressive disease can be so similar that differential diagnosis was difficult even for Bleuler, the German psychiatrist, who originated these categories. Genetic studies suggest that these syndromes can be manifestations of the same underlying biological abnormality. (See Table 4-2 and discussion in Chap. 3, Mood Disorders.) As discussed in Chap. 3, combinations of lithium and antipsychotics are often very useful for the treatment of manic-depressive disease. They can also be very useful for the treatment of other thought disorders including schizophrenia. The reason for the therapeutic overlap is probably that at the biological level one is treating the same processes.

Benzodiazepines

These agents can be useful in treating the anxiety associated with thought disorders, as well as pathological anxiety from other sources. Chapter 6

(Anxiety) discusses these medications. *Alprazolam* (Xanax) is often used in combination with an antipsychotic. In some patients diagnosed with schizophrenia, a benzodiazepine alone appears to bring the illness under control. There are reports of schizophrenics responding to relatively high doses of *diazepam* (Valium) without other medication. *Chlordiazepoxide* (Librium) was used as a primary treatment for schizophrenia when this medication was first introduced. Nowadays it is preferable to use a benzodiazepine with a shorter biological half-life, because of the possibility that these unstable people take too much of it at one time.

Anticonvulsants

The differential diagnosis between seizure disorders affecting the temporal lobe and schizophrenia and other forms of madness can be very difficult. (See Chap. 10, Disorders of Awareness.) Sometimes a psychotic patient who does not respond to other medications will respond to an anticonvulsant. Anticonvulsants can be added to the regimen of psychotic patients who have episodes of intolerable behavior, specifically of violence. Combination therapy with an anticonvulsant and an antipsychotic will sometimes help a patient who does not respond well to either alone. Care must be taken to adjust doses, because anticonvulsants can induce liver enzymes that inactivate some antipsychotics. The anticonvulsants most used to treat primarily psychiatric abnormalities are *carbamazepine* (Tegretol) and *valproate* (Depakene, Depakote). These agents are discussed with treatment of seizures in Chap. 10 (Disorders of Awareness).

TREATMENT OF ACUTE PSYCHOTIC EMERGENCIES

In the general medical setting, treatment of an acute psychotic episode is the same whether the patient ends up with a diagnosis of schizophrenia or of manic-depressive disease or of one of the other refined categories of psychosis listed in DSM-IV-TR. The discussion in Chap. 3 (Mood Disorders) applies. Typical acute treatment in an emergency room or other similar setting is haloperidol (Haldol: 10 mg by mouth or 5 mg IM, with more as necessary) and lorazepam (2 mg by mouth or IM) repeated as necessary at intervals of not less than 1 hour. Haldol has a somewhat faster onset of action than Risperdal and is therefore favored in this situation. The doses obviously need to be individualized, with less given to a smaller and less-agitated person and more to a larger and potentially violent individual.

The same considerations about further care apply more or less independently of the psychiatric diagnosis the patient ends up with. (See Chap. 3, Mood Disorders.) Medical and surgical problems need to be attended to, particularly problems with breathing and bleeding. A psychiatrist should take over management of the psychiatric problems, including making the specific diagnosis, according to the current version of DSM (Diagnostic and Statistical Manual of the American Psychiatric Association). Psychiatric hospitalization in the United States now usually requires either the consent of the patient or the signatures of two licensed physicians. The signatures of a general physician who has cared for the patient and the psychiatrist who has taken over care are adequate to get an acutely psychotic patient into a more protected setting. After that, the decision about continuing hospitalization may rest with the blunt instrument of the judicial system.

NONPHARMACOLOGICAL TREATMENTS

Chapter 3 (Mood Disorders) discusses the use of nonpharmacological techniques in patients with intractable, drug-unresponsive insanity. The same considerations apply whether the patients end up with the diagnosis of schizophrenia or of manic-depressive disease.

Social Management

A wide variety of resources to help psychotic patients exist in the community, in the United States and other developed countries. They include halfway houses, day hospitals, and of course mental hospitals. Inpatient care is usually reserved for individuals who are a danger to themselves or to others or who have medical or other problems that prevent their living in the community. Psychiatrists develop expertise in helping patients and families to choose and then use this kind of help optimally. General clinicians and their patients are usually best off if these efforts are left to trained psychiatric personnel, including psychiatric social workers.

Unfortunately, even the best intended and thought-through efforts often fail to do much for patients with this devastating group of illnesses. Perhaps half or more of the homeless in New York and other large cities suffer to a greater or lesser degree from serious mental illness. The current approach is to give these people as much freedom as is compatible with their and our safety. Whether that is the kindest way to treat them is a political issue that goes beyond the scope of this monograph.

Electric Shock Therapy

Before the discovery of chlorpromazine (Thorazine) and subsequently other antipsychotic medications, electroconvulsive therapy (ECT) was a mainstay of the treatment of schizophrenics. There are still occasional patients with this diagnosis who appear to do well receiving short courses of ECT when they have psychotic breaks. Of course, the decision for this type of treatment must rest with a psychiatrist as well as with the patient and responsible others.

Transcranial Magnetic Stimulation

This new technique may help reduce auditory hallucinations, according to recent studies.[29] At the present time, its use is restricted to academic centers where researchers are actively interested in and familiar with it. The usefulness of this noninterventive approach remains to be defined.

Psychosurgery

Psychosurgery to treat intractable insanity has a checkered past, as discussed at the end of Chap. 3 (Mood Disorders). Family physicians may be asked for their advice if such treatment is recommended. In the author's experience, it has sometimes been wonderfully successful, but not rarely the result is a depersonalized and/or neurologically disabled individual. Whatever the results, psychosurgery is irreversible.

REFERENCES

1. Nor should researchers treat them as different entities. In earlier years, researchers looking for biological concomitants to psychiatric illnesses used "depressives" as disease controls for studies of "schizophrenics" and vice versa. As noted in the text, in retrospect that decision does not seem wise.

Empirically, specific gene loci have been found that predispose to manic-depressive syndromes in some patients and schizophrenia in others, as discussed in the previous chapter on mood disorders as well as in this chapter (Table 4-2). For thoughtful discussions of these issues of classification see Kendell RE, Gourley J. The clinical distinction between the affective psychoses and schizophrenia. *Br J Psychiatry*. 1970;117:261–266.
Crow TJ, Con. The demise of the Kraeplinian binary system as a prelude to genetic advance. In: *Genetic Approaches to Mental Disorders*. (ES Gershon, CR Cloninger, eds), Washington, DC, APA Press, 1994, pp. 163–192.
For a more detailed discussion of the genetics, see
Badner JA, Gershon ES. Meta-analysis of whole-genome linkage scans of bipolar disorder and schizophrenia. *Mol Psychiatry*. 2002;7:405–411.
Crow T. Nuclear schizophrenic symptoms as a window on the relationship between thought and speech. *Br J Psychiatry*. 1998;173:303–309. This article presents a more philosophical overview.
2. Freedman R. Schizophrenia. *N Eng J Med*. 2003;349:1738–1749.
3. Kandel ER. Brain and behavior. In: ER Kandel, JH Schwarz, TM Jessel, eds, *Principles of Neural Science,* 3d edition, Elsevier, NY, 1991, p. 15. Reading this book makes it easy to understand why Kandel won the Nobel Prize.
4. A silly bureaucrat in the dean's office responded by writing the young academic a letter threatening to fire him for "moral turpitude." That administrator calmed down after receiving a letter from an M.D., on the department of psychiatry's letterhead, stating that the woman who wrote the initial letter was insane—a point that was obvious to the people sweeping the floors when she first walked in.
5. This example is based on a real clinical experience. The bracelet was of twisted copper wires. The patient knew that her husband had given it to her, and was convinced he had done so to protect her from the Martians. Since wearing it calmed her anxiety, the medical staff saw no reason to suggest that she take it off.
6. A patient once claimed to my father that the bathroom faucets in his family's home were made of gold. My father initially thought that to be a delusion, until the family told him that the taps in their apartment in New York were, in fact, of 14-carat gold. The sanity of the architect who designed their apartment or of the people who bought it was not under consideration.
7. Catatonia can lead to "plastic immobility." The patient maintains the same position almost motionlessly. If, however, someone else (like a doctor or nurse) alters that position, the patient remains motionless in the altered position.
8. Those who have struggled to computerize medical records have recognized that there must be a grab-bag category for patients who do not fit the listed diagnoses, in order to prevent contaminating the diagnostic groups included in the list with people who do not really fit any of those categories. The

acronym GORK derives from the whimsical diagnostic category, God Only Really Knows. GOMER stands for Get Out of My Emergency Room. Physicians who use GORK as a pejorative reveal how irritated they become with a patient whose illness they do not understand and do not know how to treat. Treating GORKs and GOMERs often turns out to present extraordinarily interesting diagnostic and therapeutic challenges for interested physicians.

9. Wing JK. Comments on the long-term outcome of schizophrenia. *Schizophr Bull.* 1988;14:669–673. Others have expressed other viewpoints - for instance, that the core phenomenon is deficient organization of perceptual information (e.g., Braff DL. Information processing and attention dysfunctions in schizophrenia. *Schizophr Bull.* 1993;19:233–259.).
10. Ho BC, Black DW, Andreasen NC. Schizophrenia and other psychotic disorders. In: RE Hales, SC Yudofsky, eds, *The American Psychiatric Publishing Textbook of Clinical Psychiatry,* American Psychiatric Publishing, NY, 2003, pp. 379–438. The discussion of proposed etiologies for schizophrenias is on pp. 403–408.
11. Sadock BJ, Sadock VA. Synopsis of Psychiatry: Behavioral Sciences/Clinical Psychiatry, 9th edition, Lippincott Wiliams & Wilkins, NY, 2003, p. 477.
12. Maziade M, Merette C, Chagnon YC, et al. Genetics of schizophrenia and bipolar disorder: recent success of linkage studies with evidence of specific and shared susceptibility loci. [Article in French] *Med Sci (Paris).* 2003;19: 960–966.
13. Faraone SV, Taylor L, Tsuang MT. The molecular genetics of schizophrenia: an emerging consensus. *Expert Rev Mol Med.* 2002;2002:1–13.
14. One example is phenylketonuria (PKU). A classic paper describing the syndrome of early infantile autism included, as one of the four exemplary cases, a child later found to have biochemically typical PKU.
15. Green EK, Raybould R, Macgregor S, et al. Operation of the schizophrenia susceptibility gene, neuregulin 1, across traditional diagnostic boundaries to increase risk for bipolar disorder. *Arch Gen Psychiatry.* 2005;62:642–648.
16. Maier W, Hofgen B, Zobel A, et al. Genetic models of schizophrenia and bipolar disorder: overlapping inheritance or discrete genotypes? *Eur Arch Psychiatry Clin Neurosci.* 2005;255:159–66.
17. Verma R, Mukerji M, Grover D, et al. MLC1 gene is associated with schizophrenia and bipolar disorder in Southern India. *Biol Psychiatry.* 2005;58: 16–22.
18. A famous example of frank madness after an apparent attack of encephalitis is the Roman emperor Caligula Caesar. Historians have been arguing about how crazy he was before the fever since his assassination in the first century AD.
19. That canard was preached particularly against the parents of autistic children. It added to the pain of raising a beloved, autistic child by accusing the parents of causing their child's illness by not being loving enough. Talk

therapy can be quite as painful and inappropriate as more interventive, biological treatments. The cliché that words can cut like a knife is appropriate.

20. The results of neuropathological studies of schizophrenia remain controversial. Schizophrenia has been described as the graveyard of neuropathologists. The heterogeneity of the schizophrenias may make findings variable from series to series and institution to institution.
21. Altar CA, Jurata LW, Charles V, et al. Deficient hippocampal neuron expression of proteosome, ubiquitin, and mitochondrial genes in multiple schizophrenic cohorts. *Biol Pysch.* 2005;58:85–96.
22. Davis KL, Kahn RS, Ko G, et al. Dopamine in schizophrenia: a review and reconceptualization. *Am J Psychiatry.* 1991;148:1474–1486.
23. The normal relatives of a psychotic patient can sometimes be quite weird themselves. Madness often runs in families.
24. At the time of my training in the 1960s, vomiting bright red blood. was a typical presentation of gastric ulcer disease in a schizophrenic confined to a "back ward" Schizophrenics so often complain of vague discomfort in their abdomens that it was hard to pick out those with real gastrointestinal disease from the others under the conditions in state mental hospitals at that time.
25. A recent, widely publicized article calls into question the better efficacy of the newer antipsychotics compared to older medications. (Lieberman JA, Stroup TS, McEvoy JP, et al (multicenter investigators). Effectiveness of antipsychotic drugs in patients with chronic schizophrenia. *New Eng J Med.* 2005;353:1209–1223.) In this relatively long-term study, poor compliance was taken as indicating lack of efficacy. Compliance was equally poor with both newer and older antipsychotics. Whether that study proves more than that compliance is a problem in psychotic people is a matter of interpretation.
26. Taken from Sadock BJ, Sadock VA. *Pocket Handbook of Psychiatric Drug Treatment,* 3d edition, Lippincott Williams & Wilkins, NY, 2001, p. 114.
27. A gifted Harvard medical student was once convinced that he had identified a motor syndrome of schizophrenia. What he had seen, and imitated well, was parkinsonian gait and other parkinsonian behavior presumably due to rich doses of dopamine receptor antagonists.
28. A tragic example that received extensive media coverage was a young woman with psychiatric problems who was given an injection of an antipsychotic in the emergency room and then died of neuroleptic malignant syndrome. Her father was an editor of a major newspaper. The medical staff of the university hospital was accused publicly—very publicly—of not having recognized the syndrome quickly enough.
29. Hoffman RE, Gueorguieva R, Hawkins KA, et al. Temporoparietal transcranial magnetic stimulation for auditory hallucinations: safety, efficacy and moderators in a fifty patient sample. *Biol Psychiatry.* 2005;58:97–104.

CHAPTER FIVE

Cognitive Disorders: Delirium and Dementia

This chapter discusses disorders that general clinicians will not only encounter but will also have to treat. There are too many patients with disorders of cognition for them all to be referred to the care of specialists. That is particularly true for the elderly. Furthermore, delirium is often so intertwined with medical illnesses that a key element of care is treatment of the underlying medical problems. Consultations with neurologists, psychiatrists, and neuropsychologists can still be appropriate, however, particularly for patients who present unusual diagnostic or other problems.

General physicians in the United States now tend to make a relatively sharp distinction between delirium and dementia.[1] Neurologists, however, tend to look on these two conditions as poles on a disease spectrum. Many patients have elements of both. Engel and Romano[2] pointed out that prolonged delirium can lead to dementia and that even subclinical dementia can predispose to the development of delirium. Obviously, one can, and should, treat the reversible aspects (the delirium) without losing sight of the underlying brain disease (the dementia).

INCIDENCE AND PREVALENCE

Impairments of cognition are common in medical settings. When systematic mental testing was done, about 30% of the patients on the medical and neurological wards of the Johns Hopkins Medical Institutions were seriously impaired cognitively.[3] Similar results were found 20 years later on the wards of the Burke Rehabilitation Hospital.[4] Unhappily, the nurses and doctors were not aware of disturbances of cognition in more than half of the afflicted patients, even in the rehabilitation hospital. The following is not an extreme example.

> A 72-year-old woman without previously recognized mental disability scored in the moderately impaired range on the Mini-Mental State Examination (MMSE). When an incredulous physician asked her who the president of the United States was, she answered, "What are you, crazy? Franklin Roosevelt." The correct answer at the time was Ronald Reagan. She was not acutely ill when tested. Her mental disability was presumably due to dementia rather than delirium, despite the lack of any history of dementia from her family or from the acute care hospital from which she had been transferred. This feisty lady had been functioning well in her apartment in the Bronx, partly on overlearned material about her apartment and neighborhood and partly with the help of family and neighbors. She was able to go back to her apartment, to the same support system she had had before her acute illness and rehabilitation. The staff at the rehabilitation hospital doubted that she would have lived longer or been as happy had she been forced into a nursing home or other institution to protect her.

General clinicians can be confident that a significant portion of their sick patients will develop delirium, particularly their older patients. As discussed below, regular examination of mental status particularly in the hospitalized elderly is a wise precaution by the medical and nursing staff caring for them. Delirium appears to be a very unpleasant mental state, as far as one can tell from observing these patients and from whatever memories they have of being delirious. Patients can lose all touch with reality. Terrifying hallucinations that resemble horrible but prolonged nightmares are so common as to be characteristic. The experience has been described as "like being in Hell." An example that most physicians have seen of the discomfort accompanying delirium is *delirium tremens* (alcohol withdrawal syndrome, the DTs).

Dementia is especially frequent in the elderly. An epidemiological study in Boston concluded that about half of people 80 years or older were at least mildly demented. Earlier studies requiring more severe impairment to apply the label of dementia reported that perhaps 5–10% of people over 70 should be given this diagnosis. Recently, the Finnish National Health Service reported that about 16% of the population above 85 years old in that northern European country suffered from clinically significant dementia. Whichever definition and number one chooses, the proportion of people with dementia is large and can only be expected to grow as populations age in the United States and elsewhere.

CLASSIFICATION AND DIAGNOSIS

Classification schemes have been developed for both delirium and dementias. Because these two sets of conditions are intimately related clinically and biologically, attempts to classify them independently of each other have an element of virtual reality. However, the currently conventional classifications are a good starting point for discussion.

Delirium

Delirium is defined as reversible, global cognitive impairment, typically involving orientation as well as memory and judgment. It is distinguished from stupor and coma by the depth of impairment of consciousness in the latter conditions. *Stupor* is a state of behavioral unresponsiveness resembling deep sleep, in which vigorous, repeated stimuli are needed to rouse the patient. *Coma* is a state of unresponsiveness from which the patient cannot be roused, even by vigorous and painful stimulation. There are at least two ways to classify delirium.[5] One is by etiology, the other by major clinical manifestations.

When an etiology is clear, the disorder is generally named in terms of the etiology. Examples are *hepatic encephalopathy* (from liver disease), brain hypoxia (lack of oxygen supply to the brain), or hypoglycemic confusion (from low blood sugar). Almost any intercurrent illness can present as confusion, especially in elderly people. For instance, confusion can be a classic presentation of a heart attack.

> A 79-year-old woman in good general and neurological health was participating in a multicenter trial of a medication to prevent Alzheimer disease (AD). Routine follow-up neuropsychological testing showed that she had slipped into dementia. On examination, she had rales at both lung bases. She was referred to her private physician, who admitted her to the hospital for heart failure of unknown etiology that turned out to be due to a painless myocardial infarction. Her heart disease was treated and her cardiac failure cleared. Mentally, she returned to her previous normal state. Whether or not she was in an early, "asymptomatic" state of the AD that ran in her family remained unclear. (She continued in the "prevention" study.)

The clinical manifestations of delirium are broadly divided into *apathetic delirium* and *agitated delirium.* Often patients fluctuate between these states. In apathetic delirium, the patient is relatively inactive and can appear obtunded. Such patients tend not to call attention to their cognitive problems. They cause relatively little inconvenience to the nursing staff in a hospital or nursing home. A spouse or other caregiver at home may become alarmed at the patient becoming "like a zombie," but even a family caregiver may find an apathetic person more convenient to care for than one who is more active and demanding. In contrast, patients with agitated delirium do call attention to themselves. They are typically loud, boisterous, agitated, and often suspicious. Their behavior can become very inconvenient for those caring for them. Caregivers, whether professionals or family, are likely to insist that these patients be "given something" to calm them down. (As discussed in more detail later in this chapter, such medication can be as necessary to calm the caregiver as to calm the patient.) Both apathetic and agitated delirium can have serious consequences. Apathetic patients may not eat or drink enough, avoid taking medicine, refuse to participate in their rehabilitation, or be effectively self-destructive in other "passive" ways. Agitated patients may actively hurt themselves, for instance by wandering into dangerous situations. They characteristically lack the mental organization to be dangerous to others, except by accident.

Dementia

Dementia is defined as (1) global impairment of cognition, (2) that is *permanent*, and (3) occurs in a *clear sensorium.* Global impairment of cognition in practice means impairment of memory, particularly new memory, as well as at least two other areas of cognition. (The technical terminology is "memory and at least two other cognitive domains.") Permanent in practice means for more than 3 months and, better, for more than 6 months. Patients being evaluated for dementia have usually had signs of progressive mental failure for a year or more. Clear sensorium is the most troublesome part of this definition. The requirement of a clear sensorium is meant to distinguish patients with dementia from patients with the clouded sensorium of delirium. Since patients with dementia are prone to develop delirium, this requirement is not absolute. A good history from a reliable informant can provide evidence of underlying permanent deterioration of cognition—and therefore of the diagnosis of dementia—even in a patient with a superimposed delirium. Chronic but still reversible delirium can easily be mistaken for a permanent dementia.

Diagnosis of Disorders of Cognition

The diagnosis of disorders of cognition involves at least three steps. The first is recognizing that a patient is cognitively impaired. Skill in doing so is important for general clinicians. Recognizing problems or potential problems in behavior can make patient care much smoother, easing the lives of both patients and nursing staff. Also, numerous studies in many settings have consistently demonstrated that confusion is one of the strongest predictors of mortality, particularly in older people. The second step is to make an informed judgment about the extent to which the impairment of cognition is transient (delirium) or permanent (dementia) or a mixture of the two. The third step is to determine the cause—or more likely, causes—of the cognitive disability.

Recognizing Cognitive Impairment: As discussed above, cognitive impairment tends to be under-recognized by physicians and nurses, even by skilled physicians and nurses working in first-rate institutions. The key to recognizing cognitive impairment is to think about whether or not it is present even in patients who are not inconvenient to take care of. Nursing staff, who spend more time with the patients, sometimes may recognize delirium before physicians do. As usual, it pays for physicians to listen to what nurses tell them.

There are many simple, rapid ways to test for confusion. Often simply talking with the patient shows that the patient is confused (assuming the physician is intact). But even skilled and sensitive physicians can be fooled, particularly by patients with highly developed social skills.[6]

> A lady being evaluated for AD said, with wonderful charm, "There is nothing wrong with me, doctor, but my husband worries so." The doctor replied, "That's fine—then we can get this examination over with quickly. How old are you?" She turned to her husband and asked, "How old am I, dear?" On superficial examination, she had covered her disabilities with social skills that had become deeply encoded in her brain when she was growing up as a debutante in Savannah, Georgia.

Brief mental status tests are more reliable than just conversation. There are many variants of these tests and they are described in many texts. Brief mental status testing need add little time to the examinations normally done during morning and evening rounds.[7] It can be done tactfully, without offending or frightening the patient.

One widely used test is to ask the patient to spell the word "world," first forwards and then if that is done successfully to spell it backwards. This simple exercise is a surprisingly robust screen for dementia. Simple orientation questions (time, place, and person) can also be revealing.

Factor analysis of much longer psychological questionnaires led to the development of the Mental Status Questionnaire (MSQ) by Kahn and Goldfarb and their colleagues.[7] The MSQ emphasizes orientation. Some geriatricians use this procedure routinely on their patient rounds, since confusion is such a sensitive sign of illness in the elderly. Currently the most widely used short portable mental test is the MMSE, originally developed by Folstein, Folstein and McHugh.[8] The MMSE tests not only orientation but also memory and simple skills (i.e., *praxis*). It has been translated and validated in Spanish and a number of other languages. There is a large literature about both its use and its limitations. Illiteracy tends to reduce MMSE scores even in people without other evidence of cognitive impairment. Despite such limitations, a standard way to summarize a person's mental capacities is to give their MMSE score: 29 and 30 imply more or less intact; 25–29 implies possible mild impairment; 24 and below indicates impairment. People with scores below 20 are usually obviously impaired, and people with scores below 10 are usually severely impaired. It is important to remember, however, that both the MSQ and the MMSE require language. Aphasia can cause very low scores even for people who are otherwise not cognitively impaired. Table 5-1 gives a combination form for the MSQ and MMSE that has proven useful at the Burke Rehabilitation Hospital.

TABLE 5–1
Mental status worksheet

QUESTIONS	MMSE*	MSQ†
What is today's date?		
Day (of the week)	______	______
Date	______	______
Month	______	______
Season	______	
Year	______	______
What is the name of this place?	______	______
What is the address (town)?	______	______
How old are you?	______	
When were you born?		
Month	______	______
Year	______	______
Who is the president of the United States of America?	______	______
Who was the president before him/her?	______	______
Name 3 objects. 1 second to say each.	______	
Then ask the patient all 3 after you have	______	
said them. Then repeat them until the	______	
patient learns them. Count trials and record.		
Subtract 7 from 100, and continue	______	
subtracting 7s (total of 5 times)	______	
(alternatively, spell world forward and	______	
then backward; 12 points correct for	______	
each correct letter in order backwards.)	______	
Maximum total = 5 points.		
Ask for 3 objects repeated previously.	______	
1 point for each object remembered	______	
correctly. Maximum = 3 points.	______	
Show the patient and ask him/her to name		
a pencil or pen	______	
a watch	______	
Hand the patient a piece of paper	______	
with the instructions: "take this piece	______	
of paper in your right hand, fold it	______	
in half, and put it on the floor." One	______	
point for each of the acts done correctly		
and in order. Maximum = 3 points.		

(Continued)

TABLE 5-1
Mental status worksheet (*Continued*)

QUESTIONS	MMSE*	MSQ†
Tell the patient to do what it says on the sign you will hold up, and then hold up a sign that says "CLOSE YOUR EYES."	______	
Ask the patient to write a sentence. Only a complete grammatical sentence counts—no matter how short.	______	
Show the patient a design of intersecting pentagons and have the patient copy it. The patient can keep the diagram while copying.	______	
Total score:	______ (max=30)	______ (max=10)

*Mini-Mental State Exam. Scores of 29-30 indicate normal cognition; scores <24 indicate significant cognitive impairment. Scores of 25-28 suggest following the patient to see if clinically significant cognitive disabilities develop. See: Folsterin MF, Folstein SE, McHugh PR, "Mini-Mental State"—A practical method for grading the cognitive state of patients for the clinician. *J Pyschiatr* Res. 1975:12:189-198. For a current review, see Han L, Cole M, Bellavance F, et al Tracking cognitive decline in Alzheimer's disease using the mini-mental state examination: a meta-analysis. Int Psychogeriatr. 2000;12:231-47.

†Mental Status Questionaire. Scores of 7 or less indicate significant cognitive impairment. See: Kahn RL, Goldfarb AI, Pollack M, et al. Brief cognitive measures for the determination of mental status in the aged. Amer J Psychiat. 1960;117:326-328.

Full evaluation of a cognitively impaired patient requires detailed testing by a qualified neuropsychologist. Full neuropsychological testing requires time and money, but is often invaluable in providing guidelines for patient care—specifically, for adapting the environment to the patient's remaining skills.

Knowledge of a patient's mental status is particularly important when the patient is involved in medical decision-making. The consensus in America is that patients have the right to decide what is done for (or to) them, after they have been fully informed about the alternatives In other words, informed consent is required. A person who cannot pay attention to or otherwise cannot understand the relevant medical decisions cannot give informed consent. As noted above, a clinician's impression that a patient is "all right" can be an overinterpretation of pleasant manners in someone who is too delirious or demented or psychotic to understand what is being explained. Fairness to our patients demands that we do at least brief cognitive testing before asking a sick person, particularly an old, sick person, to decide on a course of action. Documenting in the chart that the person was *compos mentis* enough to participate in decisions regarding his or her care can also protect the physician if dissatisfaction leads to later questioning on this point. Sometimes formal consultation with a psychiatrist, neurologist, or neuropsychologist is in order—for instance, if a patient refuses resuscitation or other care. The patient's decision may be entirely rational, but it behooves those caring for the patient to document that it is.

Delirium Versus Dementia

A reliable history is necessary to determine whether a confused patient is suffering from transient delirium, permanent dementia, or a combination of both. Development of confusion within a day or a few days in a previously intact person makes the diagnosis of delirium and effectively rules out dementia. A history of progressive deterioration over a year or more makes dementia more likely. Sudden deterioration in a person who has been slowly slipping mentally suggests a delirium superimposed on a "dementing" process. It is usually useful to find out why a demented patient has been brought in *now*. Did the social support system change—for instance, a new caregiver? Did a relative come to visit and insist on a "modern workup?" Has the patient developed a new behavior that is socially unacceptable? For instance, sexual disinhibitions? Did the patient develop a superimposed delirium, secondary to a new drug or an intercurrent illness? A sharp recent deterioration in behavior can suggest the latter, more "medical" possibility.

A reliable history requires a reliable informant. Confused patients are not reliable historians, by definition. Sometimes relatives are reliable and sometimes they are in such denial that their reports need to be discounted.

> The son of a severely demented 75-year-old foreign-born woman felt passionately that her score of 3 (out of a possible 10) on the MSQ was artificially low. He claimed that the "wrong questions were asked." For instance, he attributed her lack of knowledge of the name of the president to her "never having been interested in American politics." The staff's doubts about the patient's ability to live alone were confirmed when other informants were interviewed. For instance, they reported that the patient had started a fire in her house by putting meat wrapped in paper directly on the gas stove. (The son dismissed this incident saying, "My mother has always been absent minded.")

It is common to be told that an apparently demented patient was "fine" until a spouse or other caregiver died. The reason, of course, is that the dead caregiver had covered for the patient's difficulties. Troubled or otherwise contentious families often provide confusing histories, including blaming another family member for the patient's problem. Guilt frequently impairs the accuracy of an otherwise reliable historian. As always, clinical skill requires sensitivity to what is communicated nonverbally as well as to the words that are spoken.

Differential Diagnosis of Delirium

Focused treatment of a delirium requires recognition of the cause(s). That varies from straightforward to practically impossible. Classic causes of delirium include intercurrent medical illness particularly in the elderly, toxicity perhaps due to side effects of a newly ingested drug or other substance, new disease of the brain, and combinations of all three.

As noted above, essentially any concomitant medical illness can cause delirium if it is severe enough. This is particularly true in the elderly. Confusion can be the presenting first noticeable sign of an illness, again particularly in the elderly. An example in a woman with a painless heart attack is given earlier. The workup of confusion in an elderly patient is analogous to the workup of a fever of unknown origin (FUO) in a child or younger adult or chest pain in a middle-aged man. It tests the full range of the physician's diagnostic skill and knowledge. Development of delirium in a patient undergoing treatment for a medical illness is a poor prognostic sign. It may indicate that the disease is getting worse, that a new illness has also developed, or both. As noted above, confusion is an unhappily reliable risk factor for death. Concomitant medical illness can also precipitate cognitive problems in younger patients, although this scenario is less common than in the elderly. A specific and highly treatable form of delirium is the Wernicke-Korsakoff syndrome, in which confusion is typically accompanied by abnormal eye movements and staggering (*ataxia*). This highly treatable condition is discussed below and in Chap. 14 (Disorders of Conduct.)

The development of delirium after the ingestion of essentially any new substance should raise the suspicion that the new substance caused the confusion. That is true for prescription drugs, over-the-counter remedies, "holistic," "natural" nostrums, and recreational substances including alcohol. In elderly people with underlying brain disease, even one drink of an alcoholic beverage can cause confusion. A classic and tragic example is Rita Hayworth. Before her AD was diagnosed, she was called a drunk, and not only by the media types who publicized her confusion when she was getting off an airplane. If a standard, recommended dose causes confusion in a specific patient, then that standard dose is too much for that patient—of alcohol or anything else.

Common causes of delirium include sedatives of any type (including medicines for sleep, antihistaminics, and antianxiety agents); anticholinergic medications (Table 5-2); alcohol (ethanol); and "recreational drugs" (cocaine, amphetamines, LSD [d-lysergic acid diethylamide], club drugs, and designer drugs). Marijuana (cannabis) and opiates alter behavior but do not classically cause typical delirium. However, cannabis can precipitate psychosis in a susceptible individual, including a person with an underlying thought disorder that appeared to be in remission. Chapter 7 (Pain) discusses morphine and other opiates, Chap. 8 (Sleep) discusses

TABLE 5-2

Medications with anticholinergic side effects

- Antihistaminics
  - Chlorpheniramine
  - Diphenhydramine
  - Triphenylethylamine
  - Cyproheptadine
  - Promethazine
  - Hydroxyzine
- Antidepressants
  - Amitryptiline
  - Doxepin
- Muscle Relaxants
  - Carisoprodol
  - Methocarbamol
- Cardiac Medications
  - Disopyramide
- Antispasmodics
  - Propantheline
  - Hyoscyamine
  - Belladonna alkaloids in general

The list above is only partial. The Merck Manual of Health and Aging contains a much more complete discussion of anticholinergic side effects of common drugs and of other drugs that can impair cognition.

the pharmacology of sedatives, Chap. 6 (Anxiety) that of antianxiety agents including Valium, and Chap. 14 (Disorders of Conduct) of recreational drugs including alcohol and the various forms of cannabis. However, certain therapeutic traps deserve more specific discussion here.

Medications given to "calm down" a patient can also precipitate cognitive dysfunction. A vicious cycle can develop, with confused people getting more and more of a calming medicine that is in fact increasing the confusion that is agitating them. Among the drugs that can do this are *benzodiazepines, barbiturates*, and other mild sedatives. (Barbiturates can have a direct, paradoxical, exciting effect in elderly people, as they can in children.) Large enough doses of medications that depress brain function can lead to delirium even in relatively healthy, younger people. That includes alcohol and other recreational drugs of abuse.

Anesthetics can not only precipitate delirium but can probably also be followed by dementia. In general, local anesthesia, with "light sleep" if necessary, is preferable to deep general anesthesia in people at risk for delirium or dementia. Of course, local anesthesia is not always practical. However, the convenience to operating room personnel of having the patient cooperative must be weighed against the potential harm of general anesthesia in patients at relatively high risk for permanent cognitive impairment.

Prescription drugs that are not widely recognized to have potential side effects on the central nervous system can also precipitate confusion in susceptible subjects. *Digitalis in* its various forms is an important example. This side effect of digitalis glycosides is not rare in clinical practice, if the physician looks for it. Digitalis-induced confusion can contribute to digitalis toxicity in patients who become confused about how much of their medicine they have taken. That specifically includes older people and particularly those who have even mild evidence of cognitive impairment.

Over-the-counter medications that depress nervous system function are also a classic cause of delirium, as illustrated by the following example.

> A 92-year-old man was brought to the hospital with severe confusion. History revealed that the previous week he had been in good mental health and caring successfully for himself. Careful search of his home for potentially toxic agents uncovered a partly used package of an antihistaminic widely sold over-the-counter. This antihistaminic has powerful sedative and anticholinergic side effects. It turned out that he had started a cold and wanted to be free of symptoms for his great grand daughter's wedding. He went to the pharmacy, found a cold remedy vigorously advertised

by the manufacturer as safe, and took the full dose recommended for adults. His acute confusion cleared over several weeks without specific treatment, although his residual cognitive state was consistent with the diagnosis of Minimal Cognitive Impairment/early Alzheimer disease (MCI/AD). Unfortunately, he missed the wedding.

Whenever possible, a reliable relative or other caregiver should bring in all the medicines in the home of a confused patient, whether or not the relative thinks those medications are harmless. The result is often a shopping bag full of new and old (sometimes very old) prescription drugs as well as over-the-counter remedies and holistic nostrums. Careful evaluation of the potential side effects of a large number of medications can be tedious for a physician or nurse. However, taking the patient off a potentially toxic medication often precludes the need for a high-tech workup. The latter type of evaluation is typically inconvenient and often frightening for the patient. It is more expensive for the health-care system, although such high-tech studies may benefit the amortization of fixed costs in the hospital in which they are done.

Drugs of abuse can also cause delirium, and should be included in the differential diagnosis even in the elderly. (See Chap. 14, Disorders of Conduct.) Alcohol is of course a classic bad actor in this scenario, as is alcohol withdrawal (delirium tremens). But other drugs can also be involved. Steady use of a recreational drug can lead to a chronic delirium that is difficult to tell from a dementia.

A 73-year-old woman received the diagnosis of AD after an extensive evaluation in a subspecialty dementia clinic. On one-year follow-up, her daughter reported (by telephone) that her mother was now entirely well. After the daughter had found and removed the Quaaludes that her mother had hidden in a bureau drawer, the cognitive problems cleared completely. The physician who had made the original misdiagnosis of AD was both surprised and pleased.

The *Physicians Desk Reference*, in both its print and CD (compact disc) versions, is an excellent and widely available source of information on even rare side effects of prescription drugs available in the United States. When a patient has taken a medication from abroad, it is wise to obtain the foreign equivalent of the "package insert" and if necessary have it translated into English. Lists of side effects of over-the-counter medications are also listed in the appropriate volume of the Physicians Desk Reference. Relatively unregulated "natural remedies" or "holistic treatments" can contain pharmacologically active materials that can cause severe side effects, including confusion. Lists of the side effects of these remedies are becoming more available in books, on CDs, and on the Internet. Extensive medical literature is available on the side effects of recreational drugs, at least those that have been around long enough for their effects to be studied. The Merck Manual is an excellent source for information about even relatively uncommon drugs, and the Merck Manual of Health and Aging provides extensive information about medications in the elderly, including medications with anticholinergic side effects.

Differential Diagnosis of Dementias

The number of conditions that can cause dementia is large. How large depends on whether the person listing them is a "lumper" or a "splitter." At least 100–150 conditions have been proposed in the differential diagnosis. Fortunately, many of these are rare. Some are so common that they concern general clinicians.

Some of these conditions are discussed in other chapters, since most disorders of the brain that cause widespread anatomical damage can cause dementia. That is true in early and middle adult life as well as in the elderly. Head trauma and particularly repeated head trauma—for instance in professional boxers—can lead to dementia (*dementia pugilistica*) as can blood clots of the membranes lining the brain (e.g., *subdural hematomas*; see Chap. 10, Disorders of Awareness.) Subdural hematomas can occur without a good history of recent head trauma, particularly recurrent hematomas in a previously injured area. Impairment of normal drainage of the cerebrospinal fluid (CSF) surrounding the brain can lead to dementia associated with hydrocephalus (water on the brain). *Hydrocephalus* of unknown cause and with normal pressures in the brain is a well-described cause of dementia, typically accompanied by failure to control bladder and/or bowel movements and by a gait abnormality that can take the form of the patient's feet appearing stuck to the floor. The diagnosis requires confirmation by an MRI (magnetic resonance imaging) or CT (computed tomography) scan that shows large *ventricles* with compressed rather than enlarged *sulci*. The differential diagnosis between this condition and loss of brain substance from other cause (*hydrocephalus ex vacuo*) is often not easy. Accurate diagnosis is critical, since the treatment is neurosurgery (installing a shunt). The unfortunate young adults who suffer from a rapidly progressive form of multiple sclerosis typically lose cognitive abilities as the disorder gets worse. (See Chap. 13, Disorders of both Sensation and Motility.) Severe, uncontrolled seizure disorders can lead to permanent cognitive impairment. (See Chap. 10, Disorders of Awareness.) Impaired mentation frequently accompanies mild bleeds or other strokes as well as other diseases of the blood vessels (e.g., *vasculitis, disseminated lupus*, and related disorders); see Chap. 9 (Cerebrovascular Disorders). Tumors can cause dementia, often by impairing the draining of CSF (cerebrospinal fluid) and causing hydrocephalus, and often by causing brain edema (see Chap. 9). Multiple brain tumors secondary to cancer elsewhere (such as *miliary metastases*) can cause dementia because of the widespread brain damage they lead to. Tumors in the frontal lobes of the brain can cause a deficit of voluntary thought and movement (*abulia*) that can be mistaken for dementia or depression. For such patients, the path to the oncologist often runs through the psychiatrist's office. The brain damage caused by infections of the brain or the membranes surrounding the brain (meninges) can often leave residual impairments, sometimes including cognitive impairments severe enough to be labeled dementia. Prompt treatment of the acute infections is therefore essential. Infections of the meninges (*meningitis*) or of the brain itself (*encephalitis*) typically alter mental status. Acutely, they typically lead to other signs and symptoms as well—fever, stiff neck, and headache. Chronic infections of the nervous system can be harder to recognize but can lead to just as disastrous permanent damage. Optimal treatment of infections of the nervous system requires knowing the antibiotic sensitivity of the responsible agents. That tends to vary over time and often differs in different geographic areas. Consultation with specialists in infectious disease is often advisable.

Dementia is a typical manifestation of genetic inborn errors when these have a clinical onset later than childhood. Examples include the adult forms of *Tay-Sachs disease* or of *metachromatic leukodystrophy*. (See Chap. 4, Thought Disorders.)

The following discussion of differential diagnosis of dementias focuses on disorders in which dementia is a primary manifestation of the brain disease (i.e., in which the patient's dementia is usually the chief complaint). Neurodegenerative diseases occurring primarily in the elderly predominate in this group.

<ins>Alzheimer Disease (AD)</ins> This is the most common form of dementia. It occurs in more than 85% of patients with onset of dementia above age 65. Alois Alzheimer originally described AD in the beginning of the twentieth

century in terms of a clinical-pathological entity, at that time a cutting-edge way to define a disease. The characteristic pathological lesions he described are now known as *tangles* and *amyloid plaques*. The distinction Alzheimer and his colleagues made between AD and *senile dementia* was dropped in the late 1970s, since the manifestations of the condition are largely similar in people who suffer from it at any age. Both the early and late onset forms are now referred to as AD. In the last quarter century, research on this disorder has expanded enormously as have controversies about it.[9] Specific treatments have been developed, although no cures.

The original definition of AD required clinical disability as well as the characteristic neuropathological changes. When the neuropathological examination was largely limited to those who had the clinical changes, it seemed that the two were tightly linked. More recent population-based studies have shown that link to be loose. Autopsy-controlled epidemiological studies documented that a third to a half of people above age 85 have the full panoply of neuropathological changes but are not disabled cognitively. People over age 100 have been described who were entirely cognitively intact on detailed neuropsychological testing up to the time they died, despite having the full neuropathology of AD at autopsy.

For many researchers, including some outstanding clinicians, the criterion currently required for the diagnosis of AD is significant amyloid deposition in the brain at autopsy (i.e., *cerebral amyloidosis*). These workers think of people who die cognitively intact but with cerebral amyloidosis as having had preclinical AD. They assume that these individuals would have become symptomatic if they had lived to be 105 or 107. The concept of *cognitive reserve* has been invoked to explain the discrepancies between symptomatology and neuropathology. It is hard to see how to check these hypotheses experimentally, or even observationally in humans. I have therefore proposed that the term AD be used to refer to the neuropathological entity, with or without clinically significant manifestations. I've proposed using the term *Alzheimer dementia* for people who have both the neuropathological manifestations (AD) and also the clinical manifestations of dementia. This wording acknowledges that one can have AD neuropathologically without clinical dementia and clinical dementia without AD. It provides an explicit term to use in the frequent case when the two occur together.

In principle, the clinical diagnosis of Alzheimer dementia is a diagnosis of exclusion. It is made in a person with dementia who has no other evident cause for the mental disability. In practice, that definition is too confining, except for clinical research. AD does not protect against other diseases. Specifically, cerebrovascular disease is such a common concomitant that it is dangerous to conclude that demented patients with strokes do not also have AD.

Symptomatically, the onset of AD is characteristically so insidious that it cannot be dated precisely. Often relatives have also had dementia (i.e., family history is positive). The disabilities of AD tend to progress more or less steadily, but sharp exacerbations, plateaus, and even improvement are not rare and do not rule out the diagnosis. Memory impairment is thought by many to be the core phenomenon of Alzheimer dementia; it is effectively a criterion for the diagnosis. In some patients, verbal (dominant hemisphere) difficulties are prominent early in the clinical course. In others, difficulties with nondominant hemisphere functions such as spatial orientation (e.g., finding things) are more noticeable. Sometimes psychotic thinking is an early manifestation; Alois Alzheimer's index patient presented with pathological jealousy. As the disease progresses, all functions tend to become impaired, until the person is reduced to complete dependence on others for even such basic activities as eating, drinking, and bathing (i.e., is in a *chronic vegetative state*). How long patients with later-stage AD survive depends largely on how effectively they are cared for by others.

Some observers claim that patients who become psychotic from AD were often odd to begin with (specifically, had schizotypal personality disorder). This agrees with an observation made in the late 1930s, that when people become senile they become more like themselves. Learned inhibitions are lost as dementia progresses. The problem is that change in personality is also common in dementia and can be the first manifestation of AD.

The paragraph above describes typical AD. The large number of people with AD makes it likely that general clinicians will also see patients with atypical AD. For instance, primary vision is typically unimpaired in this disease. In a large database in Switzerland, however, about 0.1% of AD patients were found to have *cortical blindness* as an early manifestation.

Brain imaging sometimes helps with the diagnosis. Loss of brain substance in people under 65 ("walnut brain") tends to be significant. In older people, the correlation between cognitive function and the amount of brain substance found on imaging or at autopsy is so poor that such measurements do not aid in diagnosis, unless the loss of brain substance has been truly massive and occasionally not even then. A classic measure of the progression of AD is the overall rate of loss of brain substance over the span of half a year or a year or more. A single cross-sectional image study is much less informative, except to rule out other pathology such a tumor or *hematomas*. Proposals have been made that techniques that image brain function, such as fMRI (functional magnetic resonance imaging) or PET (positron emission tomography) scanning, can help with the diagnosis of AD by revealing a typical pattern of loss (biparietal and frontal). Whether these changes are specific enough to be useful for the clinical diagnosis has not been established. Perhaps consultation with a center where research on functional imaging in AD is going on may help to increase confidence in diagnosis of AD in difficult cases. (The effort to do so may also comfort a very concerned family.)

A number of other biological markers have been proposed to aid in the diagnosis of AD, and diagnostic kits are on the market. None of these markers has been shown objectively to improve the diagnostic accuracy of skilled and careful clinicians. Since more than 85% of demented people above the age of 65 have the neuropathological lesions of AD, it is relatively easy to achieve high diagnostic accuracy in prospective series where the presence or absence of AD is determined at autopsy.

Vascular Dementia (VaD) Impaired cognition due to cerebrovascular disease is still listed by many authors as the second most common form of dementia, but there are problems with that declaration. VaD is conceptualized as dementia due to vascular damage to the brain such as multiple strokes, without a significant contribution from neurodegenerative disease such as AD. In practice, the final decision on whether vascular damage was the major cause of clinical dementia is made by a neuropathologist. Essentially, that substitutes the subjective judgment of the neuropathologist for the subjective judgment of the clinician. Attempts to define criteria for VaD in consensus conferences have been published in the medical literature, but they still require subjective judgment.

If dementia is defined by modern neuropsychological definitions, then dementia is rare in patients with vascular disease alone, accounting for at most a few percent of elderly patients with dementia. One reason is that dementia as currently defined typically requires bilateral hippocampal damage (see below), and the nature of the vasculature of the human brain makes bilateral hippocampal damage unlikely from strokes alone. Meticulous neuropathological studies have documented that over 95% of patients with autopsy-proven AD also have enough vascular disease to account for their dementia.[10,11] Usually this includes damage to white matter of a type originally described by Binswanger (*Binswanger disease*). The term *mixed dementia* has been used for dementia caused by brain damage from both vascular disease and AD. Published data therefore indicate that mixed dementia is much more common than pure AD. This finding has direct implications for the treatment of patients with or at risk of AD, specifically in the need for close attention to the cardiovascular health of patients in the early phases of dementia. Potential interrelations between VaD, AD, and other forms of neurodegenerative dementia are discussed later under neurobiology.

VaD is diagnosed not so much by the presence of strokes in a demented person as by the historical relationship of the dementia to the strokes. As emphasized immediately above, the simple presence of strokes, clinically or by MRI or CT, does not establish that the strokes rather than AD or other neurodegenerative disease are the cause of the dementia. Dementia following a stroke suggests that the stroke caused the dementia, but a stroke can precipitate clinical dementia in a patient with previously preclinical or otherwise undiagnosed AD. Establishing that vascular disease is the sole or even the main cause of a patient's dementia is not straightforward. Fortunately, it is also not important for the patient. Vascular disease is treated in a demented patient by the same methods as it is treated in a nondemented patient, and VaD is treated with the same modalities used to treat other dementias.

Stroke can precipitate relatively focal conditions that can be mistaken for global dementia. One example is aphasia or other language difficulties following strokes that affect speech areas. A single stroke that involves the angular gyrus can lead to a set of disabilities easy to mistake for dementia in *Gerstmann syndrome*—inability to write (*agraphia*) and to do calculations (*acalculia*), with right-left confusion. (See Chap. 9, Cerebrovascular Disorders.)

One form of vascular damage to the brain that can clearly cause dementia is severe reduction in the supply of oxygen, blood sugar (glucose), and blood to the brain as a whole (*global hypoxia-ischemia*). General clinicians are well aware of how often hypoxic-ischemic brain damage occurs and of the dismal quality of life after many perportedly "successful" cardiopulmonary resuscitations. History from a reliable informant, including the police when indicated, is as always critical for making the diagnosis of hypoxic-ischemic brain damage. The reduction in blood flow or in the supply of oxygen or glucose needs to last only a few minutes, except in special circumstances that slow metabolism (e.g., near-drowning in icy water). Delayed degeneration of the brain following global hypoxia-ischemia can lead to this form of dementia becoming slowly worse over time.

Specific names exist for specific types of brain damage due to impairment of blood flow, oxygen, and blood sugar (glucose). Cutting off the supply of all three is called *hypoxia-ischemia* or sometimes just *ischemia.* Reduction but not absence of blood supply is *oligemia.* If dementia follows an episode of pure lack of oxygen without loss of circulation to the brain, it is called *hypoxic dementia*. Interference with the utilization of oxygen by the brain has effects similar to a decrease in the supply of oxygen for instance, in cyanide or carbon monoxide poisoning (forms of *histotoxic hypoxia*). Hypoglycemic dementia follows a sufficiently prolonged and severe episode of low blood sugar. In hypoglycemia, substrate for brain metabolism is lacking instead of oxygen. The effects of prolonged, severe hypoglycemia are well known to the public. A movie was made about a highly publicized case where a husband was accused of intentionally giving an insulin overdose to his wife, who continues to survive but with severe brain damage. The dementia that often follows head injury (post traumatic dementia) is thought to be mediated in large part by hypoxic-ischemic brain damage due to shear effects on blood vessels supplying the brain.

Lewy Body Dementia (LBD) This form of brain degeneration is now described by many subspecialists interested in cognitive disorders as the second most common type of dementia in the elderly. It appears to account for about 10% of the patients referred to typical American clinics specializing in memory disorders. This form of dementia is defined by its neuropathology. Lewy bodies are round inclusions in certain nerve cells that stain red with conventional tissue stains, that is, are *eosinophilic*.[24] (See Chap. 11, Disorders of Motility.) In LBD, Lewy bodies occur diffusely in the brain, in the cortex as well as in lower structures. About half the patients with LBD also have enough of the neuropathology of AD to have accounted for their dementia during life. Also, almost all patients with Parkinson disease (PD), whether demented or not, turn out to have one or more Lewy bodies in their cerebral cortex if search for Lewy bodies is done intensively using techniques that "light them up" (specifically, *immunostaining* with *anti-ubiquitin* antibodies). Patients with LBD typically have more motor signs of parkinsonism than patients with "classic" AD. The medical literature claims that they also have earlier and more prominent psychiatric manifestations, although patients with "classic" AD can certainly be quite crazy quite early in their course. The diagnostic distinction between LBD and AD can be hard to make during life, even for experienced clinicians. Fortunately, treatment for these two conditions is largely the same.

Problems with thinking are common in patients with classical PD, particularly as the disorder progresses. This can take the form of slowed thinking (*bradyphrenia*), analogous to the slowing and incoordination of motor functions characteristic of this disease. (See Chap. 11, Disorders of Motility.) Some neurologists who specialize in PD claim that essentially all of these patients will become demented if they live long enough. Certainly, the intellectual impairments can become even greater sources of disability than the motor problems. At the present time, the diagnostic term LBD is generally favored over the term *parkinsonian dementia*, at least by physicians who see these patients primarily for their dementia rather than for their motor problems.

Fronto-Temporal Dementias/Tauopathies (FTDs) FTDs are a group of dementing disorders that frequently result from genetic abnormalities in the genes encoding the tau proteins that occur in the *paired helical filaments* (PHF) discussed in more detail later in this chapter. Reports that mutations in other genes can do so as well have begun to appear. As their name implies, FTDs typically involve especially the frontal and temporal lobes. The archetype of the FTDs was until recently called *Pick disease*. In this condition, specific *Pick bodies* made up largely of tau proteins accumulate in neurons. Patients with combinations of Pick disease and Lewy Body dementia and AD have been identified. The distinction between FTD with Pick bodies and without Pick bodies is not now a crucial point in the diagnosis and treatment of these conditions.

As their name implies, FTDs tend to associate with prominent signs of frontal and temporal damage. Neuropsychology can help in making this diagnosis, since frontal damage is associated with loss of specific skills including "executive functions" and with poor performance on specific tests such as Wisconsin Card Sorting. The temporal damage can often be detected by imaging (knife-like temporal lobes). Psychiatric manifestations and aphasia are reportedly more common in FTD than in AD. However, impairments of executive function, language, and behavior are so common in AD that the differential diagnosis can be very difficult. Family history can be revealing, particularly if an autopsy or molecular genetics have documented a disorder of the *tau* gene (i.e., a "tauopathy") in an afflicted family member. Molecular confirmation in the tau-encoding gene strongly supports the diagnosis. This genetic test is available through specialized, government-sponsored Alzheimer Disease Research Centers (ADRCs).

Idiopathic Hippocampal Sclerosis Bilateral hippocampal damage is the typical anatomic substrate of dementia, as dementia is currently defined by neuropsychology. Sometimes the causes of damage to the hippocampus remain unknown even after autopsy. Replacement of neurons in the hippocampus with a glial scar for unknown reasons is referred to as *idiopathic hippocampal sclerosis*.[12] This is essentially an autopsy diagnosis. Even highly skilled clinicians with extensive experience and expertise in caring for patients with cognitive disorders regularly get this differential diagnosis wrong.

Wernicke-Korsakoff Syndrome The demented phase of this condition is also called *Korsakoff Psychosis* or *Confabulatory Psychosis*. These patients lack short-term but not long-term memory. In other words, they have trouble consolidating new memories but can retrieve well-established memories. They typically develop the habit of making up stories to cover their lack of memory of recent occurrences. They characteristically go along with whatever the examiner says is true, even if the examiner makes it up on the spot (i.e., they *confabulate*). The Korsakoff syndrome usually follows the more treatable Wernicke syndrome. As discussed below, the cause is nutritional. In the United States, the typical patient is a malnourished, "skid row" alcoholic. Other Korsakoff patients have suffered from gastrointestinal problems that lead to prolonged poor absorption of thiamin. A classic example is malignant vomiting of pregnancy (*hyperemesis gravidarum*).

Huntington Disease (HD) Patients with this hereditary disease can be referred to memory clinics, even though the earlier manifestations of this disease are usually psychiatric (often depression) and motor (choreiform movements). It is discussed in Chap. 11 (Disorders of Motility). HD is due to a well-characterized abnormality in a specific gene.[13] History of affected relatives often provides the key to the diagnosis. Confirmation by DNA (deoxyribonucleic acid) testing is widely available.

Syndrome of the Bits Didactically, it is convenient to list specific causes of dementia as if they were separate entities. In practice, they often occur together, particularly in older people. The overlaps between AD and VaD, and between AD and LBD, have been explicitly discussed earlier. The possibility that AD involves *hippocampal sclerosis* is discussed later.

In practice, many older people suffer from the "syndrome of the bits." They have a bit more plaques and tangles and synaptic loss than is good for them; a bit of vascular damage to the brain, particularly in subcortical white matter; a bit too many Lewy bodies in their substantia nigra and often in their cerebral cortex; a bit too much heart disease with resulting under perfusion of the brain, perhaps intermittently; a bit of depression; somewhat poor nutrition, perhaps including suboptimal blood levels of vitamin B_1, B_3, B_{12}, or folate; more social isolation than is good for them; and so on. The bits add up to cause significant clinical disability. The treatment of this syndrome is, of course, the treatment of each of the bits. Physicians who treat younger patients can often act as if a single disease process is superimposed on a patient's fundamentally healthy body and mind. Geriatricians rarely have that luxury. Older patients typically have multiple problems requiring multiple interventions. Skillful care of older people involves intervening gently and circumspectly to ameliorate multiple disabilities, being careful not to create more problems than are solved.

NEUROBIOLOGY OF DELIRIUM AND DEMENTIA: GENERAL CONSIDERATIONS

As pointed out, any condition that causes widespread interference with brain function is likely to cause delirium if the condition is transient and dementia if it leads to permanent brain damage. Mechanisms that lead to delirium in the short run can also lead to dementia if they are severe enough and last long enough.[2]

Impaired Brain Metabolism (Metabolic Encephalopathies)

The biological change that is most characteristic of both delirium and dementia is a reduction of the rate at which the brain burns its major substrate (i.e., the rate at which it oxidizes glucose).[14] The rate at which the brain oxidizes glucose is referred to as the CMR, that is, the Cerebral Metabolic Rate. That for oxygen is CMR_{O2}; that for glucose is CMR_{glu}. Under all but exceptional circumstances, the amount of oxygen used is that required to burn the glucose used. (Technically, CMR_{O2} and CMR_{glu} are normally stoichiometrically linked.) The rate of cerebral blood flow (CBF) is usually so tightly linked to CMR that CBF and CMR are treated as equivalent measures. For instance, brain damage identified by SPECT (single-photon emission computerized tomography) measurements of CBF is usually similar to that detected by PET measurements of CMR. My coworkers and I have postulated that the final common path and proximate cause of disorders of cognition is interference with brain oxidative metabolism.[15]

A number of lines of robustly reproduced evidence support that proposal. In both delirium and dementia, the degree of mental impairment is proportional to the degree of reduction in CMR. Superimposed events that reduce CMR lead to the type of mental disability characteristic of delirium and dementia, in human diseases and experimentally in both humans and experimental animals. For instance, both our species and other animals lose cognition when made hypoxic or hypoglycemic. In humans, the mental problems can be detected by verbal as well as by performance tests. In experimental animals, cognition has to be studied by tests of performance. Restoring CMR to normal or near normal levels restores mentation in delirious patients—for instance, providing oxygen to those with hypoxia or injecting glucose in those with hypoglycemia, if the hypoxia or hypoglycemia has not been so prolonged and severe as to have caused permanent brain damage (dementia). The same is true for experimental animals.

Neurobiological mechanisms are known by which reducing CMR can lead to mental impairments characteristic of delirium and dementia.[15] Impairing CMR leads to decreased function of those systems in the brain that use acetylcholine as a neurotransmitter. Acetylcholine is involved in arousal and attention.[16] Impairing cholinergic function impairs memory. Drugs that interfere with the function of acetylcholine in the brain are one of the most important causes of delirium and can characteristically make dementia much worse. Reducing CMR can also lead to increased release of glutamate and other neurotransmitters that can damage and kill neurons by "excitotoxicity." This effect appears to be a pathological exaggeration of a mechanism normally involved in adaptation (learning) in the nervous system. (In technical terminology, the excitotoxicity associated with impaired oxygen utilization by the brain appears to be mediated by glutamatergic NMDA (N-methyl-D-aspartate) receptors, which are involved physiologically in neuronal plasticity.) Impaired CMR also affects other forms of signaling in the brain (intracellular *second messengers* and *transcription factors*). These mechanisms can also contribute to neural cell dysfunction and death, but a detailed discussion of them is beyond the scope of this clinical monograph.

As emphasized earlier, almost any intercurrent illness can precipitate delirium, especially in older people and in those with underlying brain disease. That includes occult brain disease and specifically "preclinical" AD. Sometimes, the mechanism is decreased CMR. Sometimes the biological mechanisms linking the illness to the brain disease are less clear—for instance, when cognition deteriorates in association with an otherwise largely asymptomatic bladder infection without significant fever. (Increasing body temperature increases the metabolic demands on the brain.)

Medications and Other Drugs

Medicines that antagonize acetylcholine-mediated systems in the central nervous system are especially important potential causes of delirium. That is because of the critical role of cholinergic systems in the central nervous system in attention, awareness, and memory.[16] In prescribing treatments for medical illnesses for patients at risk of or with memory problems, it is good practice to choose the medication with the weakest anticholinergic effects if a number of effective medicines are available. That is true even if the cognitive problems are mild and subclinical.

Many medications have anticholinergic effects (Table 5-2). A minority of them are given specifically for their anticholinergic effects—for instance, *detrol* for overactive bladder or many types of eye-drops for glaucoma. Other, often more widely used medications have anticholinergic side effects. These include many centrally acting drugs including some common antipsychotics and antidepressants. They also include readily available over-the-counter medications such as the antihistamine Coricidin.

Other types of drugs can also cause delirium. Paul Greengard and his coworkers have suggested that a number of noncholinergic agents that induce bizarre behavior may act on the same intracellular mechanisms.[17]

Anatomic Brain Damage

Widespread structural damage to the brain typically leads to permanent dementia rather than to transient delirium or chronic delirium mimicking dementia.[2] The anatomic damage must have generalized effects in order to lead to the global cognitive impairment that defines delirium and dementia. That can occur if the damage is widespread—for instance, following certain head injuries or multiple sites of cancer (miliary metastases). But it can also occur with surprisingly localized damage. As discussed above, bilateral hippocampal damage can cause global cognitive impairment with severe malfunction of memory. The neurosurgical literature contains reports of a few unfortunate individuals who had both hippocampi removed in an attempt to treat their intractable epilepsy. The cognitive defects that ensued left these individuals utterly helpless to care for themselves or communicate effectively. As noted above, bilateral scarring of the hippocampi from whatever cause leads to a dementia syndrome. The importance of the hippocampus in dementias agrees with the known role of the hippocampus as an important center for learning and memory.[18]

Aging

The recognition that dementias are common in the elderly goes back to ancient times. English speakers tend to quote Shakespeare's description of the last age of man:

> "Last scene of all, that ends this strange eventful history, is second childishness and mere oblivion, sans teeth, sans eyes, sans taste, sans everything."

Aging is often assumed to be a major contributor to cognitive impairment, including AD, but close examination of that idea reveals problems. First, and perhaps most important, there is no satisfactory, widely accepted way to measure biological age. Many biological markers of aging have been proposed, and all of them have been faulted.[19] Most people, including most physicians and scientists, still use chronological age as a surrogate marker for biological age, although it is clearly unsatisfactory.[20] Modern physics reinforces the relevance of this issue, but more detailed discussion of those aspects of postrelativistic physics are beyond the scope of this monograph.[20]

Many scientists studying aging argue that there is a fundamental physiological process that underlies the development of diseases associated with later life. These scholars distinguish between the physiological process of aging and diseases of aging. That is a semantic distinction. If there is a common mechanism in many diseases of aging, then it can as well be called a disease mechanism that these diseases have in common rather than a physiological process contributing to their development. In practice, what would be useful is to find out what this putative mechanism(s) consist(s) of, whether that be accumulation of errors (i.e., increasing entropy) or genetic programming or some combination of those, perhaps along with other mechanisms. At the present time, we are debating what to name something when we don't know what it is.

At the practical clinical level, there are a number of diseases that are much more common in the elderly population than in younger people. The increased prevalence of these disorders in older patients can help with making the clinical diagnosis, although as always it is dangerous to use statistical frequency to justify jumping to a conclusion.[21] These disorders include a number of specific types of dementia including AD.

PATHOPHYSIOLOGY OF SPECIFIC FORMS OF DEMENTIA

Research on dementias and specifically on AD has accelerated remarkably during the last 25 years. That reflects in part the recognition by governments and private organizations that dementias and specifically AD will cause immense social problems in our aging population, unless science identifies a "technical fix." The growth in information reflects the funding that has been made available to try to find such a solution. A clinically valuable consequence is that people who have to deal with these sicknesses in their families or themselves tend to feel less isolated than they did 30 years ago. Another valuable clinical consequence is that the increased information on the pathophysiology of specific diseases now allows more focused if still unsatisfactory treatment. That is specifically true for AD.

Alzheimer Disease (AD)

Alzheimer described this condition in terms of a clinical-pathological correlation. Despite extensive research, the disease is still defined basically in terms of its neuropathology.

The earliest part of the brain that is affected by visible neuropathology in Alzheimer disease tends to be the entorhinal cortex, which connects to (projects to) the hippocampus. Imaging studies have confirmed that hippocampal shrinkage is a good anatomic sign for dementia in AD. It has even been proposed that frank dementia begins when hippocampal atrophy can first be detected by specialized analyses of MRI images. Changes in another part of the brain, the entorhinal cortex, may occur even earlier, but attempts to image the smaller entorhinal cortex have been less successful.

Examination with a microscope is necessary to identify the lesions that define AD. They are amyloid plaques, neuritic tangles made up of paired helical filaments, loss of synapses, and either shrinkage or loss of neurons with increase in glia (*gliosis*) with overall loss of brain substance. Other lesions that have been described are not needed for the autopsy diagnosis.[22] The chemical composition of the plaques and tangles has been much studied. The plaques contain many proteins, but the most important appears to be an amyloid-forming fragment resulting from the breakdown of another specific protein. The fragment is a 40-42 amino acid residue called Aβ, and the protein from which it is formed is called the Alzheimer amyloid precursor protein (APP). Mutations in the gene encoding APP, or more commonly in the genes for presenilin proteins that act on APP, can lead to the rare, early onset familial form of AD. Neurofibrillary tangles are made up primarily of an aggregated form of a family of proteins involved in cell motility, namely tau protein(s). The aggregates are in the form of specific structures called paired helical filaments (PHF). The tau proteins in PHF have been robustly found to contain more phosphorous than most tau isolated from human brain post mortem. The reason may be less efficient removal of phosphorous from the tau in PHF (put technically, less agonal and postmortem dephosphorylation of PHF tau compared to normal tau.) Many other changes have also been described in the cells that shrink and/or die in AD. These include robust demonstration of mitochondrial damage and evidence of disordered metabolism of oxygen free radicals (ROS), with oxidative damage to proteins, lipids, and DNA. A form of chronic inflammation of the brain is also characteristic (specifically, a noncellular, complement-mediated process).

The most characteristic deficiency in communication between cells in the AD brain is in the neurotransmitter acetylcholine. Abnormalities also occur in other chemicals involved in signaling (i.e., in information processing). The deficiencies in the neurotransmitters norepinephrine and perhaps serotonin have been associated statistically with the development of manifestations of depression.

The causes of AD are debated. Most workers currently think that it is a heterogeneous disease to which a number of factors contribute. The most prominent hypothesis at the present time puts amyloid and Aβ at the center of the "Alzheimer story" (the *amyloid cascade hypothesis*). The arguments about this hypothesis have become unpleasantly bitter, and will not be reiterated here.[23]

A reduction in CMR is as characteristic of AD as it is of other dementing disorders. The reduction in CMR invariably accompanies the clinical disorder and progresses in parallel with clinical worsening. The correlation is so close that reductions in CMR (and/or CBF) are used to map the parts of the brain most affected by AD in individual patients. Aβ can itself damage mitochondria and catalyze the formation of ROS leading to oxidative stress. Thus, the amyloid cascade hypothesis and the metabolic or oxidative hypothesis are mutually supportive rather than mutually exclusive. For clinicians caring for these patients, the critical question is whether these or other abnormalities in AD provide clues to treatments that will help patients. That jury is still out.

Vascular Dementia

This condition is due to impaired circulation to the brain with permanent brain damage. The cause is circulatory compromise severe enough to kill brain cells (specifically, the cells that do not regenerate, i.e., neurons). Chap. 9 (Cerebrovascular Disorders) discusses the mechanisms of brain damage due to impaired blood supply.

The total supply of blood and therefore of glucose or oxygen to the brain can become inadequate for the needs of the organ even without direct damage to the blood vessels of the brain—for instance, when heart disease prevents adequate pumping of blood (i.e., when cardiac output falls below a critical threshold). The extent to which dementia can be caused by repetitive episodes of inadequate perfusion of the brain due to irregularities of the heartbeat (*cardiac arrhythmias*) has been debated. Current thinking is swinging back to the view that this is likely to be an important mechanism. The most severe form of impaired perfusion of the brain is when the heart stops beating effectively at all. In such situations, the heart sometimes restarts itself (e.g., in *Stokes-Adams attacks*). Sometimes medical personnel restart it (cardiopulmonary resuscitation, CPR). People who survive CPR sometimes regain the bulk of their faculties. Often they end up dreadfully impaired even if the resuscitation is successful in terms of maintaining life. Other causes of impaired blood supply to the brain are mentioned earlier, for instance, shear effects secondary to brain trauma.

Impairment of the supply of sugar (glucose) from the blood and interference with the utilization of oxygen or glucose in conditions such as carbon monoxide (CO) poisoning lead to effects similar (although not identical) to those of cutting off the supply of blood or oxygen.

Severe brain damage can also occur when the demands of the brain for oxygen and sugar increase to the point where they outrun what can be supplied by the circulation. This is a classic danger in the repetitive seizure activity *of status epilepticus*. (See Chap. 10, Disorders of Awareness.)

The hippocampus, whose role in memory is discussed above, is particularly sensitive to damage when the circulatory supply to the brain, becomes inadequate for the needs of the organ.

Lewy Body Dementia/Parkinsonian Dementia

This disorder is defined by the presence of Lewy Bodies at neuropathology. These are round inclusions in susceptible neurons that are red after standard (*hematoxylin/eosin*, H&E) staining.[24] The main protein making up Lewy bodies is synuclein. Associated with it is the protein ubiquitin, which is involved in the breakdown of other proteins. Among the materials present in Lewy bodies are neurofilament proteins and various amounts of fats (lipids). The cause of deposition of synuclein and other materials in Lewy Bodies is not known. Nor are specific mechanisms linking the clinical dementia to the accumulation of these structures. As discussed in Chap. 11 (Disorders of Motility), specific mutations identified in a familial form of PD suggest that the accumulation of Lewy Bodies can be related to mitochondrial damage, but the evidence is not compelling, at least not yet. As also discussed in more detail in that chapter, historical evidence suggests that one of the causes of accumulation of Lewy Bodies is environmental pollution (*environmental toxicants*).

Frontotemporal Dementias/Tauopathies (FTDs)

A major known cause of these disorders is mutations in the gene encoding the tau proteins. However, as studies of this condition accumulate, it is becoming evident that mutations in other genes can also lead to this pathological entity. A recent report indicates that a mutation in a presenilin gene normally associated with early onset familial AD can also cause a frontotemporal tauopathy without any accumulation of Alzheimer amyloid.[25] The reason for these different clinical and pathological manifestations of mutations in the same gene is not known.

Tau isoforms are *microtubule-associated proteins* and are involved in cell motility. That includes the transport of organelles including mitochondria within the cell. Presumably, mutations in tau that cause FTDs interfere with important aspects of these cell functions. Increased in vivo phosphorylation of tau has been suggested to be a mechanism impairing tau function in these diseases.

Idiopathic Hippocampal Sclerosis

The cause(s) of loss of neurons and gliosis in the hippocampus are unknown by definition in this "idiopathic" syndrome. Among areas of the brain, the hippocampus is particularly sensitive to impairments in oxygen utilization. A speculation about this syndrome is that it can result from repeated episodes of inadequate perfusion of the brain, perhaps secondary to heart disease, in people who lack the genetic predisposition to form Aβ in their brains and are therefore by definition free of the pathology that defines AD.

Wernicke-Korsakoff Syndrome

Thiamin deficiency causes this entity. The mechanisms of brain damage due to thiamin (vitamin B_1) deficiency have been the subject of intensive investigations for many years. This vitamin is converted to a cofactor (TPP [thiamin pyrophosphate]) that is necessary for the activity of three enzymes in mitochondria as well as to a form (TTP) associated with membranes. Experimental thiamin deficiency leads to the accumulation of a form of the APP associated with AD. Thiamin deficiency classically leads to highly localized brain damage in both humans and experimental animals, but the reasons for the selective vulnerability of the affected regions are not known. Wernicke-Korsakoff syndrome is only one of several clinical manifestations of thiamin deficiency. Others include *peripheral neuropathy* and heart failure. Genetic factors have been proposed to play a role in determining which of these syndromes a thiamin-deficient person develops.

Other Vitamin Deficiencies

Deficiencies of other vitamins can also cause dementia. Dementia is one of the four "D's" classically associated with deficiency of niacin (vitamin B_3): dermatitis, diarrhea, dementia, and death. The fortification of flour has almost eliminated this disorder in the United States and other developed countries, except in people who persist in eating a bizarre diet because they are psychotic or for other reasons. Deficiency of vitamin B_{12} or of folic acid (folate) can cause dementia, but in recent experience in the United States dementia is rarely the complaint that brings them to clinical attention. (For instance, these conditions were rare among the thousands of patients studied in the Alzheimer Disease Research Centers). About 0.1% of patients referred to the dementia clinic directed by the author had B_{12} deficiency, and they were easily recognized by routine blood examination (i.e., they had *macrocytic anemia* and *hypersegmented polymorphonuclear leukocytes* on complete blood count (CBC). None of over 2000 patients tested had deficiencies of folic acid.

Huntington Disease

Huntington disease is caused by mutations in a specific gene, as discussed in Chap. 11 (Disorders of Motility).

TREATMENT

One of the reasons that many clinicians distinguish between delirium and dementia, despite their overlaps in clinical signs and symptoms and in neurobiologic mechanisms, is that the treatments for these entities differ.

Treatment of Delirium

The treatment of delirium has several parts: treating the underlying, often medical, cause; supportive care; treatment directed at the manifestations of the delirium itself; and, sometimes antidotes to specific, identified causes of the delirium.

Treatment of the Underlying Illness: This is, of course, part of ordinary good medical care. The development of confusion during a medical illness is a sign of worsening of the illness. It is particularly ominous in older people. Unhappily, improvement in a medical illness is often beyond the scope of even the most devoted and up-to-date medical care, particularly in the terminal stages of sickness.

Delirium generally gets better with appropriate treatment of the underlying medical condition. Hypoxia requires treatment with oxygen. Hypoglycemia requires treatment with glucose. Impairments of circulation that lead to inadequate perfusion of the brain require appropriate clinical management including repletion of volume in patients in shock, treatment of cardiac arrhythmias in patients where irregularities of heart beat impair cardiac efficiency, and improving the function of heart muscle if possible when the heart is simply too weak to pump blood adequately. The confusion that accompanies kidney failure usually gets better when dialysis brings body chemistries back to or nearly to normal. Reversal of liver failure, when possible, improves hepatic encephalopathy. In some patients, dramatic improvements in hepatic delirium follow treatment with mixtures of materials that help to reduce ammonia levels (*branched-chain α-keto acids*). All patients with this condition do not respond, but in those who do the results of treatment can be very gratifying to the patient, the family, and the medical personnel caring for them. Successful liver transplant can alleviate confusion as well as other aspects of liver failure.

The acute delirious phase of Wernicke-Korsakoff syndrome (Wernicke syndrome) constitutes a medical emergency. Prompt treatment with thiamin (vitamin B_1) is necessary to minimize permanent brain damage. Thiamin is given intravenously (IV) by push. A typical dose is 100 mg thiamin. (The minimum daily requirement for thiamin is 3 mg/day orally). The response is typically prompt and dramatic if the syndrome is treated early enough. There are essentially no side effects. In caring in an emergency situation for patients who are severely confused and for whom a history is not available, this dose of thiamin is often administered empirically, even in the absence of other signs of Wernicke syndrome (eye signs and/or incoordination). That is particularly true in caring for confused alcoholics or others at risk of vitamin deficiency. The injection of thiamin is often followed by an IV push of 50 g of glucose, given even before a value for blood sugar is known but after a sample of blood has been obtained for determination of blood sugar and other relevant measurements. The rate of brain damage in Wernicke-Korsakoff syndrome (or in hypoglycemia) can be rapid enough that these essentially harmless empirical treatments are not contraindicated in this situation. The reason for giving thiamin before giving glucose is that the coenzyme form of thiamin is important in the major pathways of glucose utilization. Increasing carbohydrate load in a thiamin-deficient person or animal can exacerbate the damage due to the vitamin deficiency.

Delirium due to a medication or other ingested substance typically clears as the substance is removed by the body, by being metabolized or excreted or both. Sometimes this occurs quickly. For barbiturates and ethanol in otherwise healthy people, that can take hours or a day or two. Sometimes clearing a toxin is inconveniently slow, particularly in older people and in those with liver or kidney disease. Further exposure to the offending substance should of course be stopped if at all possible. The large variety of medications now available for many disorders makes it easier than in previous years to find a regimen that will treat the patient without inducing mental changes. For instance, digitalis glycosides are still often useful in the treatment of heart failure and arrhythmias. However, if they make a patient confused, other medications are available to remove water and salt and to control arrhythmias.

Antidotes are available for some toxins that impair mental function (for instance, opioids; see Chap. 7 [Pain]). Two general principles should be mentioned in regard to antidotes. First, it is unwise to try to titrate the dose of antidote too closely. Enough antidote to keep the person out of trouble is enough to let the body and brain do the rest of the healing itself. Overdoses of antidotes can be as or more harmful than the original toxin. Second, poison control centers are valuable resources for information about what specific toxins do and what can be done to ameliorate their bad effects.

Certain **common toxins** are such frequent causes of delirium that discussion of them is in order here.

Alcohol (Ethanol) Alcohol remains the most widely used substance of abuse in the United States and most of the rest of the Western world. Simple, transient alcoholic delirium is conventionally called drunkenness. The usual remedy is to let the drunk sleep it off. On occasion a boisterous drunk will become so potentially violent that a sedative is needed. Depending on the circumstances, an antipsychotic or benzodiazepine can be used. Either if used should be given in judiciously low doses. Benzodiazepines and ethanol can have synergistic interactions, so short-acting drugs are advisable in no more than the doses necessary to calm the patient down.

Complications of alcohol abuse that require prompt and active medical intervention are thiamin deficiency and hypoglycemia. These can occur independently but can also occur together. They tend to be found in chronic, skid row alcoholics rather than in social drinkers. Both are included in conventional emergency treatment for a confused skid row alcoholic for whom a medical history cannot be obtained. The treatment protocol is discussed above (obtain a blood sample for glucose and other measurements, give 100 mg of thiamine intravenously by push, then 50 to 100 gm of glucose by intravenous push). Treatment with thiamin is essentially innocuous, and treatment with glucose is usually not harmful, even in patients who are already hyperglycemic.

People who drink alcohol heavily enough to come to medical attention may have drunk other things as well. That may include methanol, paraldehyde, and ethylene glycol (antifreeze). Sometimes they may not know they have drunk these poisons. Sometimes they may not know they are poisons. Sometimes they don't care. Sometimes they are consciously attempting suicide. The characteristic clinical findings in people who have ingested these materials are visual disturbances ("blind drunk") and dangerous dysregulation of blood acidity (severe *metabolic acidosis*). With adequate treatment of the acidosis, patients can survive without sequelae. They can also die—sometimes with striking speed—despite prompt and skilled medical attention. The behavior of people who are pathological drinkers, like that of other people with psychiatric diseases, can be confusingly unpredictable. It is essentially impossible to know for sure what they have ingested. Their treatment is generally symptomatic. The physician needs to stay alert and not be nonplused by surprising developments in their clinical illness. In these circumstances, a significant proportion of treatment failures are inevitable.

Alcohol withdrawal (*delirium tremens*, DTs) is a common and potentially life-threatening condition. This condition is most commonly seen in alcoholics who have stopped or sharply cut down on their drinking. It can, however, also occur in people who are withdrawing from barbiturates or other sedatives. A similar condition can develop postoperatively in people who have no history of alcohol or sedative abuse. Magnesium deficiency or other abnormalities of blood chemistry may contribute. The characteristic clinical picture is tremulousness, delirium typically with unpleasant visual hallucinations, and sometimes seizures. The condition tends to clear within a week. Treatment consists of the minimum necessary doses of sedatives, (typically short-acting benzodiazepines), and supportive care. Sometimes addition of a magnesium salt, orally or by injection into muscle (IM) helps, particularly with shaking (tremulousness). The end point of drug treatment is reasonable calm, not abolition of all signs of the condition. Too much benzodiazepine can kill a patient with DTs, particularly if it is a long-acting benzodiazepine such as librium.[26] In most of the recent hospital-based series, mortality has been less than 5% and often 0%. On the other hand, death rates above 20% have also been reported.

<u>Opiates</u> Opium derivatives characteristically depress brain function rather than excite it. They can be associated with delirium but more often with stupor and coma. (See Chap. 7, Pain.)

Antidotes for opioid overdose include *naloxone* (Narcan), and also *nalorphine*, *levellorphan*, and *naltrexone*. The doses of these antagonists needed to counteract opioids are relatively small; 1 mg of injected naloxone (IV, IM, or even SC [subcutaneus]) counteracts 25 mg of heroin. A dose of 0.5 mg naloxone injected IM can precipitate withdrawal symptoms in an opiate-dependent person. As discussed in more detail in Chap. 7 (Pain), treatment of opioid overdose requires only enough naloxone or other antagonist to keep the patient out of danger. The body can then safely eliminate the rest of the toxic opioid. In people whose circulation is depressed because of opiate overdose or from other causes, opioid antagonists may be relatively slowly absorbed after IM or SC injections. Lack of response can lead to repeated injections of naloxone or other antagonist. The total antagonist administered can then precipitate acute withdrawal when the antagonists reach the brain and act to restore blood pressure. This is not a problem with IV injections.

Opioid antagonists are safe. These drugs normally have no effect in people not exposed to opiates, except when there are unusually high levels of endogenous materials acting at opiate receptors (e.g., *endorphins*; see Chap. 7, Pain). These medications have no significant addictive potential themselves. Rare cases of pulmonary edema have been reported following treatment with naloxone.

"Mind-Altering" Drugs Cocaine, amphetamines, and club drugs are mind-altering substances. These drugs act by similar mechanisms (primarily as agonists on dopamine receptors, although some club drugs act on other receptors as well). It is therefore logical to treat delirium due to these agents with dopamine receptor antagonists such as risperidone or haloperidol (Haldol). These antipsychotic agents are also standard treatments for delirium in general. Starting doses are similar to those given for other types of delirium. However, people poisoned with such mind-altering drugs of abuse can be dangerously crazy, including paranoia. They need to be kept from hurting themselves or others, sometimes including hospital personnel. That consideration reinforces the third part of the general rule of treatment with drugs: start low, go slow, but give enough.

Nonspecific Pharmacological Treatments of Delirium: The most widely used treatment for agitated delirious patients is now a "calming" antipsychotic. Resveratrol and sometimes haloperidol are widely used. (See Chap. 4, Thought Disorders). Other "calming" medications can also be used, notably antianxiety agents such as benzodiazepines. (See Chap. 6,

Anxiety.) Benzodiazepines with shorter biological half-lives are preferable for this purpose. Patients who have been exposed to toxic amounts of a drug or other material can become delirious before the full dose of the toxin has been absorbed. They can then slip into more clouded states of consciousness with more severe suppression of brain functions. In this case, one does not want to have given them a full dose of a long-acting medication.

The rule for dosage of sedatives for agitated delirium is the same as that for medications for other conditions—give enough but not too much. That can obviously vary among patients and among different causes of impairment of cognition. For risperdal and haldol, doses of less than a milligram every 4–6 hours as needed can have surprisingly gratifying results. If patients need more in order not to be a danger to themselves or others, it is appropriate to give them more. Sometimes it is necessary to give them more to allow them to receive optimal medical care—for instance, if they pull out the IV lines through which they are receiving life-saving antibiotics or other medications. Eventually enough antipsychotic medication or benzodiazepine will immobilize anyone, let alone people who are sick and elderly. Too much can be dangerous. As noted previously, apathetic delirium is rarely treated even though it appears to be just as unpleasant for the patient as the agitated form.

Extensive studies have indicated that functional deficiency of the neurotransmitter acetylcholine is frequently the direct cause of delirium, as discussed earlier. This raises the possibility that delirium could be treated with cholinergic agonists such as the cholinesterase inhibitors discussed below that are used in the treatment of AD. Some of these, like *donepezil* (Aricept), have not shown significant clinical side effects on the function of the heart or lungs or kidneys, even in patients with serious medical illness affecting one or more of these organs. Case reports of successful treatment of delirium of various causes with donepezil and other cholinesterase inhibitors have begun to appear in the literature. A large, appropriately designed, well-conducted, prospective, placebo-controlled study could be useful. A safe treatment for this unpleasant complication of medical illness would be a welcome addition to the modern clinician's armamentarium.

Supportive Care is Critical for Confused Patients: They can rarely take care of themselves. Supportive care includes such standard procedures as maintaining nutrition and adequate fluid intake, intravenously if necessary, and keeping these patients clean and free of bedsores. It sometimes includes medication, particularly for agitated delirium. It definitely includes keeping them from getting themselves or others into trouble with potentially damaging ordinary activities, such as driving a car or using knives or a gas stove. That sometimes requires effectively constant observation of the patient by a dedicated observer, or by several observers working in shifts. Such one-on-one care is expensive but is essentially custodial rather than medical. People with low levels of education can often do it very well. Kindness, empathy, and common sense can be more important for this responsibility than technical training.

Treatment of Stupor and Coma

Delirium can progress to states where arousal is more difficult, namely stupor and coma. The treatment of these conditions involves keeping the patient alive (i.e., maintaining physiological functions) while treatment for the underlying disorder progresses. That subject goes beyond the scope of this monograph, but excellent discussions are available in specialized texts.[27] Some decades ago, it was common to attempt to wake such patients up with stimulants such as picric acid. Careful studies indicated that such maneuvers were more likely to harm the patients than to help them. Pharmacology does have a role in preventing complications and in treating some causes of stupor and coma, including opiate overdose (discussed in Chap. 7, Pain) and brain *edema* (see Chap. 9, Cerebrovascular Disorders).

Treatment of Dementia: General Considerations

Certain general principles apply to the treatment of dementias, apart from the more specific treatments recently introduced to treat the cognitive aspects which are the putative core of these disorders.

General Care: As dementia develops, patients lose the ability to care for themselves. That eventually includes such basic biological functions as eating, drinking, toileting, and keeping clean enough to reduce the chance of skin infections. The health of these disabled people—indeed, their survival—depends on how well they are taken care of.

Assuming those responsibilities can severely strain their caregivers. Caregiver burden has been much studied and a variety of support mechanisms for caregivers have been developed. Caregivers typically need someone to whom they can complain without feeling guilt; family members and clergy sometimes fill that role but often do not. In designing a clinical service for demented people, it is wise to have a designated sympathetic person to handle the stream of telephone calls that are likely to come in. Sometimes these calls represent all too real problems. Sometimes they are simply cries for support and sympathy from overloaded caregivers.

In the United States, local chapters of the Alzheimer Association almost always provide useful information in terms that are culturally congruent for the different parts of the country. Similar organizations exist in Britain and in a number of other countries. Alzheimer Association chapters often supply other important services as well. These include support groups, availability of professional legal counsel on relevant "elder law," other aspects of case management, and often individual counseling by appropriately trained social workers. The Alzheimer Association chapters can usually also help in finding Day Hospital and Respite Programs. We like to think that day hospital programs benefit patients, at least by providing a social setting where they can interact with others in the same boat. Day Hospital programs certainly give family caregivers some time off without incurring too much guilt. Full time respite is often an entryway to full time placement. Caregivers often find that the person they are devoted to is actually happier and less stressed in the institutional setting, and full-time placement in a nursing home or similar settings therefore becomes a more attractive alternative.

Other community supports are also available. Most counties and many cities also have Offices of the Aging. There is also a National Institute of Aging (NIA/NIH) Web site. Some clergy provide invaluable assistance to caregivers; others are uncomfortable with illness. In the author's experience, that is a function of the individual clergyperson rather than of the faith tradition. As with patients, some caregivers respond to some interventions, others to other interventions, some to almost any intervention, and some not to anything. Both instrumental and internal psychological mechanisms contribute to caregiver stress. Sometimes improvement in a patient's cognition can increase stress in the caregiver.

> A 69-year-old woman with AD responded dramatically to treatment with a cholinesterase inhibitor, with an increase in her MMSE score from 22 to 30. Her husband, who had been caring for her, developed a suicidal depression, which responded well to

> treatment with a standard (SSRI) antidepressant. Their marriage had been severely troubled for decades. (Divorce was not considered on religious grounds.) As she lost cognition, the wife plagued the husband less. As her cognition returned, she went back to making him miserable more effectively. The extent to which his tendency toward developing depressions contributed to their marital problems remained unclear, even after counseling.

Eisdorfer's rule states that "When the main caregiver gives out, the care system gives out."

Clinicians should be alert to the possibility that the stressed caregiver, who is in a difficult and sometimes nearly impossible situation, must be offered medication as well as social support. Sometimes the best thing a physician can do for a patient is to prescribe an antidepressant or antianxiety medication to a caregiver.

When to place a patient in a full-time care facility is an individual issue. On the Burke service, two situations almost always led us to recommend placement. First, if the patient no longer recognizes the caregivers, people who work 8-hour shifts and then go home might as well provide the care. Second, if the major caregiver has accelerating health problems, physical or mental, placement becomes advisable. A husband may declare passionately that he will "never" place his wife in a nursing home, even as he is popping nitroglycerin for his worsening angina. Unfortunately, when he is delivered to the hospital with a serious or fatal heart attack, the wife will be placed on an emergency basis in whatever facility is then available. Better that she enter in good time into a carefully chosen setting that will continue to be as pleasant as possible for her even if her husband succumbs to his illness.

<u>Nutrition:</u> Extensive studies have been done to define optimal nutrition in people with AD and related dementias. These patients often lose weight, although it is not clear that AD actually increases their requirements for calories. Their nutritional problems may reflect a loss of interest in eating and ability to eat (eating apraxia). Burning off calories due to agitation or pacing seems to play less of a role quantitatively.

> A 63-year-old former wine importer with moderately severe dementia was found to have the cracks at the corners of his lips that are characteristic of vitamin B complex deficiency (perleche). The examining physician jumped to the erroneous conclusion that the man was malnourished due to alcohol abuse. Actually, he had

> never drunk excessively, and he had cut back sharply on wine when his memory problems began. Both he and his wife had been very interested in food, and she had taken advanced *cordon bleu* courses in cooking. As his dementia progressed, he became a more picky eater. She tried to tempt his appetite by making more and more elegant and more and more complex meals. He, however, had lost the ability to eat complicated dishes. His nutrition improved dramatically when she started to serve him simpler meals (e.g., hard boiled eggs he could take into his hands instead of *oeuf en gelée*). Vitamin pills helped, too.

Probably it is wise for demented patients to take a vitamin supplement each day, since it is too much to expect that they will eat a balanced diet. In the later stages of dementia, patients may tolerate only a few simple foods. Feeding them ice cream is often a good answer. Ice cream contains nutritionally complete milk protein (casein), fats (lipids) including essential fatty acids, sugar (carbohydrates), and calcium (from the milk). Most Americans eat ice cream with pleasure, even if they are in their "second childhood." Patients can live well on a diet composed primarily of ice cream, with supplemental vitamins and adequate intake of fluids. Such a diet is not "heart healthy," but long-term protection against atherosclerosis is a secondary consideration in a patient who would otherwise under-eat to the point of clinically significant malnutrition.

Intake of alcohol is problematic in patients with dementia. On the one hand, extensive epidemiological studies indicate that the equivalent of up to three glasses of wine a day tends to slow AD. Reports that red wine is healthier than other forms of alcohol have not been robustly confirmed in larger studies. Many investigators think that the apparent superiority of red wine reflects that it is a typical beverage in cultures where wine is drunk regularly and in moderation. On the other hand, the damaged brain is typically sensitive to chemicals that act on the brain, including ethanol. Very little alcohol sometimes makes AD patients appear drunk. (The example of Rita Hayworth is discussed earlier.) As always, patient care must be individualized and judgment exercised.

Treatment of intercurrent illnesses can be important for patients with dementias, particularly patients in the earlier stages of a dementing disease. These people are sensitive to induction of delirium due to concurrent illness and resulting metabolic encephalopathy. They also have difficulty learning to adapt to the demands of an illness. A person who is struggling to remember where the toilet is does not benefit from also having frequency and urgency due to an under-treated bladder infection. A person struggling to remember the details of ordinary life is not helped by being distracted by pain or indigestion. On the other hand, meddlesome medicine is as always to be avoided. The diagnostic curiosity of doctors and families does not always have to be satisfied, if doing so harms rather than benefits the patient.

Behavioral Medication: Behavioral problems are characteristic in AD and other dementias. Judicious use of psychotropic drugs is one of the greatest benefits a physician can offer these patients and their families. The rule is start low, go slow, give enough. Often the brain damage in these patients makes them sensitive to medications active on the nervous system, but sometimes they need full doses comparable to those given to much younger people.

Depression is common in AD and a number of other dementing illnesses. Whether this is "true depression" or "depressive manifestations" is a semantic issue. Probably the same neurotransmitters are functionally deficient in AD depression as in endogenous depression. Depressed AD patients are suffering. They can attempt suicide, sometimes successfully. The standard treatment is the same antidepressants used in people with "primary" mood disorder. (See Chap. 3, Mood Disorders.) Nowadays the usual starting drug is an SSRI. Low doses may be surprisingly effective. A regimen found useful on our unit is to start with Zoloft at 25 mg/day, taken at bedtime. If the patient does not show side effects, the dose is increased by increments of 25 mg/day to a total of 75 mg/day and if necessary even more. The end point is relief of the depression without significant side effects. The patient's response is more important than whether the "full doses of antidepressants" recommended in review articles and textbooks have been achieved. In the author's experience, larger doses are relatively rarely needed in patients whose primary diagnosis is AD. Sometimes patients and their families state that the patient does not respond to or tolerate Zoloft but does respond to another SSRI or to another type of antidepressant. Often objective scores on depression rating scales support their conclusions. It is generally wise practice to use the medication that the patient and family feel works best, unless there is a clear contraindication.[28]

Hallucinations and delusions are both common in AD and other dementias, as are illusions and other psychotic manifestations. As discussed in Chapter 4 (Thought Disorders), the vigor with which psychotic manifestations need to be treated depends on whom they harm. Crazy ideas certainly deserve to be treated, if they make the patient miserable, lead to unacceptably antisocial behavior, or otherwise threaten the stability of the care system. Hallucinations that bother neither the patient nor the caregivers do not need to be treated, particularly not with drugs that can have unpleasant and sometimes permanent side effects. (See Chap. 4, Thought Disorders.)

The standard medications to treat psychotic manifestations in dementias are the same as those used to treat other psychoses. They are discussed in Chap. 4 (Thought Disorders). Risperidone is widely used in demented patients at the present time. Sometimes amazingly low doses of risperidone (or of haloperidol) can be effective in patients with AD and other dementias. Doses as low as 0.05–0.10 mg/day (i.e., one to two drops of risperidone solution) have been reported by caregivers to be fully effective in calming psychotic manifestations in patients with AD. Whether this is a placebo effect that works by empowering the caregiver or by an actual physiological effect on dopamine-mediated pathways in the patient's brain is relatively unimportant. What matters is that the patient appears to be doing well, and is on a dose of medication too low to be likely to induce serious side effects such as dyskinesias. On the other hand, sometimes larger doses are necessary and if so should be prescribed. Also, some patients respond much better to some medications than they do to others. One of our patients responded to full doses of thiothixene (10 mg twice a day) even though he had not responded to either low or full doses of risperidone, haloperidol, short-acting benzodiazepines, or to lower doses of thiothixene. The general principle is, as always, that treatment of an individual patient is fundamentally empirical, although standard doses of standard medications are usually a good place to begin.

Antisocial behavior including what is referred to as "violence," is often a problem in patients with AD and other dementias. Unacceptable behavior can lead to long-term placement more rapidly than do unappetizing events such as fecal incontinence. How serious "antisocial behavior" is depends in large part on how much it upsets the caregivers. For instance, the same sexual disinhibitions may be tolerated in demented people in relatively easygoing settings but be totally unacceptable in other settings, even though no one is actually harmed physically (for instance, by an older demented lady lifting her skirt in public). Aberrant behavior must, however, be taken seriously if it threatens or causes physical harm to the patient, caregiver, or others. That includes other residents in a nursing home.

In the author's experience, few patients with AD or other dementias are truly violent. Unlike patients with primary psychoses, demented patients usually lack the mental organization needed to carry out focused violence. On the other hand, their frustration and confusion can lead to them doing things that seem violent. A large, athletic man with diminished verbal skills may shake a small female caregiver because he is frustrated at being unable to communicate with her. The caregiver can become appropriately frightened even if the patient really didn't mean to harm her. She naturally enough wants others to recognize that her bruises are real and hurt, and does not want a similar event to happen again. Potentially harmful behavior calls for treatment similar to the treatment of unacceptable psychotic manifestations discussed in the previous paragraph. Similar medications are used and similar considerations apply. Surprisingly low doses of an antipsychotic such as risperidone can be effective, particularly if they succeed in making the caregiver feel safer.

Treatment of Specific Dementias

Research over the last 25 years has introduced relatively specific treatments for some dementias, notably AD.

Alzheimer Disease (AD) Two treatments at the neurotransmitter level have been introduced for the memory disorder that is thought to be the core phenomenon in Alzheimer dementia. One type of treatment acts on acetylcholine-mediated systems, the other on a glutamate receptor.

Cholinesterase Inhibitors The medications currently used most widely to treat AD modify the deficiency in acetylcholine function. They do so by reducing the activity of the enzyme that breaks down acetylcholine, that is, they are cholinesterase inhibitors. Their action increases the chemical activity[29] of acetylcholine in the presynaptic cleft of appropriately innervated neurons. Attempts to treat AD with compounds that directly stimulate cholinergic receptors have not led to clinically useful medications, at least as yet. Extensive clinical studies of such agents (e.g., drugs that act directly on *muscarinic cholinergic receptors*) showed no more than mild, clinically unexciting benefits.

Four cholinesterase inhibitors that act on the brain are now approved in the United States for treatment of AD: donepezil (Aricept), rivastigmine (Exelon), galantamine (Reminyl, also available in extended-release capsules under the name Razadyne), and the older and now less used tacrine (THA, Cognex). Another, physostigmine, is not widely used because it has such a narrow and variable range of beneficial compared to toxic actions. (In other words, its therapeutic window is too narrow for convenient clinical use.)[30] Both anecdotal experience and objective data[31,32] indicate that the therapeutic benefits of donepezil, galantamine, and rivastigmine are approximately the same in most patients, if the drugs are properly prescribed and administered. Table 5-3 presents the conventional dosage regimens and ranges for these medications, and side effects more or less specific to each of these drugs. Gastrointestinal and other side effects characteristic of cholinesterase inhibitors as a group are discussed in the text below.

Both short-term and long-term benefits of cholinesterase inhibitors in AD have been examined.[31,32] Treatment with donepezil replicably benefits performance on the most robust and widely used simple test of cognition, the MMSE, even after 2 years.[32] Studies in the United States have concluded that the improvements are clinically meaningful. Treatment with cholinesterase inhibitors has been reported to delay institutionalization in the United States but not in the United Kingdom.[32] Whether it is worth the cost depends on one's viewpoint. The British health-care system requires clear cost-benefits in addition to measurable medical benefits for medications paid for by the National Health Service. American health care emphasizes doing as much as possible for that portion of the population whose medical care is paid for. A "hands across the sea" debate about this fundamentally political issue is unlikely to be illuminating medically.

TABLE 5-3

Central cholinesterase inhibitors used to treat AD

Name	Trade name	Usual dosage	Comments
Tacrine	Cognex	10–40 mg 4id	Liver damage (transaminitis)
Donepezil	Aricept	10 mg/day	Most commonly used; most extensively documented
Rivastigmine	Exelon	3-6 mg bid	Titrate up to full dose
Galantamine	Reminyl (Razadyne)	12 mg bid	Titrate up to full dose; long-acting (once per day) form available

Side effects on the nervous system of these medications tend to be minor. Occasional patients have very unpleasant dreams while taking donepezil. Sometimes these nightmares become so unpleasant that the medicine must be stopped. Whether this will be a problem with the other cholinesterase inhibitors is not clear, since these have not been as extensively prescribed. It was not recognized to be a problem with the first cholinesterase inhibitor to be widely used, namely tacrine (THA; Cognex). In research studies, treatment of patients with bipolar disease with cholinergic agonists has proven capable of precipitating depression, but this has not proven to be an important problem with therapeutic doses of these agents.

Gastrointestinal (GI) side effects are common with all four of the cholinesterase inhibitors now used to treat AD. These side effects are a consequence of their mechanism of action. Acetylcholine is a transmitter not only in the central nervous system but also in the periphery, including specifically the GI system. Clinically, the resulting side effects range from vague GI discomfort to stomach cramps, diarrhea, and nausea and vomiting. These side effects can be so intolerable that the medication needs to be stopped. They tend to be more evident at larger doses, and can often be overcome by reducing the dose of medication. Often the dose can then be slowly increased to previous levels without the GI side effects returning. Galantamine and rivastigmine are marketed in functionally lower doses than donepezil. As a result, they can be started at effectively lower doses than donepezil, and families can therefore decide that their relative tolerates these medications better. Tolerance can usually be achieved with donepezil as well, by starting it at 5 mg every other day or every third day and then working up incrementally to the dose tolerated by the patient. Often this “start low, go slow” approach ends up with patients tolerating a standard full dose of 10 mg every day.

Side effects of these cholinesterase inhibitors on other organ systems are generally rare, even though acetylcholine affects heart rate, bronchial dilation, and is the neurotransmitter at the neuromuscular junction. Recommended doses of the newer centrally acting cholinesterase inhibitors have not been documented to precipitate cardiac arrhythmias or bronchospasm, despite their wide use in sick elderly people.

NMDA Blockers Memantine (Namenda), which was approved for use in AD first in Europe and then in the United States, acts by a different mechanism than the cholinesterase inhibitors. Memantine appears to slow the progress of AD in both the milder and later stages. It benefits activities of daily living even in severe disease.[33] Projections suggest that it will be cost-effective even by the standards of the nationalized Swedish or the British health services, particularly in mild to moderate disease (MMSE ≥10).[34]

Memantine is a relatively weak blocker (antagonist) of a specific receptor for the neurotransmitter glutamate. This NMDA receptor[35] is present on many neurons in many parts of the nervous system. It appears to be involved in normal learning (plasticity). Overstimulation of the NMDA receptor leads by well-documented mechanisms to cell damage and then death. This effect has been termed *glutamatergic excitotoxicity*. Fast excitotoxicity results when the load of glutamate is so large as to overwhelm even a normal cell's ability to regulate itself (i.e., to maintain homeostasis). Slow excitotoxicity occurs when a neuron cannot maintain itself even when challenged by normal levels of glutamate or other transmitters. Excitotoxicity via NMDA receptors is a major mechanism of neuronal death when oxidative/energy metabolism is impaired, which it characteristically is in AD and other dementias. Both fast and slow excitotoxicity can result when an excitable cell cannot produce energy (i.e., ATP [adenosine triphosphate]) fast enough to meet the requirements imposed on it. In other words, excitotoxicity can reflect relative deficiencies in energy metabolism.

The dosage of memantine is normally increased over the course of 3 weeks to the full maintenance dose of 10 mg twice a day. The recommended dosage schedule is: 5 mg once a day for 1 week; then 5 mg twice a day for the next week; 15 mg a day for the third week, as 10 mg in the morning and 5 mg in the evening; thereafter 10 mg twice a day. The manufacturer offers a titration pack to be used for the first month, to make this incremental dosage easier for the patient and caregiver.

Memantine appears to be safe. The major reported side effects are confusion, dizziness, headache, and constipation. These occurred in 1–2% more of the treated patients than in those on placebo. Deaths have not been reported. The pharmacology of NMDA antagonism suggests that excitation would be an expected side effect of memantine. Anecdotal clinical experience indicates that caregivers often report patients on this medication to be more "roused" or "a little more irritable." Manufacturer-supported studies, however, recorded excitation as occurring more often in placebo-treated patients than in those on the active drug. The difference may lie in part in the stringency of the definition of excitation. In contrast to the safety of this low-affinity NMDA antagonist, high-affinity antagonists such as PCP (phencyclidine) or MK-801 (dizocilpine) are dangerous. They can cause psychosis, coma, and death. PCP is used as an anesthetic in veterinary medicine. Unfortunately, humans sometimes use it as a recreational drug. (See Chap. 14, Disorders of Conduct.) The effects of genetic variation on drug actions suggest that some humans will not be able to tolerate even the conventional doses of memantine, but experience so far suggests there are not many of them.

Memantine and cholinesterase inhibitors, specifically including donepezil, can be used safely together. When and for whom combined therapy is better than treatment with either approach alone needs to be determined by appropriate and appropriately large prospective studies. Available data suggest that addition of memantine can benefit AD patients already on full doses of donepezil.

Other Medications A number of other pharmacological approaches have been tested in AD, with less-encouraging results.

Anti-inflammatory agents seemed a reasonable approach to the treatment of AD, because the brains of AD patients show signs of chronic inflammation. Unfortunately, despite encouraging information from retrospective epidemiological studies, direct interventions have shown little benefit. Even dosages of 20 mg of prednisone a day did not alter the course of AD. The possible benefits of non-steroidal anti-inflammatory agents (NSAIDs) may have had more to do with their effect on vascular disease than on the AD process itself.

Antioxidant therapy seemed reasonable because of evidence of oxidative stress in AD brain. Unfortunately, prospective studies including epidemiologically based prospective studies have not given consistent support for this approach, neither in AD[36–39] nor in milder forms of cognitive impairment. Research in this area continues, however. Other dietary constituents are also being studied, such as the ω-3 and ω-6 fatty acids that appear to protect against the development of disease of the blood vessels. (See Chap. 9, Cerebrovascular Disorders.)

Larger and more rigorous studies have not borne out enthusiastic early reports that treatments with *statins* protects against the development and progression of AD.[40] at result is disappointing, since statins do protect against vascular disease, which is a risk factor for AD.

Vaccination against amyloid (Aβ) has become an area of intensive research that has been widely publicized in both the lay and professional media. Vaccination clearly benefits transgenic mice who overexpress disease-causing human genetic variants of the Alzheimer precursor protein (APP). These results and the prominence of the amyloid cascade hypothesis of AD have encouraged studies in human patients. Whether this procedure helps or harms humans with AD is an area of intense controversy. Vaccination does appear to clear amyloid from the brains of AD patients,[41] but clear-cut clinical benefits to human patients have not been reported. Endogenous antibodies to amyloid do not appear to benefit patients with AD.[42] Prof Roger Nitsch in Switzerland has described slowing of the progress of AD in some of his patients for 2 years after vaccination, but others have questioned the statistical significance of those observations. In other trials, statistically significant benefits on neuropsychological testing have not been found in patients who made antiamyloid antibodies compared to those who have not.[43] Some of the vaccinated patients developed inflammatory encephalopathies after vaccination. These have usually responded well to treatment with steroids, but a few percent of patients have had irreversible brain damage. A few have died.

Loss of brain substance as measured by MRI was statistically significantly greater in AD patients who made antibodies compared to those who did not, in a large, multicenter, collaborative investigation by a consortium of workers in the United States and at the National Hospital for Neurological Diseases in Queen Square (London); quantitation of the amount of brain was done blind at the latter location.[43] On face value, this disturbing finding argues against amyloid-directed therapies. Loss of brain substance by MRI has classically been considered perhaps the most characteristic biological concomitant of progression in AD. Explanations of this worrisome finding are possible, some of which would indicate benefit (e.g., removal of amyloid and of resolution of related inflammatory edema.) The greater loss of brain substance in people who make antiamyloid antibodies does, however, raise the question of whether amyloid is more protective than harmful even in the later stages of the disease.

Despite these worrisome observations, enthusiasm for vaccination against amyloid remains great. Anecdotal experiences continue to be widely publicized. Hopefully, adequately large and rigorous placebo-controlled double-blind trials will eventually allow clear-cut consensus conclusions about whether this form of treatment is helpful, harmful, or harmless but useless. The same is true for enthousiastic reports in the press and other media claiming that hyper-immune human globulin benefits people with AD.

Anti-amyloid treatments by other methods are in the experimental stage. These include inhibitors of the enzymes involved in the processing of APP to Aβ (β-secretase and γ-secretase). Theoretical arguments about whether these approaches are likely to be helpful or harmful can be made similar to those about vaccination against amyloid. Data on humans with AD are not available.

Caveats about reports in the media of "exciting new treatments" need to be kept in mind. The development of new and better treatments for AD is passionately desired by affected families as well as by those of us who have devoted our research to this area. Unfortunately, the desire for "something that works" can become so great that people lose their judgment. The media and commercial interests can fan unreasonable enthusiasms to further their own interests. Twenty-five years ago, many families were eager to obtain "therapeutic" preparations of algae from Lake Klamath in Oregon, encouraged by blurbs about the purity of the water there. When memantine was introduced, some Americans who could not get this drug for affected members of their families became guilt-ridden. Wanting to do so was not unreasonable, but the expectations that their relatives were being denied a "miracle medicine" were unrealistic. Among other reasons, the European data did not support that view. In our catchment area, where many people are involved in international commerce, care givers set up an organization to get this medication promptly "despite the medical-industrial complex." One of the duties of physicians caring for the stressed families coping with AD is to help them keep a level head about "miraculous new therapies." Sometimes sending the family to talk with experts at an Alzheimer Disease Research Center (ADRC) or other specialized center can calm their enthusiasms and assuage their guilt.

Vascular Dementia The treatment of dementia in patients with prominent cerebrovascular disease is essentially the same as that for patients with AD. Obviously, optimal treatment of the cerebrovascular disease is a key component. This is discussed in more detail in Chap. 9 (Cerebrovascular Disorders). Cholinesterase inhibitors including donepezil appear to be as useful in demented patients with strokes as in those without strokes.[44] Dosages are the same. Controlled clinical trials have confirmed beneficial effects of donepezil, galantamine, and rivastigmine not only on memory but also on other disabilities in patients with dementia and stroke.[44]

Lewy Body Dementia/Parkinsonian Dementia (LBD/PD) These two conditions are now considered by many clinicians and investigators to be different clinical forms of the same disorder. In some patients, dementia is an earlier and more prominent manifestation, in others the motor manifestations. The accepted treatment for the cognitive disorder is cholinesterase therapy, similar to that for AD. A recent study documenting the effectiveness of the cholinesterase inhibitor rivastigmine in *Parkinson disease dementia* also described it as increasing tremor, as well as nausea and vomiting. Sometimes cholinesterase therapy also benefits psychiatric manifestations such as hallucinations. Case reports have, however, been appearing of unusual side effects of donepezil in these patients, including a case of neuroleptic malignant syndrome. (See Chap. 4, Thought Disorders, for a discussion of this syndrome.)

The motor disorders in Lewy body dementia are treated the same way as for other forms of Parkinson disease. These patients are, however, typically sensitive to the psychic effects of treatment with Sinemet or other dopaminergic agonist. Fortunately, hallucinations induced by dopamine antagonists often do not induce the terror or other unpleasant feelings that typically accompany endogenous hallucinations.

Patients with LBD/PD are typically hypersensitive to the motor complications of dopamine blockers, including the relevant antipsychotics. This makes sense, since they have an endogenous functional dopamine deficiency. Even very low doses of medications such as risperidone or haloperidol can exacerbate motor symptoms and signs. In these patients, benzodiazepines or other psychiatric medications that do not act on dopamine receptors may be more useful.

Frontotemporal Dementia (FTD) This condition is often treated with donepezil or another cholinesterase inhibitor, because of its clinical and neuropathological overlaps with AD. The differential diagnosis can be difficult. Objective data from clinical trials to support this form is treatment is almost absent, however. Other treatments for the prominent behavioral symptoms of FTDs have concentrated on agents that act on serotonin-mediated systems. These have included trazodone and SSRIs. Beneficial results in short series have been reported in some studies and refuted in others.

Idiopathic Hippocampal Sclerosis This is in practice treated as if it were AD, since the differential diagnosis between these two conditions is so difficult before the patient comes to autopsy. AD even in its variant forms is much more common than idiopathic hippocampal sclerosis, which is a rare disease. The conservative course is to treat the patients for the former even if the latter is raised in the differential diagnosis. In theory, cholinesterase inhibition might improve the function of hippocampal neurons innervated by the septal-hippocampal system, since that system uses acetylcholine as a neurotransmitter. Data on the response to cholinesterase inhibitors of a series of patients with Idiopathic Hippocampal Sclerosis is not available.

Wernicke-Korsakoff Syndrome Treatment of the acute (Wernicke) phase of this disorder is discussed earlier. No treatment has been shown to be effective for the short-term memory defect of chronic Korsakoff Psychosis. That includes large doses of thiamin or of chemical derivatives of thiamin that cross into the body and brain more readily than thiamin itself. Treatment is symptomatic and often requires some form of custodial care, even if that care is given in a family setting.

Huntington Disease (HD) No effective treatment is known for HD. Recent studies in transgenic mouse models raise the possibility that cystamine might be helpful, but this has not yet been tested adequately in the human disease. Treatment is therefore symptomatic. These patients develop psychiatric illness that puts them at risk for suicide. This risk appears to be greater for patients with HD than for patients at high risk for other disorders diagnosed by studies of their DNA (i.e., by molecular genetics).

Other Neurological Disorders The treatments for other neurological disorders that cause dementia as one of their manifestations are discussed elsewhere in this monograph with the discussions of those disorders. As expected from the pharmacology of the cholinesterase inhibitors and from the role of acetylcholine-mediated systems in the brain, cholinesterase inhibitors are also proving useful for memory impairments associated with a variety of brain diseases, including for instance, multiple sclerosis.[45] Recent studies suggest that genes that predispose to other neuropsychiatric disorders may also predispose to the development of signs and symptoms of these disorders in Alzheimer patients,[46] providing modern, molecular genetic information to support the use of antipsychotic medications for people with AD who develop the relevant symptoms. Tentatively, it seems likely that the same may well be true for less common dementias, but relevant studies are not yet available.

REFERENCES

1. For instance, when the editors of the *Textbook of Geriatric Medicine and Gerontology* were planning for the fifth edition, most of the internist editors preferred separate chapters on delirium and dementia to a single chapter on disorders of cognition.
2. Engel GL, Romano J. Delirium, a syndrome of cerebral insufficiency. *J Chronic Dis*. 1959;9(3):260–277. Engel and Romano used EEG (electroen-

cephalogram), then a relatively new technique, to buttress their argument. Slowing on the EEG often occurs in delirium and in dementia, but is now considered a nonspecific finding.

3. Folstein MF, Folstein SE, McHugh PR. Cognitive defect in medical illness. *Ann Intern Med.* 1977;86:827–828.
4. Garcia CA, Tweedy JR, Blass JP. Underdiagnosis of cognitive impairment in a rehabilitation setting. *J Am Geriat Soc.* 1984;32:339–342.
5. The correct Latin plural of "delirium" is "deliria." The anglicized form is used here for simplicity.
6. Social skills tend to be learned early and encoded deeply and redundantly. For a time, our clinical service included a day hospital program for demented people. Having lunch with our patients was the epitome of a certain type of New York dinner party. The forms of polite conversation were elegantly maintained although without any content.
7. Kahn RL, Goldfarb AI, Pollack M, et al. Brief objective measures for the determination of mental status in the aged. *Am J Pyschiat.* 1960;117:326–332.
8. Folstein MF, Folstein SE, McHugh PR. "Mini Mental State.": a practical method for grading the cognitive state of patients for the clinician. *J Psychiatr Res.* 1975;12:189–2000.
9. Bagley S. Scientists world-wide battle a narrow view of Alzheimer's cause. *Wall Str Jl.* 2004;April 16: p. 9.
10. Blass JP, Ratan RR. "Silent" strokes and dementia. *N Engl J Med.* 2003;348:1277–1278.
11. Brun A, Englund E. A white matter disorder in dementia of the Alzheimer type: a pathoanatomical study. *Ann Neurol.* 1986;19:253–262.
12. This impressive name is, of course, just a statement of the phenomenon in long words of Greek and Latin origin. The English translation is "scarring of the hippocampus of unknown cause." Using a term coined from classic languages should not foster the belief that we know what we are talking about.
13. These mutations are pathologically long (>35–40) CAG repeats in the *HTT* gene that encodes the huntingtin protein.
14. The clinical importance of the human brain's ability to oxidize materials other than glucose is limited. Ketone bodies substitute effectively for glucose during prolonged starvation but do not do so during acute diabetic ketoacidosis.
15. My longtime colleague, Gary Gibson, and I did much of the work described in the subsequent paragraphs. I apologize to readers who find this discussion self-serving.
16. "Awareness uses a serial attention mechanism consisting of high-frequency (40-Herz), synchronized oscillations that transiently "bind together" widely distributed cortical neurons related to different aspects of a perceived object...Direct application of [acetylcholine] ... induces just such fast, synchronized activity in hippocampal slice preparations ... It seems likely that

the action of [acetylcholine] ... in the cortex and thalamus is central to the normal maintenance of conscious awareness." Hardman JG, Limbird LE, Gilman AG. *Goodman & Gilman's The Pharmacological Basis of Therapeutics,* 10th edition, McGraw-Hill, NY, 2001, p. 327.

17. Svenningsson P, Tzvarra ET, Carruthers R, et al. Diverse psychotomimetics act through a common signaling pathway. *Science.* 2003;302:1412–1415. Among the components of this pathway are the DARPP-32 protein, CREB(CREB), and c-Fos.
18. This effect of damage to the hippocampus does not prove that memories (*engrams*) are stored there. The hippocampus can have a central role in the control of mental traffic even if its function is more that of a "switching yard" than of a storage hall.
19. Many prominent researchers in "aging" are now convinced that telomerase and its effect on DNA has more to do with cancer than with aging.
20. It is common experience to see someone go through a tragic experience and suddenly seem much older, e.g. "The divorce has aged him by at least ten years." It is equally common to see someone who appears to be rejuvenated by a happy event, e.g. "Since he fell in love with his new wife and remarried, he seems at least ten years younger." The obvious question is whether the potential for the biologic appearance of age to change rapidly and reversibly indicates that biologic age itself can actually change rapidly and reversibly.

    Isaac Newton's "arrow of time" is now recognized to be a practical but theoretically incomplete approximation, rather like the rest of Newtonian physics. In the relativistic/quantum mechanical universe that we have lived in for most of the last hundred years, time is reversible and variable. If we define aging as "biological change over time," what do we mean by time? Newtonian time? Relativistic or quantum mechanical time? In other words, how do we define the denominator? We now measure time either by the movement of planets (specifically, the Earth around the Sun) or by the decay of a radioactive element in an atomic clock. Stephen Hawking, among others, has suggested that the link between biology and the apparent arrow of time lies in the physical chemistry (thermodynamics) governing our own bodies. Specifically, it arises from the tendency of things left to themselves to become random (of entropy to increase).

    "Our subjective sense of the direction of time, the psychological arrow of time, is therefore determined within our brain by the thermodynamic arrow of time...Disorder increases with time because we measure time in the direction in which disorder increases." [Hawking SW. *A Brief History of Time,* Bantam Books, NY, 1988, p. 147.]

    Unfortunately, Hawking's profound analysis does not clarify the intimate mechanisms that lead to or link together the ways we measure time to the molecular and cellular events we try to associate with "aging."

21. There are many teaching jokes to illustrate the flaw in depending too heavily on statistical likelihood. An economist taught me that a statistical description of nine pregnant women and a virgin is that each pregnant woman is 1/10 a virgin and the virgin is 9/10 pregnant. A New York story expressing the same idea is the fabled Mrs. Rabinowitz. She named her children Daniel, Joseph, Miriam, and Lee Hung Chang, because she had read that every fourth child born in the world is Chinese.
22. Other neuropathological findings have been described as also being characteristic in AD—for instance Hirano bodies and neural threads. A detailed discussion of the neuropathology of AD is beyond the scope of this monograph, and is readily available in standard textbooks and reviews.
23. An example is accusations about the narrow mindset of devotees of the church of the Holy Amyloid, and contemptuous dismissal of reformers who challenge the formulations favored by bishops of that church. One is reminded of previous unfortunate episodes in the history of biology, when personal issues became too important compared to data. For instance, Justus von Liebig dismissed the concept of the tetrahedral carbon atom as the speculation of Dutch snot-noses. That concept is fundamental to all of organic chemistry and therefore to biochemistry. OttoWarburg said of the young Hans Krebs that he had no future as a scientist but would do well treating heart disease in wealthy German Jews. Krebs and Warburg both won Nobel Prizes.
24. Presumably, Lewy Bodies are more or less spherical in vivo but look round after they have been cut during tissue sectioning.
25. Dermaut B, Kumar-Singh S, Engelborghs S, et al. A novel presenilin 1 mutation associated with Pick's disease but not beta-amyloid plaques. *Ann Neurol.* 2004;55:604–606.
26. As an intern, I was taught to treat delirium tremens (DTs) by giving increasing doses of a long-acting benzodiazepine until the patient's tremors stopped. I did so to a patient who quieted down to the point where he died. Review of the case by the medical staff of the hospital concluded that the patient had been treated entirely appropriately, and had died of his basic illness and not from my treatment. Nevertheless, I subsequently tolerated more tremulousness in my patients being treated for DTs. Happily, none of the rest of them died during my treatment.
27. A classic work is Plum F and Posner JB. *The Diagnosis of Stupor and Coma*, 3d edition, Oxford University Press, NY, 1982. Although this book is almost 25 years old, the discussion of the clinical aspects is still up-to-date.
28. At least in our catchment area, patients and families who are refused a medication will usually shop around until they find a doctor who prescribes the medicine they want.
29. Physical chemistry distinguishes between chemical activity and concentration. Detailed discussion of that difference is beyond the scope of this monograph.

30. Physostigmine was used as an arrow poison, and it can still kill people.
31. Ritchie CW, Ames D, Clayton T, et al. Meta analysis of randomized trials of the efficacy and safety of donepezil, galantamine, and rivastigmine for the treatment of Alzheimer disease. *Am J Geriatr Psychiatry*. 2004;12:358–369.
32. Courtney C, Farrell D, Gray R, et al. Long-term donepezil in 565 patients with Alzheimer's disease (AD2000): randomized double-blind trial. *Lancet*. 2004;363:2105–2115.
33. Doody R, Wirth Y, Schmitt F, et al. Specific functional effects of memantine treatment in patients with moderate to severe Alzheimer's disease. *Dement Geriatr Cogn Disord*. 2004;18:227–232.
34. Jones RW, McCrone P, Guilhaume C. Cost effectiveness of memantine in Alzheimer's disease: an analysis based on a probabilistic Markov model from a UK perspective. *Drugs Aging*. 2004;21:607–620.
35. The term *NMDA receptor* reflects that this receptor is selectively activated by n-methyl-D-aspartic acid.
36. Luchsinger JA, Tang MX, Shea S, et al. Antioxidant vitamin intake and risk of Alzheimer disease. *Arch Neurol*. 2003;60:203–238.
37. Zandi PP, Anthony JC, Khachaturian AS, et al. Cache County Study Group. Reduced risk of Alzheimer disease in users of antioxidant vitamin supplements: the Cache County Study. *Arch Neurol*. 2004;61:82–88.
38. Petersen RC, Thomas RG, Grundman M, et al. Alzheimer's Disease Cooperative Study Group. Vitamin E and donepezil for the treatment of mild cognitive impairment. *N Engl J Med*. 2005, Jun 9;352(23):2379-2388.
39. The author has a patent and pending patents on an approach to treatment of the oxidative/cerebrometabolic lesion in AD. Discussion of it in this monograph would obviously be inappropriate, until adequate data about it have been gathered by people free of financial interest in its efficacy.
40. Rea TD, Breitner JC, Psaty BM, et al. Statin use and the risk of incident dementia: the Cardiovascular Health Study. Arch Neurol. 2005;62: 1047–1051.
41. Nicoll JA, Wilkinson D, Holmes C, et al. Neuropathology of human Alzheimer disease after immunization with amyloid-beta peptide: a case report. *Nat Med*. 2003;9: 448–452.
42. Nath A, Hall E, Tuzova M, et al. Autoantibodies to amyloid beta-peptide (Abeta) are increased in Alzheimer's disease patients and Abeta antibodies can enhance Abeta neurotoxicity: implications for disease pathogenesis and vaccine development. *Neuromolecular Med*. 2003;3:29–39.
43. Fox NC, Blasck RS, Gilman S, et al. Effects of Aβ immunization (AN1792) on MRI measures of cerebral volume in Alzheimer disease. *Neurology*. 2005;64:1563–1572.
44. Erkinjuntti T, Roman G, Gauthier S. Treatment of vascular dementia-evidence from clinical trials with cholinesterase inhibitors. *Neurol Res*. 2004;26: 603–605.

45. Krupp LB, Christodoulou C, Melville P, et al. Donepezil improved memory in multiple sclerosis in a randomized clinical trial. *Neurology*. 2004;63: 1579–1585.
46. Caimi L, DiLuca M, Padovani A, et al. Catechol-O-methyltransferase gene polymorphism is associated with risk of psychosis in Alzheimer disease. *Neurosci Lett*. 2004;370:127–129.

CHAPTER SIX

Anxiety

Anxiety is common in patients in general clinical practice. Sometimes the patient or a family member complains of it. Sometimes the patient and family deny being anxious even when their anxiety is palpable. The practical questions for the clinician are: when has anxiety reached a level where it needs treatment; and if so what should that treatment be, who should give it, and who should get it. (Sometimes treating a relatively healthy caregiver who is anxious about the patient's "agitation" is better medical practice than adding yet another medication to a patient's already complex regimen.)

A variety of medical and neurological disorders characteristically leads to anxiety as a major symptom. Treatment of these conditions is that of the underlying disease. For instance, anxiety due to hyperthyroidism is treated by treating the excess thyroid activity. Episodes of acute fear that are manifestations of temporal lobe epilepsy are treated by treating the seizure disorder. (See Chap. 10, Disorders of Awareness.) Adjunct, relatively short-term use of a medication to reduce anxiety may, of course, help the patient to be more comfortable during the time needed for treatment of the underlying disease to become effective.

Reasonable amounts of anxiety are part of normal healthy life and can be useful. For instance, some actors and actresses say they need a degree of performance anxiety to maintain their edge while on stage or before the camera. So do some medical academics before they give a presentation. Caring about something can reasonably rouse anxiety even when the event is unlikely to have longer-term significance. An example would be concern about how one's child will succeed in a grade school concert or other performance. Anxiety about whether or not children are admitted to the college of their – or their parents – choice is widespread, but in most instances is not considered pathological.[1]

Illness is a stressor that typically arouses anxiety even in normal people. The ability to provide reassurance is an important therapeutic skill, as every general clinician knows. However, discussion of that clinical skill is beyond the scope of this monograph, as are psychotherapeutic and other techniques for treatment of anxiety in a general practice setting.[2] This discussion focuses on pharmacological agents.

American psychiatry now makes a distinction between fear – which has a rational cause – and anxiety, which does not. Freud did not make this distinction, and many psychiatrists in other countries do not consider it particularly useful. Fear can be debilitating and make a person miserable even if it has a rational basis.[3] Some patients with terminal illnesses develop an overwhelming fear of death. The suffering their fear arouses can sometimes be reduced by treating them with an antianxiety medication, even though their fear is of a real event.

CLASSIFICATION AND DIAGNOSIS

The discussion of anxiety in this chapter focuses on anxiety in patients seen in general clinical practice. This discussion differs in a number of ways from the classification of anxiety disorders in the current version of DSM, DSM-IV-RT. As always, the pressing clinical question is less what to call an illness than how to treat it.

Mild Anxiety

General clinicians often see patients in whom anxiety leads to discomfort that is not severe enough to deserve the label of an anxiety disorder as classified by DSM-IV-RT. Survey data indicate that anxiety is one of the most common reasons people see their physicians. Medical illnesses typically induce anxieties in patients, and some medical illnesses such as hyperthyroidism typically present with anxiety as a prominent symptom. General clinicians also frequently encounter patients suffering primarily from anxiety who however complain of a physical problem instead of their other worries. Among the more common forms of such "somatizations" are back pain and headache. Clinical judgment is required to decide when a patient needs medication to bring anxiety down to a tolerable level.[4] Not surprisingly, factors related to the physician as well as to the patient affect the decision on when to treat with talk therapy, when with medication, and when with both.[5] Physicians comfortable with talk therapy tend to rely on it more heavily.[6,7]

Sometimes a person is in a situation that rationally evokes a high level of anxiety and cannot be objectively alleviated. One example is a dying patient.[3] Another example is a parent caring for a child with an incurable disease—medical or psychiatric. The parents of a child with a psychiatric problem may themselves carry a genetic predisposition to psychiatric illness that exacerbates their anxiety. Sometimes a person will declare that the anxiety aroused by a situation is "more than I can bear." The clinician must decide whether such a statement calls for further reassurance, for pharmacological treatment, for referral to a psychiatrist, or for some combination of the three. Severe enough anxiety is a risk factor for suicide, particularly when the anxiety is associated with depression.

Generalized Anxiety Disorder/Somatoform Disorder

Although DSM-IV-RT treats these conditions as separate entities, they are discussed together here because their presentations to the general clinician often overlap. Studies have shown that patients with generalized anxiety disorder (GAD) tend to complain to their general physicians about pain or other somatic disorder rather than about generalized anxiety.

The first consideration for the general clinician in evaluating an anxious patient with a somatic complaint is whether that complaint arises from a medical or surgical illness. The fact that a patient seems excessively anxious does not mean that he or she is not also physically ill. In the 1960s, a fifteen-year follow-up study of patients diagnosed as hysteric found that half of them were dead of the disease that had been misdiagnosed as hysteria. This study was done at a hospital world famous for the diagnostic acumen of its staff, namely the National Hospital for Neurological Diseases on Queen Square in London, England. The rate of misdiagnosis in specialty centers has been reported to have fallen to a much more acceptable 4% in the current century, purportedly because of more thorough evaluations rather than because of the availability of modern diagnostic techniques including imaging (CT [computed tomography] and MRI [magnetic resonance imaging] scans).[8] The author's own recent experience in New York does not, unfortunately, agree with that optimistic analysis.

Having a brain disease does not protect against having disease in other organs. Neuropsychiatric illnesses often interfere with the affected people taking good care of themselves. Many medical illnesses lead to pathological anxiety or other neurological or psychiatric abnormalities among their major clinical manifestations. Examples include not only endocrine diseases such as thyroid abnormalities but also diseases of the heart or lungs or other organs. The discussions in this monograph assume accurate medical diagnosis and appropriate medical and surgical care of patients who may also need pharmacological treatments directed at their nervous systems. That care includes recognition and treatment of medical illnesses with neurological and/or psychiatric manifestations.

Patients with *generalized anxiety disorder* (GAD) are so chronically anxious that they often cannot remember a time when they were not worried. If they find nothing else of concern, they will often worry about their anxiety (or, if partially treated, about the return of their anxiety). Often they will focus on a physical manifestation and therefore suffer from a *somatization disorder.* Table 6-1 gives the major criteria from DSM-IV-RT for GAD. Table 6-2 lists criteria for somatization disorder and gives its subclassifications. (DSM-IV-TR distinguishes between generalized anxiety disorder and somatization disorder as separate categories of illness.)

The drugs discussed below (see Treatment) and notably the benzodiazepines can reduce anxiety even in people with major medical disorders. Short-term treatment to "tide a patient" over an episode of excessive anxiety can be a useful part of general medical care. However, consultation with a psychiatrist is part of good medical practice, particularly if such treatment is prolonged beyond 2 weeks or if it is instituted for a psychiatric disorder such as GAD with or without somatization. Chronic pain for which no adequate somatic cause can be found is a common and difficult problem in general clinical medicine. Referral to a specialist is indicated, even though this problem often eludes successful treatment by specialists as well. Pain and its treatment is the subject of the next chapter in this monograph (Chap. 7, Pain).

Anxious Depression: Anxious depression can be difficult to distinguish from anxiety with depressive features. The distinction between these diagnostic categories is often more theoretical than practical. Some 60% of patients with GAD also meet criteria for depression (see Chap. 3, Mood Disorders). Psychiatrists use antidepressants as first-line treatments for GAD. General clinicians need to be sensitive to the possibility that medically serious obesity can result if someone with one of these disorders eats "to calm down." Loss of appetite with severe weight loss may also occur. Since many antidepressants can take weeks to have a meaningful clinical effect, optimal

TABLE 6–1

Diagnostic criteria for generalized anxiety disorder

A. Excessive anxiety and worry (apprehensive expectation occurring more days than not for at least 6 months, about a number of events or activities (such as work or school performance).

B. The person finds it difficult to control the worry.

C. The anxiety and worry are associated with three (or more) of the following six symptoms (with at least some symptoms present for more days than not for the past 6 months). Note: only one item is required in children.

1. Restlessness or feeling keyed up or on edge
2. Being easily fatigued
3. Difficulty concentrating or mind going blank
4. Irritability
5. Muscle tension
6. Sleep disturbance (difficulty falling or staying asleep; or restless unsatisfying sleep)

D. The focus of the anxiety and worry is not confined to features of an Axis 1 disorder, e.g. as in Panic Disorder, Social Phobia, Obsessive-Compulsive Disorder, Separation Anxiety Disorder, Anorexia Nervosa, Somatization Disorder, or Hypochondiasis, and the anxiety and worry do not occur exclusively during Post-traumatic Stress Disorder.

E. The anxiety, worry, or physical symptoms cause clinically significant distress or impairment in social, occupational, or other important areas of functioning.

F. The disturbance is not due to the direct physiological effects of a substance (e.g., a drug of abuse, or a medication) or a general medical condition (e.g. hyperthyroidism) and does not occur exclusively during a Mood Disorder, a Psychotic Disorder, or a Pervasive Developmental Disorder.

Adapted with permission from *Diagnostic and Statistical Manual of Mental Disorders*, 4th ed., Text Revision (DSM-TV-TR), American Psychiatric Association, Arlington VA, 2000, p. 476. DSM-IV-RT also gives specific diagnostic criteria for subtypes of somatization disorder: undifferentiated somatoform disorder, conversion disorder, pain disorder, hypochondriasis, body dysmorphic disorder, and somatoform disorder not otherwise specified.

treatment may include "tiding the patient over" the initial phase of therapy with a benzodiazepine or other antianxiety drug. Feeling better after taking a *benzodiazepine* does not rule out a concomitant depression. It does not rule out the possibility of suicide. As emphasized in Chap. 3, Mood Disorders, depression and specifically anxious depression is unpleasant and can predispose to suicide. That includes patients who start

TABLE 6–2
Diagnostic criteria for somatization disorder

A. A history of many physical compaints beginning before age 30 years that occur over a period of several years and result in treatment being sought or significant impairment in social, occupational, or other important areas of functioning.

B. Each of the following criteria must have been met, with individual symptoms occurring at any time during the course of the disturbance:

1. Four pain symptoms
2. Two gastrointestinal symptoms
3. One sexual symptom
4. One pseudoneurological

C. Either (1) or (2):

1. After appropriate investigation, each of the symptoms in Criterion B cannot be fully explained by a known general medical condition or the direct effects of a substance (e.g., a drug of abuse, a medication).
2. When there is a related medical condition, the physical complaints or resulting social or occupational impairment are in excess of what would be expected from the history, physical examination, or laboratory findings.

D. The symptoms are not produced intentionally or feigned, as in Fictitious Disorder or Malingering.

Adapted with permission from *Diagnostic and Statistical Manual of Mental Disorders*, 4th ed., Text Revision (DSM-IV-TR), American Psychiatric Association, Arlington VA, 2000, p. 490.

to feel better on medication and then have the drive and mental organization to kill themselves successfully. Depression presenting as anxiety can be a psychiatric emergency requiring hospitalization of an actively suicidal patient. (See Chap. 3, Mood Disorders.)

Other Anxiety Disorders

DSM-IV-RT lists a number of other types of anxiety disorder in addition to GAD. In general, psychiatrists rather than general clinicians should treat these conditions. When patients who need psychiatric care refuse to see the specialist, consultation with a psychiatrist is still in order and should be documented in the patient records. Sometimes when the patient's anxiety recedes during treatment with a benzodiazepine or other appropriate medication, their reluctance to see a psychiatrist diminishes as well.

Since these conditions optimally fall outside of the realm of treatment by general clinicians, their characteristics are reviewed only briefly here.

Panic: A panic attack is, according to DSM-IV-RT, a discrete period of intense fear or discomfort, typically associated with a number of physical manifestations. Panic disorder is characterized by recurrent panic attacks and persistent worrying following an attack. Panic disorder can occur with or without the patient having a *phobia*, and specifically *agoraphobia*. The FDA (Food & Drug Administration) has approved the SSRI antidepressant paroxetine (Paxil) for treatment of panic disorder. Although the FDA has also approved the benzodiazepine *alprazolam* (Xanax) for this indication, its use is not favored by most psychiatrists because of the serious side effects that can ensue.

Phobias: A phobia is a pathological fear of some object or situation. Epidemiological studies indicate that phobias are the most common form of psychiatric disease in the United States. That, of course, raises the question of how much fear a person has to have for it to be pathological. Classically, the lady standing on a stool because she has seen a mouse is not considered crazy. People who grow faint at the sight of blood are not treated as insane, even though they have a recognized phobia that can be a disability in specific circumstances. On the other hand, people so afraid of dirt that they scrub the skin off their hands should get psychiatric help. Specific phobias have names derived from classical languages (Table 6-3).

The word *agoraphobia* comes from the Greek words for fear and market place. It is defined as anxiety about being in places or situations from which escape might be difficult (or embarrassing) or in which help may not be available. Sometimes people can deal with agoraphobia by being with another person on whom they rely. This disorder tends to be chronic but in the majority of cases becomes manageable.

Social phobias are also called social anxiety disorders. People with this condition have a pathologically intense fear of humiliation in common social situations. Examples include fear of public speaking, fear of social encounters with the other sex, and even fear of urinating in a public restroom ("shy bladder"). Again, where to draw the line between odd

TABLE 6–3
Types of phobias

Agoraphobia	Fear of crowds and of social situations where a means of escape does not appear obvious to the patient
Acrophobia	Fear of height
Ailurophobia	Fear of cats
Hydrophobia	Fear of water
Claustrophobia	Fear of closed spaces
Cynophobia	Fear of dogs
Mysophobia	Fear of dirt
Ophidiophobia	Fear of snakes
Pyrophobia	Fear of fire
Xenophobia	Fear of strangers
Zoophobia	Fear of animals

The Internet site http://www.phobialist.com provides a much more exhaustive list of phobias.

behavior and pathological fear can be difficult. Common sense argues that if the fear interferes with life or even if it just makes a person miserable, it is a disability that deserves treatment.

Treatment of phobias optimally involves behavioral techniques, often including "flooding" or other forms of desensitization. Insight therapies are claimed to have helped some people. Drugs have also proven useful–specifically the SSRI antidepressants—but are not the optimal form of treatment if used by themselves. Phobias that need treatment should be treated by psychiatrists.

Obsessive-Compulsive Disorder (OCD): By definition, obsessions are thoughts and compulsions are actions (behaviors). In obsessive-compulsive disorder (OCD), intrusive, repetitive thoughts lead to compulsive behaviors that may or may not soothe the anxiety induced by the thoughts. There are people who claim that their lives are made meaningful by religious or political rituals that others find insane.[9] Whether these people are considered mad or inspired is largely determined by the social and political situation in which they find themselves (see Table 6-4). OCD is

TABLE 6–4 Common manifestations of obsessive-compulsive disorder
Terror of dirt or other forms of contamination
Pathological doubt (*folie de doute*)
Intrusive thoughts
Excessive exactitude such as a fixation on excessive symmetry
Religious or political obsessions
Hair pulling (trichotillomania)
Nail-biting

now distinguished from obsessive-compulsive personality. (See Chap. 14, Disorders of Conduct.)

Extreme, pathological obsessive-compulsive behavior can be as debilitating as any other form of madness. The differential diagnosis of OCD includes schizophrenia and depression as well as phobias, tics (e.g., Tourette syndrome), temporal lobe epilepsy, and obsessive-compulsive personality disorder (See Chap. 14, Disorders of Conduct).

Both behavioral and pharmacological therapies are used to treat OCD. Generally the combination is more effective than either alone. First-line drugs include antidepressants: SSRIs (selective serotonin reuptake inhibitors), clomipramine, venlafaxine (Effexor), and MAO inhibitors such as phenelzine (Nardil). Some patients with OCD have been reported to respond to antiseizure medications such as *valproate* (Depakene) or *carbamazepine* (Tegretol); they may have been misdiagnosed patients with epilepsy with primarily behavioral manifestations. (See Chap. 10, Disorders of Awareness). Electroconvulsive treatments (ECT) can sometimes rescue patients from disabling, drug-refractory OCD. In patients who do not respond even to ECT, psychosurgery may be called for—specifically, *cingulotomy*. Again, the degree of disability and suffering has to be great enough to warrant the irreversible intervention of opening the skull and cutting the brain. Sometimes patients who did not respond to treatment with drugs before cutting the *cingulum* will respond to those same drugs after surgery.

Patients with OCD severe enough to require specific treatment need to be treated by psychiatrists or other specialists.

Post-traumatic Stress Disorder and Acute Stress Disorder: This condition is well known to the general public as well as the general medical profession (see Table 6-5). It is common both in survivors of combat and in

TABLE 6–5

Criteria for post-traumatic stress disorder

1. The person has been exposed to a traumatic event
2. The traumatic event is persistently experienced
3. Stimuli associated with the trauma are persistently avoided
4. Persistent symptoms of increased arousal are present
5. The disturbance lasts more than a month
6. The disturbance causes clinically significant distress

women who have been raped or otherwise assaulted, and we have an abundance of people in both those categories in the United States. It also occurs in victims of torture, including psychological torture such as brainwashing.

Many of us – most of us – remember bad things that have happened to us, and sometimes those bad memories come up at inconvenient times. In post-traumatic stress disorder, the bad thing was typically very bad and the intensity and frequency with which the memories come back are disabling. Table 6-5 lists the DSM-IV-RT criteria for post-traumatic stress disorder. Acute stress disorder by definition lasts less time than post-traumatic stress disorder. According to the current definition, the acute condition occurs within 4 weeks of the trauma and lasts between 2 days and 4 weeks.

Post-traumatic stress disorder tends to respond to a combination of behavioral and pharmacological therapy. The first-line medications for treating it are the SSRI antidepressants. (See Chap. 3, Mood Disorders). Other antidepressants that have been useful include buspirone (BuSpar), the tricyclic drugs imipramine (Tofranil) and amitriptyline (Elavil), MAO inhibitors such as phenelzine (Nardil), and trazodone (Desyrel). This pharmacology suggests that these environmentally triggered conditions involve neurobiological mechanisms similar to those of depressive disorders. Previous generations of clinicians might have called these conditions "reactive depressions," Specific patients with post-traumatic stress disorder have benefited from treatment with anticonvulsants such as those used to treat OCD.

General clinicians are likely to see patients who have some form of post-traumatic stress disorder. Optimal clinical management requires referral to a psychiatrist or at least collaboration with a psychiatrist familiar with these disorders.

Theoretically, it is interesting to speculate about how many of the "neuroses" described by Freud were forms of post-traumatic stress disorder, in which the stress was repressed from verbal memory but still influenced behavior. Of course, in Freud's cases, the stress was less violent than combat or rape, and it was not readily available to conscious (verbal) memory. It may have been an otherwise innocuous event—the Viennese equivalent of seeing "Mommy kissing Santa Claus underneath the mistletoe last night." *Catharsis* classically included recognizing and dealing with stress in terms of adult, verbal consciousness. The point is, of course, that different people can respond to the same stress in different ways. That is also true of the horrible stressors that classically precipitate post-traumatic stress disorder.

NEUROBIOLOGY

The mechanisms underlying the anxiety disorders are complex. Joseph LeDoux at New York University has recently defined an *emotional learning system,* using as a main paradigm classical Pavlovian fear conditioning.[10,11] Emotional conditioning can occur early in life and be powerful and long-lasting. A specific part of the brain, the amygdala, is heavily involved in fear and therefore presumably in what in humans is considered anxiety. Emotional conditioning may underlie some of the nonverbal anxiety disorders discussed earlier. It does appear to underlie post-traumatic stress disorder and has been invoked in OCD.

Different anxiety disorders may involve different mechanisms.[12] Family and molecular genetic studies implicate inherited predispositions in many patients with these disorders. Attempts to link susceptibility to anxiety disorders including OCD to genetic variations in specific genes have not yet yielded compelling associations.[13] Specific molecular loci have not been defined to the point where they can be useful for clinical diagnosis and practice.

Neuroanatomically, a number of brain structures have been associated with specific anxiety disorders. These typically involve the *limbic system*, which contains parts of the brain that subserve emotion. (The limbic system is relatively well developed even in animals we consider far below us in the evolutionary tree. It has also been called the "crocodile brain.") The *amygdala* is part of the limbic system. So is the *hypothalamus*, which was once considered the "head ganglion of the autonomic system." The involvement of the hypothalamus in anxiety disorders agrees with the presence of peripheral signs of *autonomic nervous system* action in these disorders. Abnormalities of the caudate nuclei have been found in patients with OCD.

At the neurotransmitter level, anxiety disorders as a group tend to be associated with a relative overactivity of circuits mediated by the neurotransmitter *norepinephrine* and a relative functional deficiency of *GABA* and *serotonin*-mediated systems. This formulation agrees with the relative overactivity of norepinephrine-mediated functions in the periphery of patients with anxiety disorders. Examples include alterations in autonomic functions, that is, rapid heartbeat, sweating, and increase in blood pressure. This formulation also agrees with the known role of GABA as primarily an *inhibitory* neurotransmitter. It also agrees with the ability of drugs that act like norepinephrine (*α-adrenergic agonists*) to make anxiety worse and of drugs, which act on serotonin systems (e.g., SSRIs) or on GABA receptors (e.g., benzodiazepines) to treat anxiety disorders. The pharmacology is rational if not yet fully understood.[12]

TREATMENTS

The practical problems facing the general clinician who is treating an unusually anxious patient are matters of clinical judgment.

The first problem is whether the anxiety needs treatment[4,5] Apparently "excessive" anxiety can be normal ("ego congruent"). In some patients that may be a matter of personality style and in others of social conformity. The latter can apply particularly to women of certain backgrounds.[5]

A second problem is to determine whether or not the patient is anxious because of a medical or surgical condition that makes him or her feel sick and frightened. Answering that question is the stuff of medicine and surgery, including family practice and specialized geriatric practice. Anxiety does not protect against other illness. Treating an underlying illness effectively often, although certainly not invariably, reduces the patient's anxiety to a manageable level.

A frequent practical problem is whether or not to treat the patient with a benzodiazepine or other antianxiety agent to "tide the patient over" while diagnosis and treatment are instituted. There are simply too many people in that unpleasant position to refer all of them to psychiatrists. However, sustained treatment of anxiety or treatment for a more severe anxiety disorder does call for a consultation and often for continuing collaboration with a psychiatrist. Severe anxiety disorders are not only unpleasant and disabling but can be physically dangerous, particularly if they produce suicidal or other destructive behavior. According to current standards, chronic treatment with a benzodiazepine (e.g., Valium) incurs significant risks including charges of malpractice, and antidepressants may take too long to start having significant effects (to "kick in"). The psychiatrist may not have more success treating a patient with a recalcitrant anxiety disorder than the general clinician does, but calling in a psychiatrist at least makes it clear even to lawyers or other hostile outside observers that "standards of good medical practice for the area" were complied with.

A fourth problem is to decide whether or not the anxiety reaches the level of a mental illness. Some phobias and compulsions are common and can be relatively harmless. If the anxiety reaches the level of a mental illness, the diagnosis and treatment is the province of the psychiatrist rather than the general clinician. When a patient refuses to see a psychiatrist, attempts should still be made to obtain advice from a psychiatrist or other expert and to document in the medical records the attempts to get specialist treatment for the patient. Distinguishing disabling anxiety from suicidal depression calls for a specialist with established expertise, for both clinical and medicolegal reasons.

Antidepressants: In general, psychiatrists now prescribe antidepressants and specifically SSRIs as the first-line drugs for anxiety disorders. (See Chap. 3, Mood Disorders.) That specifically includes GAD. The FDA has approved paroxetine (Paxil) and escitalopram (Lexapro) for this indication. Fluoxetine (Prozac) is not the optimal SSRI for treating a disorder in which anxiety is a major component, since it can increase anxiety in the early stages of treatment. The tricyclic antidepressants doxepin (Sinequan, Adapin) and imipramine (Tofranil) have been reported to be relatively effective in panic disorders with agoraphobia. The doses of SSRIs and cyclic antidepressants used to treat people diagnosed with anxiety disorders are the same as those used to treat those with mood disorders. Since antidepressants typically do not take effect immediately, prescribing a more rapidly acting medicine such as a benzodiazepine or *bupropion* may be necessary to carry the patient until the effects of the antidepressant kick in.

As previously discussed, the differential diagnosis between anxiety disorder with depression or anxious depression can become rather theoretical. A personal or family history of a mood disorder, somatic signs of depression such as difficulty maintaining weight or sleeping, and depressed affect when the patient is encouraged to talk about his or her mood can tilt toward the latter diagnosis. Clinically, what is important is to find the right modality or combination of modalities to help the patient. As noted in Chap. 3 (Mood Disorders), suicide can be a serious risk in such patients, who are often extraordinarily uncomfortable. It pays to ask not only if the patient is considering suicide but also how he or she would do it. If they deny suicidality but have detailed plans, they have obviously been thinking seriously about it. The appropriate conclusions should be drawn including, where necessary, emergency admission to a facility where the patients can be protected from their own self-destructive urges.

Other antidepressant medications have also proven useful in treating anxiety but have their own potentially serious side effects. Trazodone (Desyrel) has sedative effects and can be particularly useful in the treatment of GAD. In the author's experience, surprisingly low doses of trazodone (50 mg h.s., repeat x1 h.s. p.r.n for sleep) can reduce anxiety to a manageable level in older people with mild cognitive problems. Excess sedation can be a problem and, much more rarely, permanent erections in men (priapism). Venlafaxine (Effexor) has been reported to be useful for treating GAD. Typical doses are 100–200 mg of the delayed release preparation. Venlafaxine can be physically habituating and can cause significant medical side effects, notably including a rise in blood pressure. It can also cause troublesome sexual side effects and in some patients can cause anxiety. Nefazodone (Serzone) has been found useful for both GAD and panic disorder, but it can cause hypotension including symptomatic postural hypotension in the elderly. Venlafaxine and Nefazodone can both cause paradoxical agitation. Nefazodone has even been reported to precipitate mania in perhaps one percent of the people who take it.

Good clinical judgment and luck are needed in deciding when to add an antianxiety medication to an antidepressant in the regimen of a patient with an anxious depression as well as when to taper and stop it. On the one hand, easing a patient's anxiety and helping with sleep may reduce suicidal inclinations. On the other, the central nervous system depressing effects of a benzodiazepine can itself depress affect in some individuals and thereby increase the risk of suicide. Longer-term therapy with buspirone is preferable to that with a benzodiazepine.

Benzodiazepines: Benzodiazepines are the first-line drugs for treatment of acute anxiety. Psychiatrists now tend not to use them to treat more chronic anxiety because of the risks of habituation and dependence.

The benzodiazepines act on receptors for the inhibitory neurotransmitter *γ-aminobutyric acid* (GABA). A large variety of these agents are available.

Table 6-6 lists the properties of some of those in common use for treating anxiety. The dosage ranges in that table are on the low side of those recommended in psychiatric texts. Since the benzodiazepines are relatively safe drugs, a larger dose than those listed in Table 6-6 can be used when a patient requires it. The larger doses of course incur larger risks of side effects. In the author's experience, doses used for psychiatric illness in otherwise healthy young people can be too high for medically ill people, particularly sick elderly people. Benzodiazepines are widely and appropriately used by physicians in general clinical practice to treat milder and transient episodes of anxiety. The use of benzodiazepines for sleep is discussed in

TABLE 6–6
Properties of specific benzodiazepines

Name	Common name	Dosage
Short half-life (<6 hours)		
Triazolam	Halcion	0.125-0.250 mg h.s.
Clorazepate	Tranxene	12-30 mg/day
Halazepam	Paxipam	20-160 mg/day
Prazepam	Centrax	30 mg/day
Intermediate half-life (6–20 hours)		
Lorazepam	Ativan	1-6 mg/day
Oxazepam	Serax	15-60 mg/day
Chlordiazepoxide	Librium	5-40 mg/day
Alprazolam	Xanax	0.50-4.00 mg/day
Long half-life (>20 hours)		
Diazepam	Valium	2-30 mg/day
Clonazepam	Klonopin, Rivotril	0.5 mg 3id

Except for triazolam (Halcion), which is normally taken at bedtime, the short half-life benzodiazepines are best administered as divided doses during the day. The intermediate and long half-life drugs can be administered in divided doses during the day or as a single dose at bedtime. Clonazepam is a highly potent, long-acting benzodiazepine originally used to treat epilepsy, which has come to wider use by psychiatrists.[15]

As noted in the text, the dosage ranges indicated here tend to be low compared to those recommended in a number of psychiatric texts. The benzodiazepines are relatively safe drugs, and the larger doses discussed in the psychiatric literature may certainly be indicated in some patients, particularly in younger patients and patients without concomitant medical illnesses. Contrariwise, even lower doses than those described here may be adequate, particularly in the elderly.

Chap. 8 (Sleep), for delirium tremens in Chap. 5 (Cognitive Disorders), for acute psychosis in Chap. 4 (Thought Disorders), and for epilepsy in Chap. 10 (Disorders of Awareness).

The usual considerations relating to longer-acting and shorter-acting medicines apply to benzodiazepines. Those with shorter half-lives are safer in the sense that the effects of excessive doses wear off more quickly. However, the short-acting drugs need to be taken more often, and compliance cannot always be depended on in patients distracted by their anxiety. Rebound anxiety is a significant risk when the effects of shorter-acting—but not longer-acting – benzodiazepines wear off. The major risk with longer-acting benzodiazepines is that they can build up in the body. The minimal effective dose when treatment is started may lead to an accumulation over time that leads to such side effects as sedation. A middle way is to use benzodiazepines with intermediate half-lives (6–20 hours), such as lorazepam (Ativan) or oxazepam (Serax).

Chronic benzodiazepine use can lead to habituation and dependence. These can occur within 2 weeks. Careful clinical judgment is required to decide whether these potentially disastrous side effects are worth risking in a specific patient. Psychiatrists dealing with anxiety disorders are now widely convinced that the risks outweigh the benefits. Some patients with chronic anxiety, however, respond better to benzodiazepines than to any other class of drugs. As mentioned previously, there is fragmentary evidence that some patients with anxiety disorders have hereditary variations at the molecular level that appear to predispose to their anxiousness.[13] Speculatively, patients who require chronic treatment with benzodiazepines might have a functional deficiency of the neurotransmitter GABA. From this viewpoint, they require chronic treatment with a GABA agonist just as many depressed patients require chronic treatment with a serotonin agonist or insulin-dependent diabetics require chronic treatment with insulin. If treated with longer-acting benzodiazepines, the patient does not crash if he or she misses a single dose. At the proper dosage, he or she does not develop side effects from build-up of the drug in his or her body, but does remain at high risk of habituation and its consequences. Of course, the correct dose for a specific patient depends on that person's genetic makeup and other characteristics, and must in the end be adapted to each individual. "Standard" doses do, however, indicate a good place to start. Committing suicide is harder with benzodiazepines than with tricyclic antidepressants.

Side Effects Side effects of benzodiazepines are common. By far the most common is drowsiness. Sedative action is inherent in the mechanism of action of the benzodiazepines. Somnolence is usually not dangerous for a patient at home but can be dangerous for a patient driving a car or operating other machinery. Benzodiazepines are also used as sleep medications. (See Chap. 8, Sleep.) Taking the daily dose of an intermediate- or long-half-life benzodiazepine at bedtime can not only help an anxious patient to sleep but can also avoid some of the riskier aspects of benzodiazepine-induced drowsiness. However, even with such a regimen enough of the side effects of the drug may last during the next day to cause a "sleep hangover" with attendant risks. Although benzodiazepines and alcohol have different mechanisms of action, they can have surprisingly similar behavioral effects. (Valium has been called "a martini in a capsule.") A person with too much of a benzodiazepine can act "drunk," including mental dulling or frank confusion, blunting of inhibitions, slurring of speech, and ataxia severe enough to lead to falls—even to hip fractures in older people. The combinations of a benzodiazepine and other central nervous system depressants including alcohol can be dangerous. Besides causing other signs of being "very drunk," they can lead to depression of breathing and to shortness of breath. High-potency benzodiazepines sometimes cause a paradoxical increase in aggression, sometimes to dangerous levels. That reaction has been particularly noted with *triazolam* (Halcion). The British banned this drug over 10 years ago.

Benzodiazepine use requires caution in patients with liver or kidney damage, *porphyria*, *myasthenia gravis*, cognitive impairment or other types of depressed brain function, and in pregnant women. Benzodiazepines have been known to precipitate *hepatic coma* in people with compromised liver function.

Habituation and withdrawal are significant risks with these drugs. Chronically anxious people easily become psychologically and eventually physically dependent on these medications.

Physical habituation results in part from the physiology of receptors. As with other agents that act directly on receptors, benzodiazepine usage can lead to a change in the number of receptors in the membranes of the relevant postsynaptic neurons. As a result, sensitivity to the drug decreases. These mechanisms can lead to "tolerance," with a need for increasing doses to maintain the same "therapeutic" effect.

Withdrawal can occur even in patients on stable doses of benzodiazepines, if they choose to stop taking the drug or no longer have access to it. Risk of an acute withdrawal syndrome is particularly great with benzodiazepines with short half-lives. In fact, careful observation often reveals the occurrence or more or less minor degrees of withdrawal syndrome occurring even after single doses of a short-acting benzodiazepine. A delayed withdrawal syndrome can occur as much as 2 weeks or more after stopping a benzodiazepine, if accumulated body stores of the drug are slowly metabolized. The risk of a withdrawal syndrome is, not surprisingly, higher in people who have been taking higher doses of benzodiazepines for longer periods of time and/or have been taking medication with a longer half-life. The withdrawal syndrome includes the recurrence of anxiety and such manifestations of anxiety as restlessness. Typically, it also includes physical changes such as tremor, sweating, irritability, and trouble with sleep. Abrupt withdrawal of a benzodiazepine can precipitate an acute syndrome with characteristics of alcoholic delirium tremens, including delirium, seizures, paranoia, or depression. Treatment with the benzodiazepine antagonist *flumazenil* can precipitate an acute withdrawal syndrome.

The dosage of a benzodiazepine should if possible be reduced at a rate of no more than 25% per week, at least initially. Some specialists favor concomitant prescription of the anticonvulsant carbamazepine (Tegretol) at about 400–500 mg/day, particularly in patients at risk of seizures. (See Chap. 10, Disorders of Awareness.) Withdrawal from alprazolam (Xanax) can be particularly difficult. Sometimes that can be facilitated by switching the patient from alprazolam to clonazepam (Klonopin), a benzodiazepine used to treat seizure disorders, and then tapering the patient's dosage of clonazepam.

An *antidote* to benzodiazepine overdose is available, namely, flumazenil. This antagonist is given intravenously (IV). The starting dose is 0.2 mg (2 mL of the standard dosage form) over about 30 seconds. If the effects of that dose are inadequate, repeat doses can be given at 1-minute intervals until a maximum dosage of 3.0 mg is reached. A dose of 1 or 2 mg is adequate in most people with benzodiazepine overdose. If no significant benefit is seen with a dose of 3.0 mg, then the patient probably is suffering from some other condition, often enough including overdose of some other drug, sometimes in addition to a benzodiazepine. Flumazenil does not counteract overdoses of opioids, alcohol, or barbiturates. The biological half-life of flumazenil is 7 to 15 minutes, and patients who have benefited from treatment with it may slide back into stupor or coma when the initial dose wears off. In that case, more of the drug may be injected, but not more than 1 mg at a time and no more than 3 mg in any hour.

Treatment with flumazenil can itself have significant side effects. Seizures are one of the most common. That is not surprising, since one of the actions of benzodiazepines on the relevant receptors is to suppress seizures. A potentially fatal side effect of flumazenil treatment can be loss of the beneficial results of benzodiazepine treatment on other organs including the heart. Patients who have taken a mixed overdose of a potentially cardiotoxic drug such as a tricyclic antidepressant as well as a benzodiazepine can develop cardiac arrhythmias when the effects of benzodiazepines are blocked by flumazenil. Minor side effects of flumazenil include nausea and vomiting, fatigue, impairments of vision, headache, and pain at the site of injection. As expected, blocking benzodiazepine actions with flumazenil can lead to recurrent anxiety and to such manifestations of anxiety as agitation.

The general rule with flumazenil is not to overtitrate. That is of course true for most antidotes and indeed for most medications of any type. Patients suffering from an overdose of a benzodiazepine do not have to be brought back quickly to a "normal" state of "full" consciousness. It is quite adequate for them to be awake enough to be safe while their bodies get rid of the rest of the poison. As usual, a physician in too much of a rush risks harming the patient he or she is trying to help. The rushed physician thereby also risks having to spend more time than originally necessary, to take care of the patient he or she has gotten into trouble by giving too much antidote too fast.

Buspirone (BuSpar) can be a useful medication for chronic, generalized anxiety disorder. It has been reported to benefit many women with "premenstrual tension," although whether that condition should be considered an anxiety disorder is arguable. This medication is typically ineffective in panic disorder or social phobias and of distinctly variable use as an antidepressant. It can, however, help reduce anxiety in patients also being treated with primary antidepressants.

The mechanism of action of buspirone is poorly understood, but it does seem to act on serotonin receptors and more weakly on dopamine receptors. It has a relatively short half-life, and dosing three times a day is necessary. Food does not interfere with its absorption after oral doses. It is not addictive. The fatal dose is so much larger than the therapeutic dose that no human fatalities have been recorded. It has few significant interactions with other drugs, except that it can cause high blood pressure in combination with monoamine oxidase inhibitors (MAOs). The MAO should be stopped for a minimum of 2 weeks before administering buspirone.

Two to three weeks of treatment with buspirone are needed before the desired clinical effect is achieved. Thus, it is not a good treatment for acute anxiety. A widely accepted way to switch patients who have been on a benzodiazepine to the less-habituating BuSpar is to keep them on full doses of the benzodiazepine for several weeks while they are also on the BuSpar, and then to taper the benzodiazepine over several weeks.

The usual starting dose of buspirone is 5 mg, two to three times a day. The dose is increased by 5 mg/day about every 4 days until an adequate therapeutic response is achieved. Usual daily doses are about 15 mg a day but in psychiatric treatment it can be as high as 60 mg/day.

Antipsychotics: The treatment of severely agitated people who appear acutely psychotic typically is with a dopamine receptor antagonist (e.g., risperidone [Risperdal] or haloperidol [Haldol]), sometimes by injection, as well as concomitant treatment with a benzodiazepine. These treatments are discussed in Chap. 3 (Mood Disorders) and Chap. 4 (Thought Disorders). Chapter 5 (Cognitive Disorders) discusses the treatment of agitated delirium, often with the same drugs.

Anithistaminic Medications: Anithistaminic medications usually have greater or lesser sedating effects, as discussed in Chap. 8 (Sleep). They can therefore be somewhat effective against anxiety, although in most patients they are less useful than the antidepressants or benzodiazepines or buspirone. Antihistaminics prescribed for anxiety include *hydroxyzine* (Atarax, Vistaril) and *promethazine* (Phenergan). In occasional patients, antihistamines can cause paradoxical excitation.

In the author's experience, over-the-counter combinations of an anti-inflammatory with an antihistaminic taken at bedtime can help people with relatively mild levels of anxiety. In some people, they also seem to have a more specific antianxiety effect than just providing a good night's sleep. Such medications typically have "PM" appended to their usual name, for example, Tylenol PM. The usefulness of such preparations for this indication has not, however, been formally studied.

Older Agents: Meprobamate and Barbiturates: A number of older medications that were once used to treat anxiety disorders have been largely replaced by newer, safer drugs, where the effective doses are not so close to the doses that induce important side effects (i.e., by drugs with higher "*therapeutic indexes*"). The older drugs, which include barbiturates and meprobamate, are sedating and potentially addicting. Nevertheless, general clinicians may see patients who have been taking one of these drugs for years and are wedded to that "therapy." The author has seen patients who have been taking meprobamate for over 3 decades and emphatically rejected suggestions that they might no longer need it. Usually these patients have integrated "their" medication into their lives and do not suffer excessively from side effects, although side effects may develop if they become physically ill or even just with aging. In practice, it may be close to impossible to wean such patients from the medicines "that have worked for them" onto newer and safer ways of dealing with their anxiety.[14] Attempting to do so may just lead them to find another clinician who will prescribe what they want.

REFERENCES

1. Moviemakers have found the response of parents and children to this "normal" stress in American society to be a good subject for drama and comedy.
2. Proudfoot J, Ryden C, Everitt B, et al. Clinical efficacy of computerized cognitive-behavioral therapy for anxiety and depression in primary care: randomized controlled trial. *Br J Psychiatry*. 2004;185:46–54.
3. A decorated American soldier once said about fear, "Everyone is scared. It's what you do when you are scared that counts." Shakespeare's wording was more elegant, "The coward dies a thousand times, The brave man faces death but once."
4. Dr Robert Loeb taught generations of Columbia medical students the adage, "Don't just do something, young man; stand there."
5. As a medical student in New York, I learned that the enormous anxiety some Hispanic women appeared to mobilize around their illness was just a show for their husbands and other men in their family. When alone with me, the same women were as tough as any steel magnolia. One of them who put on a particularly dramatic show for her husband, taught me "hospital Spanish" during the period every day when I was dressing her wound, which had dehisced. Her show of anxiety was a way of supporting her devoted husband, who was very worried about her (and who spoke less English than she did). This form of behavior is not, of course, limited to women from South America.
6. Anxiety in doctors or nurses is not dealt with here.
7. Kisely S, Linden M, Bellantuono C, et al. Why are patients prescribed psychotropic drugs by general practitioners? Results of an international study. *Psychol Med*. 2000;30:1217–1225.
8. Stone J, Smyth R, Carson A, et al. Systematic review of misdiagnosis of conversion symptoms and "hysteria". *Brit Med J*. 2005;331:989. EPub 2005 Oct 13. Comments in *Brit Med J*. 2005;331:1145 and *Brit Med J*. 2005;331:1145.
9. The distinction between religious and a political rituals is often arbitrary.
10. LeDoux J. The emotional brain, fear, and the amygdala. *Cell Mol Neurobiol*. 2003;23:727–738.

11. LeDoux J. Fear and the brain: where have we been, and where are we going? Biol Psychiatry. 1998; 44:1229–38.
12. Burghardt NS, Sullivan GM, McEwen BS, et al. The selective serotonin reuptake inhibitor citalopram increases fear after acute treatment but reduces fear with chronic treatment: a comparison with tianeptine. *Biol Psychiatry.* 2004;55:1171–1178.
13. Feusner J, Ritchie T, Lawford B, et al. GABA(A) receptor beta 3 subunit gene and psychiatric morbidity in a post-traumatic stress disorder population. *Psychiatry Res.* 2001;104:109–117.
14. These patients often speak in the most glowing terms about the physician—often retired or dead—who gave them the original prescriptions that allowed them to become addicted to their medication of choice.
15. Chouinard G. Issues in the clinical use of benzodiazepines: potency, withdrawal, and rebound. *J Clin Psychiatry.* 2004;65(suppl)5:7–12.

CHAPTER SEVEN

Pain

Pain, like anxiety, is an important physiological mechanism. The sensation of pain serves to protect us in the dangerous world in which we live. For instance, people with defective pain reflexes tend not to yank their hand away from hot objects fast enough to avoid burns. One of the ways to recognize patients who suffer from congenitally inadequate pain sensation (*hypoalgesia*) is by their scars. Those typically include scars on their hands. Fortunately, congenital lack of pain sensation is rare.

On the other hand, excessive or prolonged pain is common. Pain has been reported to be the most frequent single reason that patients see doctors. Like excessive or prolonged anxiety, excessive and prolonged pain typically leads to medical consultation and often to treatment. Whether pain is "excessive" and "prolonged" depends not only on the nature and intensity of the pain but on the patient's reaction to it. The experience of pain is not just a matter of peripheral stimulation of *pain receptors* but also of the processing of that information in higher brain structures, including the thalamus and cerebral cortex. Pain inevitably has "psychological" elements.[1] It is not optimal medical practice to treat pain as a neurophysiological or neuropharmacological phenomenon without dealing with each patient's individual reactions to his or her pain.

CLASSIFICATION AND DIAGNOSIS

A useful if simplistic classification of people seeking relief from pain is into four categories. (1) Those with an identifiable and treatable organic lesion that causes pain, who need pain medication to tide them over the acute illness. (2) Those with an identifiable lesion that cannot be successfully treated, who need pain medicine in order to be able to function as well and as long as possible despite their illness. Osteoarthritis in old people is a well-known example of such a disorder. (3) Those with painful end-of-life conditions including cancer. Their treatment has become the new subspecialty of *palliative care*. Relief of pain has a major role in palliative care. Unfortunately, humane care at the end of life has needed defense against politicians and voters who are committed to legislating rules to protect us poor, ordinary Americans against moral impurity. Fortunately kindness has always been part of good medical care, even when hysteria about opiate addiction was at its height.[2] (4) People who complain of pain but without an identifiable lesion that accounts for their pain. These categories are not iron-clad, and patients can move from one to the other. A classical example is the patient who has had pain associated with a seriously damaged leg, and who continues to have "phantom limb" pain even after that leg has been amputated. Attempts to explain the anatomical basis of pain from a leg that is no longer there have not been notably successful, at least not yet. Although some of the same medications are used to treat all four groups, the constraints on the use of these medications and the therapeutic goals differ in important details.

Diagnosing and treating the medical and surgical disorders that can cause pain involves knowledge of the whole of general medicine and surgery. For instance, the differential diagnosis of chest pain is one of the key areas of knowledge of the general clinician. The differential diagnosis of belly pain is the subject of surgical texts on the *acute abdomen*. Attempts to summarize that body of knowledge here would be both ridiculous and superfluous. For painful chronic illnesses, managing the illness well is an important step in ameliorating the pain. Osteoarthritis is an excellent example. Occasionally only one joint is involved, and surgical replacement with a prosthesis is possible. An example would be osteoarthritis of a knee after an athletic injury or damage from an auto accident. Unfortunately, most of us who have earned our osteoarthritis by using and overusing our joints over many years have arthritic pain in multiple sites. Keeping fit and keeping down inflammation helps keep down our pain. Often medication is also needed—fortunately usually relatively mild pain medications.

In palliative care, including hospice care, biologically effective therapy of the underlying illness is no longer possible, by definition. (Otherwise, the patient should be treated actively, not palliatively.) When effective biological treatment is no longer possible, the paradigms of medical care change. Relief of suffering becomes the primary goal. Giving terminal patients mild therapies that allow them to maintain hope makes sense even if such therapy has no realistic chance of modifying the biological course of their diseases (for instance, small doses of methotrexate to a patient whose metastatic cancer no longer responds to methotrexate). There is an emerging consensus in the United States and the rest of the Western world that in this situation, what a Pope has called "extraordinary means" to prolong a suffering life are not appropriate. Effective pain medication becomes a central facet of care. There is a widespread and increasing agreement in the United States and other Western countries that effective pain medication is indicated in dying patients even if it carries with it some risk of a somewhat earlier death.

A number of patients have syndromes where pain is the most important manifestation, without other evidence for biological dysfunction. Sometimes these syndromes have identifiable biological causes, but often not. Medical management for these individuals becomes management of the pain. These patients can be very difficult and time-consuming to care for. Sometimes their pain ends up being classified as a "somatization" of a psychiatric illness. In these cases, consultation with a specialist and where necessary with a pain clinic is advisable.

Some pain syndromes are so common that general physicians will have to treat patients suffering from them. They include common forms of headache and of backache as well as fibromyositis (fibromyalgia).

Headaches

Headaches have been classified in a variety of ways. Table 7-1 presents an attempt at a classification useful for general clinicians. The key point is whether a patient has developed new headaches or new types of headaches or is struggling with a long-standing condition.

A new headache or new type of headache can be a manifestation of acute, life-threatening disease. It can be a sign of a bleed into the meninges or into the brain that poses immediate threat to life. That can include a bleed into a tumor or a subarachnoid hemorrhage. It can be a sign of a thrombotic stroke, more often due to an embolus than to an endogenous blood clot in a vessel in the brain. It can be a manifestation of brain swelling and potentially deadly pressure on lower brain structures (*herniation*, or in medical slang "*coning*"). It can be a manifestation of an infection of the *meninges* or the brain, bacterial or viral. It can be a sign of *temporal arteritis* or of *acute angle glaucoma*, which threaten irreversible loss of eyesight. The differential diagnosis and work-up of new onset headache is far too long to belabor here.

TABLE 7–1
Classification of headaches

I. New onset headaches
   1. Tumors
   2. Vascular accidents
      a. Bleeds
      b. Emboli
      c. Other
   3. Temporal arteritis (acute)
   4. Glaucoma (acute)
   5. Sinusitis (new onset)
   6. Other injuries to the blood vessels, meninges, or other cranial structures

II. Chronic headaches
   1. Migraine headaches
      a. Without other neurological signs
      b. With other neurological signs
   2. Tension headaches
   3. Cluster headaches
   4. Arthritis
   5. Temporal arteritis (subacute)
   6. Glaucoma (subacute or chronic)
   7. Mood disorder ("depression") presenting clinically as headache

Head pain, like pain in the belly or the chest, is often a sign of serious and acute illness. Examination of the eyes is mandatory to see if the optic discs are being pushed forward, a sign of increased intracranial pressure (and sometimes of a mimic of increased intracranial pressure, i.e., of *pseudotumor cerebri*). In treating new onset headaches, consultation with a neurologist or neurosurgeon is indicated, if the delay in obtaining the consultation is not too long. (See discussion of herniation [coning] in Chap. 9, Cerebrovascular Diseases.)

On the other hand, headache is often a chronic condition for which a clear medical or surgical cause cannot be identified. Table 7-1 lists some of the more common types of chronic or recurrent headaches. In many patients, headaches seem to shift among types. As always, effective treatment is more important than diagnostic labels. Some patients are convinced that they can identify "triggers" for their headaches. As discussed below, such triggers can include certain foods, fatigue, menstruation, and other experiences. Often a mechanism linking the head pain to the trigger cannot be identified by "objective criteria." The headache may even be a conditioned response to the stimulus. (Conditioned responses to foods, called *visceral conditioning*, can be very strong and long lasting, as documented in the work of John Garcia and subsequently others.) Common sense indicates that when avoiding such putative "triggers" helps the patients avoid headaches, they should do so. The best way to prevent "red wine headaches" is not to drink red wine.

Tension Headaches: Tension headaches are the most common types of headaches. They can be occasional, frequent, or even daily. Some unfortunate people are bothered by them for years. When tension headaches develop a throbbing quality or are associated primarily with one side of the head, they merge into migraines. Tension headaches can be the major manifestation of a disorder that responds to antidepressant treatment. Whether the headaches should then be considered a "depressive equivalent" or a "manifestation of an underlying mood disorder" is a semantic issue.

Recently, the terms *daily headache* or *rebound headaches* have been applied to headaches that occur every day despite chronic and sometimes excessive use of over-the-counter medications. Most current articles on this subject agree that over-medication with resulting rebound pain is a major mechanism in this type of headache. Most current writers also agree that discontinuation of pain medication including over-the-counter medication is critical to treating these headaches successfully. Treatments of daily headache are discussed later.

Migraines: Migraines are periodic, recurring, throbbing headaches that usually affect only half of the head. (The word *migraine* is a corruption, through the French, of the Latin *hemicranium.*) The condition is common. Among Caucasians, it affects perhaps 5% of men and perhaps 15% of women. Specialists make a distinction between *common migraine*, which affects perhaps 80% of victims of this condition and *classic migraine* that affects the rest. The former is characteristically not complicated by other neurological manifestations. Classic migraine, also known as *neurological migraine*, is associated with other neurological signs.

A prodrome characteristically precedes both common migraine and classic migraine. In common migraine, the nature of the prodrome varies, but most patients learn to recognize their own signal that they are getting a migraine. They frequently volunteer this information and almost always provide it if asked. In classic migraine the prodrome by definition consists of neurological manifestations that constitute a true *aura*. These are most frequently visual. The classic "*scintillating scotoma*" is an enlarging blind spot with flashing lights around its edges. It is only one of the forms the auras of neurological migraine can take.[3]

Classic migraines can be associated with other neurological phenomena that can make one think of a stroke, including numbness and weakness in an extremity. They do, in fact, appear to be associated with an increased incidence of clinically silent abnormalities in deep white matter in women with migraine headaches. The extent of that increase appears to relate to the frequency of the migraines.[4] The fact that classical migraines are bilateral perhaps 30% of the time can make the differential diagnosis more difficult. The neurological symptoms and signs almost always clear when the migraine is over. Fortunately, for each patient the neurological manifestations tend to take the same form in each attack. The patient and the doctor can therefore learn that they are part of the migraine pattern *in that patient*, and therefore have less dire implications than when they occur in association with a new or new pattern headache. A rare neurological syndromes accompanying migraine occurs in *basilar migraine*, in which the patient (usually a young woman) has an episode of *quadriplegia* or coma lasting about half an hour followed by a severe headache. Other types of migraine, more common in children, are *ophthalmic migraine*, in which there is weakness of one or more of the eye muscles and *hemiplegic migraine*, in which weakness can last after the headache is over. Unfortunately, some migraines in adults are associated with complete strokes with permanent neurological impairment.

The causes of migraine are still unclear. Most theories emphasize vascular involvement, typically involving spasm and dilatation. That accords with the characteristically throbbing pain and with the presence of pain innervation in cerebral blood vessels but not in the brain itself. As mentioned above, some patients learn that specific stimuli including certain foods can cause their headaches. The responsible foods vary among patients, and include red wine ("port wine headache"), chocolate, and some cheeses. Fermented foods often contain tyramine, a derivative of the amino acid tyrosine; the literature on tyramine migraine is extensive. Some women suffer from migraines before they menstruate, but the relation between the hormone shifts of the female cycle and the head pain is not clear. Classic migraine shows familial clustering, and specific loci and specific genes have been identified in a few families. These include a gene for a Na^+/K^+ ATPase (sodium-potassium-adenosinetriphosphatase) (*ATP1A2*) and a gene for a component of a calcium channel (*CACNA1A*).[5] Migraine headaches can be mistaken for sinus headaches, and sinus headaches for migraines.

Cluster Headaches: Cluster headaches are headaches that recur repetitively, usually at night but sometimes during the day, for a limited period—often 6–12 weeks, but sometimes longer. Among other names for this syndrome are *histamine headache*, *migrainous neuralgia*, and even *paroxysmal nocturnal cephalalgia.*[6] In perhaps one out of ten patients, these headaches continue for more than 3 months. If they appear permanent, they can be classified as a form of daily headache. They are most frequent in adult (not elderly) men. The pain is typically one-sided and centered around the eye, but generalizes around the affected side of the head and even the neck. A runny nose, a blocked nostril, tearing, a small pupil, and flushing of the face and neck frequently accompany attacks, all on the affected side. As discussed below, this symptom complex may respond to treatment with antihistaminics. The temporal artery on the affected side may become enlarged and tender during an attack, allowing confusion with *temporal arteritis.* A number of named syndromes known to neurologists are associated with the same type of headache but with more neurological signs and symptoms. A related type of headache known as *chronic paroxysmal hemicrania* is more common in women than in men, occurs many times a day, can persist for decades, and characteristically responds to the NSAID (nonsteroidal anti-inflammatory drug) *indomethacin.*

Temporal Arteritis: Temporal arteritis, also known as *giant cell arteritis,* is an inflammatory disease that typically affects the temporal artery and sometimes other cranial arteries. It is a disease of the elderly, rarely if ever seen in someone under 50. The pain can start suddenly or slowly. It is typically described as aching rather than throbbing, typically lasts more or less continuously through the day and becomes worse at night, and usually affects only one side of the head although it can affect both. The temporal arteries on the affected side(s) are usually thick, tender, and do not pulsate. This condition can lead to sudden, irreversible blindness in the eye on the affected side. Suspicion of this disease requires prompt treatment with steroids and biopsy of the affected artery. As noted above, temporal arteries can also be enlarged and tender during cluster headaches.

Tic Douloureux: Tic douloureux causes perhaps the worst pain human beings suffer. The pain occurs in the face, in the territory of Cranial Nerve V. The human head is a sensory knob, and the fifth nerve carries sensory information from the face. The representation of Nerve V in the sensory cortex is appropriately large, and pain from neuralgia of the fifth nerve is correspondingly intense. The pain can be so severe that it leads to thoughts of suicide in rational people who are not depressed but just cannot stand the pain. Involvement of the second and third branches of nerve V is much more common than involvement of the first branch, which carries sensory input from the eye. The pain in *tic douloureux* tends to be short lasting but recurrent. In many patients, onset of pain is associated with stimulation of sensory nerve endings in the face. Triggers tend to be relatively specific for each patient. They can include such common activities as eating, brushing one's teeth, or yawning. Treatment of this condition is classically with anticonvulsants, notably Tegretol, and where necessary by nerve block or simply cutting the nerve. Almost everyone prefers lack of feeling in the face to the almost unbearable pain.

Other Headaches: Other headaches including *glossopharyngeal neuralgia* and other forms of facial neuralgia are the province of specialists. The general clinician is wise to seek consultations for non-typical headaches even if they are long standing. Head pain can of course arise from disease of the teeth, *temporomandibular joint*, sinuses, or other parts of the head, or from osteoarthritis of the cervical spine. The diagnosis and treatment of these conditions are part of general medicine and dentistry.

Back Pain

Back pain affects most of the population at one time or another. It may result from the hubris of our species in walking on only our two hind limbs, but there is no prospect of most of us going back on all fours. Again, a critical distinction is between new onset pain or other pain that signals a medical emergency and chronic back pain that requires less acute but still sensitive and knowledgeable care. Table 7-2 lists common causes of backache.

TABLE 7–2
Classification of back pain

I. Acute back pain
II. Chronic back pain
1. Back strain
2. Prolapsed disc disease
3. Arthritis

New forms of back pain require prompt work-up, just as new types of headaches do. Such back pain can signal acute disease that needs prompt intervention. Fractures of the spine, including fractures related to osteoporosis, are typically painful. Back pain can come from a vascular lesion or other cause of pressure in the spinal cord that can lead to death of the relevant segments of the cord and subsequent paralysis.

Chronic backache can be due to arthritis, to cancer of the spine, or to other conditions that are well-known to general clinicians. Pain in the shoulder, arm, and hand, often accompanied by some degree of muscle wasting, can result from *spondylosis*, a degenerative disease that leads to compression of the spinal cord, often in the neck (*cervical spondylosis*). Such upper limb pain can also arise due to a "cervical rib," to other musculoskeletal conditions, or to vascular abnormalities that lead to pressure on the roots of the brachial plexus and lead to "*thoracic outlet syndromes*." Neurologists have special training in recognizing the less common forms of backache.

Back Strain: Back strain is the most common form of back pain, both in the general clinician's office and outside it. Back strain ("back sprain") generally results from minor injury to muscles, connective tissues, or joints (to *musculoskeletal* tissues). The cause is usually over-exertion or other unfortunate movement ("straining"). The pain is typically in the lower back (*lumbar region*), and people often call it "low back pain." Pre-existing spinal arthritis or disk disease can predispose to and complicate this condition. Usually, lower back pain is self-limited and responds to relatively mild pain medications and appropriate exercise and other activities, as discussed below. It can become chronic, however, particularly in people with concomitant degenerative disease of the spine. Some degree of degenerative spine disease is common in older people.

Pain that radiates beyond the buttock and peripheral weakness or sensory loss has typically been attributed to disk disease rather to back strain. *Prolapse* (slippage) of an intervertebral disk (disk disease; *herniated nucleus pulposus*) is a complex problem, conceptually as well as clinically. Identification of the disk, the roots, and the nerves involved falls within the area of expertise of the neurologist and neurosurgeon. This syndrome can not only cause pain in the back but also pain and/or weakness in the area served by the nerve roots on which the herniated disk is pressing. Disease in the cervical spine (neck) can be particularly unpleasant and potentially dangerous, because of the importance of the nerves that originate there. Before the wide availability of MRI scans of the spine, the accepted concept of disk disease was relatively simple. When the substance of an intervertebral disk slipped out of the ligaments that normally contained it and pressed on the spinal roots of sensory and/or motor nerves, it was presumed to set up a vicious cycle: nerve root compression → pain → muscle spasm → more compression → more pain → more muscle spasm → a debilitating downward spiral. This formulation led to a set of maneuvers designed to replace the vicious cycle with a virtuous cycle going in the opposite direction. Often although certainly not always, medical and/or surgical treatment based on this concept allowed the patient to return over time to a more or less normal life. The problem with this satisfying formulation is that prolapsed disks that cause no symptoms are common by MRI. Attempts have been made to provide criteria to distinguish "pathological" disk disease from "benign disk disease."[7,8] Retrospective studies have suggested an intuitively attractive conclusion: the worse the disk disease looks radiologically, the more likely it is to be symptomatic and the more likely surgery is to help. However, a prospective study in patients who meet explicit, prestated criteria for disk disease is needed before firm conclusions about biological criteria that make a herniated disk "pathological" are possible. Truly pathological herniation of a disk may turn out to be relatively uncommon—but we don't know yet.

Fibromyositis

Fibromyositis is a relatively general term to refer to disorders where multiple muscles and joints are painful. Not rarely, the pain is debilitating. This condition has also been appropriately called *fibromyalgia*, since there are few if any signs of inflammation.

Fibromyositis/fibromyalgia is a mysterious condition.[9,10] The common forms are not associated with other, more objective signs of disease. Blood tests including ESR (*erythrocyte sedimentation rate*) are typically normal, as are brain scans including PET scans. Current speculations focus on hypersensitivity to pain due to a poorly defined "sensitization state" of the central nervous system. That speculation implies the further speculation of a possible functional abnormality in pain-mediating pathways that use endorphins or serotonin as neurotransmitters. (See discussion of Neurobiology of Pain, below.) As discussed below, fibromyositis/fibromyalgia tends to respond better to serotonergic "antidepressants" than to pain medicines such as NSAIDs. It is not even clear whether the appropriate specialty to care for these patients is Rheumatology, Neurology, or Psychiatry.

A clinical picture similar to that of fibromyositis/fibromyalgia can arise from other, relatively well-defined clinical entities. *Polymyalgia* rheumatica is an inflammatory disease that can do so. It is often associated with temporal arteritis (giant cell arteritis) and with a significant risk of blindness (See above.) In polymyalgia rheumatica, blood tests characteristically reveal an elevated erythrocyte sedimentation rate (ESR) with normal creatine kinase levels. In *polymyositis*, with which polymyalgia rheumatica can be confused, the damage to muscle cells themselves is extensive enough to elevate blood levels of creatine kinase. General clinicians are usually familiar with the treatment of these inflammatory diseases with anti-inflammatory agents. *Ehlers-Danlos syndrome* refers to a group of inherited disorders that can sometimes mimic fibromyositis/fibromyalgia. The abnormal genes are thought to encode proteins found in ligaments, tendons, and joints (in connective tissues). This is thought to be a rare group of disorders found particularly in people of Scandinavian or North German origin, but a systematic search for such abnormalities has not been made either in the general population or in people with fibromyositis.

NEUROBIOLOGY[1]

Pain is part of the body's alerting system. It interacts with other types of information the organism uses to protect itself in dangerous or potentially dangerous situations. Those interactions can be clinically beneficial or contribute to clinical disability, depending on the person, the situation, and the nature and degree of the pain.

Although pain is not identical with the sensation of a damaging, "noxious" stimulus (*nocioception*), the two usually go together. Nocioceptive stimuli that are perceived as pain motivate us to do something to avoid or heal the source of the unpleasant stimuli. Sometimes the something we do is driven by a reflex, sometimes very quickly. However, nocioception can occur without pain and pain without nocioception. The "Central Pain Syndromes" are examples of the latter. For obvious reasons, the neuroanatomy and neurophysiology of pain have been studied in more detail in experimental animals than in humans. The principles summarized below do, however, appear to apply to our species as well.

The sensory end organs for painful stimuli (*nocioceptors*) are predominantly "bare" nerve endings. Some structures are rich in nocioceptors. They include the eye, the skin and particularly the skin of the face, and the meninges and blood vessels feeding the brain. Other organs have few nocioceptors. Brain tissue itself contains no pain sensors; cutting the brain itself at neurosurgery is painless.[11] Injury can lead to the release of a number of small molecular weight substances that are involved in nocioception. *Bradykinin*, *histamine*, *serotonin*, and potassium stimulate nocioceptors; *prostaglandins*, *leukotrienes*, and *substance P* act as sensitizers for these sensory endings.

Painful stimuli are transmitted through peripheral nerves to the dorsal roots of the spinal cord. (The dorsal roots are also known as the sensory roots and mediate other sensations as well.) Information then travels as nerve impulses through the spinal cord to higher brain centers. The five major spinal pathways transmitting painful stimuli to the brain are: the spinothalamic tract, the spinoreticular tract, the spinomesencephalic tract, the spinocervical tract, and pain fibers among the other fibers in the dorsal columns of the spinal cord. There are also pain-suppressing fibers that extend into the spinal cord. Sensory stimuli from cranial nerves are transmitted directly to the brain itself.

In the brain, the thalamus appears to be a major location for processing noxious stimuli and transmitting them to higher centers that mediate the perception of pain. Stimulating the spinothalamic tract can cause pain, as can certain irritating lesions of the thalamus. Some tumors of the thalamus cause a *central pain syndrome*. The thalamus connects widely (*projects widely*) to the cortex and to other brain centers including the basal ganglia, to which it sends information. The cortical perception of pain is relatively poorly understood. In humans, pain perception persists after damage to large areas of the sensory cortex (more precisely, to the *somatosensory* cortex).

At least two normal mechanisms in the nervous system can reduce and even abolish pain. One is a descending tract and the other the phenomenon of *gating*. Both have proven clinically useful.

The descending pathway that reduces pain starts in the nerve cells that line the compartments of the brain that contain cerebrospinal fluid (CSF), that is, neurons of the periventricular and periaqueductal gray matter. They connect to other neurons in the base of the brain (in the rostral medulla). This second group of neurons connect to parts of the spinal cord that transmit pain sensations. They use serotonin as a neurotransmitter. That is one of the reasons that agents that act on serotonin systems can be useful in relieving pain, including a number of "antidepressants." Electrical stimulation of the primary neurons in this system relieves pain. Also, these neurons are one of the primary sites of action of opiates, both endogenous *endorphins* and exogenous morphine and its derivatives. The presence of an opiate-blocking drug (*naloxone*) in this area of the brain increases pain. The opiates are discussed in more detail later.

Gating is a phenomenon by which a strong enough sensory stimulus that is not painful blocks the simultaneous perception of a painful stimulus. Only so much information can get through the neurobiological "gate" at one time. The anatomical basis of this phenomenon is well understood. To summarize it, (*myelinated*) fibers that do not carry pain impulses activate an interneuron that turns off the signals from other (*unmyelinated*) pain fibers. This phenomenon has been turned to clinical use. An elegant example is electrical stimulation of the appropriate myelinated fibers to reduce pain in chronically ill people. A technically simple example is the U.S. Navy World War II system for giving injections. The person giving the injection slaps one buttock hard, and then immediately gives the injection into the other buttock. If done properly, the patient does not notice the injection.[12] Pain can, of course, be poorly localized. Pain arising from internal organs (*viscera*) often is—for instance in a patient presenting with an "acute abdomen." Skill is often needed to find the source of a patient's pain.

Thus, the experience of pain involves the central nervous system and specifically the cerebral cortex and thalamus, although the reception of painful sensory stimuli involves both peripheral and central nervous system components. General anesthesia provides a straightforward demonstration of the requirement of the central nervous system for the perception of pain. Patients rendered unconscious by an anesthetic do not feel pain. They can undergo surgical procedures the pain of which would throw them into shock if they were conscious. Jessel and Kelly[1] have summarized the complexities of the pathophysiology of pain concisely.

Pain is a highly complex perception. More than any other sensory modality, it is influenced by emotions and the environment. Because it is so dependent on experience, and therefore varies from person to person, pain is a difficult clinical problem. Moreover, our current understanding of the anatomy and physiology of specific pain circuits is still fragmentary. Nevertheless, recent advances in understanding the basic physiology of pain mechanisms have led to some effective pain therapies.[1]

TREATMENT

Treatment of a disease that causes pain of course includes the most effective possible treatment of the underlying disease. Doing that does not preclude treating the patient's pain at the same time. Often effective treatment of the underlying disease requires treatment of the pain. A classic example is the use of morphine in the treatment of heart attacks (myocardial infarctions).

There are many treatments for pain. The mainstays of pain treatment are, however NSAIDs (Non-Steroidal Anti-Inflammatory Drugs) including aspirin, acetaminophen (e.g., Tylenol; in the UK, paracetamol), and opiates including morphine and codeine. Other useful medications include antidepressants and anticonvulsants. There are also treatments that are reasonably specific for a particular type of pain. Examples of the latter include the *triptans* for migraine headaches or steroids for polymyalgia rheumatica. Of course, whether or not a treatment helps a specific patient must always be tested empirically in that patient, even if the choice of medication has been guided by more or less effective theory. The principle has been put forward well in an article on pain for older lay people.

> "When I started in pain management, apart from narcotics and anti-inflammatory drugs there were only two medications commonly used—Tegretol and Elavil," says Russel Portnoy, M.D., chair of the Department of Pain Management and Palliative Care at Beth Israel Medical Center in New York City. " Now I have more than 50 medications to pick from. I have no way of knowing which a patient will respond to, so my approach is one of trial and error."[13]

Whether to give pain medicine as needed (p.r.n.) or at regular intervals depends on the patient and the situation. Patients who are in control of their own pain medication in general take less than if they depend on getting relief promptly from busy nursing staff or other caregivers. That holds true for most patients taking opiate derivatives, as discussed below. On the other hand, some patients do overuse pain medicine if they have the chance. Overuse of NSAIDs, for instance in people with chronic headaches, can lead to a characteristic form of potentially fatal kidney disease. Recent studies indicate that it can predispose to other fatal conditions as well, notably disease of the heart. Regular doses of pain medicine are better treatment than medication taken only when the pain is severe for conditions where the pain itself contributes to the damage to tissues (i.e., where pain is part of the pathophysiology of the disease process). An example discussed below is spinal disk disease. According to many pain specialists, overuse of pain killers is less of a problem in the United States than underuse of pain medication out of fear of inducing medical addiction. (See discussion of opiates, below.)

NSAIDs

Table 7-3 lists the Non-Steroidal Anti-Inflammatory Drugs (NSAIDs) now in common use. The original and archetype of this widely used

TABLE 7–3
NSAIDs in common use

Name	Common name	Usual dose	Specific side effects
	Nonselective, COX I + COX II inhibitors		
Salicylates	Aspirin Bufferin Ecotrin	650 mg, up to q 4 hours	–
Acetaminophen	Tylenol Other trade names	650 mg, up to 4 gm/day	–
Ibuprofen	Motrin		
Naproxen			
Indomethacin			granulocytopenia
	Selective COX II inhibitors		
Rofecoxib	Vioxx	withdrawn from market	heart attacks, strokes
Celecoxib	Celebrex	–	–

group of agents is aspirin (acetylsalicylic acid; ASA). Nowadays a whole panoply of these agents is available (Table 7-3). General clinicians are so familiar with this group of medicines that an extensive discussion here is unnecessary.

The NSAIDs are generally available over-the-counter, without prescription. Some patients report that they respond equally well to any of these. Other patients report that they respond much better to one than to the others.

> A 63-year-old, highly educated man insisted that his occasional headaches responded to a specific preparation of buffered aspirin (Bufferin) but not to other forms of aspirin or other NSAIDs. His young physician tried patiently but with no success to convince him that the different formulations of aspirin were equivalent, and that milk or other antacid would be as effective as the buffer in Bufferin. Eventually the young physician realized that there was no medical reason for the patient to try anything but the medicine that already worked for him—despite the theoretical pharmacology the doctor had recently learned in medical school.

A simple maneuver often helps a patient find an effective NSAID to relieve his or her pain. The patient is instructed to go to the local pharmacy and buy the smallest possible amount of each of the over-the-counter pain medicines available. The patient then tries them one after the other, decides which is most effective for himself or herself, and then sticks to that one. A theoretical justification for this approach can be constructed from speculations about unknown genetic variations among patients in the structure of cyclooxygenases (COX I or COX II) enzymes. Another theoretical justification can be constructed from the rapid, hard-wired, "visceral conditioning" described by John Garcia, in which an ingested material can become associated with either getting sick or getting well.[14] In any case, this maneuver can be gratifyingly effective. It empowers the patient, and it usually convinces patients that their doctor listens to and respects them.

The NSAIDs act by inhibiting the COX enzymes that synthesize prostaglandins. The latter increase sensitivity to pain, as well as participating in other parts of the inflammatory response. There are two cyclooxygenases—COX I and COX II. Most of the NSAIDs inhibit both. Recently a new group of these medicines have been synthesized that inhibit COX II more effectively than they do COX I. Post-marketing studies have implicated some COX II inhibitors as increasing the risk of cardiovascular disease, and this group of drugs is falling out of favor.

All NSAIDs can reduce pain, fever, and inflammation. Treating inflammation successfully generally reduces the pain associated with it—for instance in arthritis. However, discussion of the anti-inflammatory actions of the NSAIDs is beyond the scope of this monograph. The NSAIDs as a group are well absorbed after being taken by mouth and achieve satisfactory levels in blood and tissues. For some of these drugs, related forms are available for injection or in suppositories, but these are seldom necessary when NSAIDs are prescribed for pain relief.

Aspirin, or acetylsalicylic acid (ASA), is quantitatively the most used NSAID in the United States.[15] The acetyl group of aspirin modifies the structures of COX enzymes (covalently), and its effects are therefore long-lasting. Acetaminophen (Tylenol) is also widely used. It does not generally act effectively on inflammation, since inflammation typically is associated with high levels of peroxide produced by inflammatory cells, and peroxides inhibit the action of acetaminophen on COX enzymes. Acetaminophen does, however, act effectively in the brain where peroxides are normally low. *Ibuprofen* and *naproxen* can sometimes relieve pain where other NSAIDs do not. *Indomethacin* is an effective anti-inflammatory medication that is relatively little used because of its side effects, which sometimes include serious damage to the production of blood cells in the bone marrow (*agranulocytosis*). Indomethacin can be very useful in special situations such as headaches precipitated by sex ("coital headache"), but its use requires monitoring of blood counts.

Combinations of NSAIDs with other drugs are available. Over-the-counter preparations include the combination of an NSAID with caffeine. (Preparations containing aspirin, phenacetin, and caffeine (APC) are no longer on the market.) Combinations of NSAIDs with a sleep-inducing (*soporific*) antihistamine are widely available. Examples are Tylenol PM or Excedrin PM. These can be very useful for headache or other pain that awakens a patient at night, or for inducing restful sleep in patients with chronic tension headaches. Combinations of NSAIDs with the mild opiate codeine are also available, for example, Tylenol 3 (15 mg codeine/tablet) or Tylenol 4 (30 mg codeine/tablet) or preparations of aspirin with codeine. The toxic effects of chronic use of these combination medications are more likely to be due to the side effects of the NSAID than those of the accompanying antihistamine or opiate.

Certain side effects are common to the NSAIDs as a group. With the exception of acetaminophen, all cause more or less gastric irritation. The frequency of unacceptable gastric side effects varies somewhat among these agents, but it is high enough for all of them (except acetaminophen) that patients taking these medications with any regularity need to be warned about and observed for evidence of gastrointestinal irritation and bleeding. NSAIDs other than acetaminophen are contraindicated in patients with history or evidence of gastric or duodenal ulceration or other bleeding problems. The COX II inhibitors may cause fewer gastrointestinal problems, but as mentioned above, they appear to predispose to the development of symptomatic heart disease and stroke. That has led to the withdrawal of the COX II inhibitors *rofecoxib* (Vioxx) and *valdecoxib* (Bextra) from the market, and an FDA caution on the use of *celecoxib* (Celebrex) in patients with fluid retention or other sign of cardiovascular disease. Whether the use of any "selective" COX II inhibitor is now warranted except in special circumstances remains to be determined by extensive post-approval monitoring. The NSAIDs typically interfere with platelet function and thus prolong bleeding time. This effect is, of course, the basis of the use of low-dose aspirin and related drugs to prevent clots in people with atherosclerosis. (See Chap. 9, Cerebrovascular Disorders.) Large doses of NSAIDs over long periods of time can lead to severe kidney damage, including *papillary necrosis* and *interstitial nephritis*. The mechanism of this effect is unknown. NSAID use has also been associated with inability to empty one's bladder (*urinary retention*). Some patients are hypersensitive to aspirin and other NSAIDs. For them, these drugs are very dangerous and can lead to *anaphylactic shock*. This hypersensitivity can cross among the NSAIDs. Allergy to any of the NSAIDs including aspirin strongly contraindicates the use of all NSAIDs.

The NSAIDs are widely available and are relatively frequent choices in suicide attempts. Treatment of aspirin overdose includes ridding the body of the drug by emptying the stomach and by alkalinization of the urine, and support of the cardiovascular system and respiration. A dose of 10 gm of aspirin can be fatal, although some people have survived much larger doses. Acetaminophen overdose can cause severe and even fatal liver damage, probably by depleting *glutathione*. Treatment of acetaminophen poisoning requires a *sulfhydryl agent*, usually *acetylcysteine*, as well as supportive measures. In the United States, acetylcysteine is available only in a foul-tasting and foul-smelling oral preparation. In Britain and Europe, where suicide attempts with acetaminophen are more common, a preparation of acetylcysteine is also available for intravenous use. (Acetaminophen is called "paracetamol" in Britain.) Treatment of poisoning with aspirin or acetaminophen is part of general medical knowledge and does not need to be belabored here.

The NSAIDs are a mainstay of the control of milder forms of pain. However, like all other medications and indeed all chemicals, they can have serious bad effects if too much is given to the wrong person. Overuse of NSAIDs can be as dangerous as overuse of opiates. Patients can become dependent on both and commit suicide with both, but prolonged over use of opiates does not kill people from kidney damage or heart failure.

Opiates

Opiates have been used medically for over two thousand years. The general opinion of physicians during that time has been that the opium poppy and the chemicals in its juice are one of God's greatest gifts to man. Sydenham wrote, "Among the remedies which it has pleased Almighty God to give to man to relieve his sufferings, none is so universal and so efficacious as opium." Sir William Osler described opium as "God's own medicine." These physicians were just as aware as we are of the potential side effects of opiates, including addiction. They appear to have been more sensitive than we have been to how much the benefits of opiates outweigh the risks. Modern research has shown and modern texts emphasize that addiction due to medical use of opiates is a rare event.[16] As discussed below, the phenomena of tolerance and dependence can develop and can typically be easily treated without significant risk of addiction. As noted in Chap. 14 (Disorders of Conduct), the large majority of people who become addicted to opiates suffer from other psychiatric diseases as well.

Studies over the last 25 years have revealed that morphine and other opioids act on receptors for a family of endogenous, normally occurring materials in the brain. These endogenous materials are peptides. They include three families: the endorphins, enkephalins, and dynorphins. Each of these families is derived from a distinct polypeptide encoded on a distinct gene. The receptors for these molecules are of three types, referred to as μ (M) receptors, κ (K) receptors, and δ (D) receptors. The latter are divided into δ_1 and δ_2 receptors. The receptors primarily responsible for reducing the sensation of pain are the μ and also the κ receptors. The μ receptor is the classical morphine-binding receptor. These receptors are widely distributed within the nervous system, but each type of receptor has a different set of locations in the human brain. The μ receptors in the periaqueductal and periventricular gray matter appear to have a major role in reducing pain sensation. Blocking the action of either endogenous or externally derived substances at these receptors increases the sensation of pain, as discussed above. Thus, the opioids are a set of naturally occurring plant chemicals (alkaloids) that mimic the action of an endogenous system in the brain, by binding to and activating the same receptors that the endogenous compounds do.

Habituation, Dependence, and Addiction: A major limitation on the use of opiates in the United States has been fear of inducing addiction. Currently, the general consensus among specialists in this area is that the fear of addiction has been overblown in America.

Habituation and dependence, which occur in most patients on chronic morphine therapy, do *not* equal addiction. Habituation is the need for an increasing dose to retain the same effect. It arises by a number of mechanisms, including replication of receptors. (See discussion of the biological mechanisms of habituation in the section on benzodiazepines in Chap. 6, Anxiety.) Dependence is the development of physical signs and symptoms when a drug that has been used chronically is abruptly withdrawn rather than tapered. Many medicines can cause both habituation and symptoms on withdrawal. Withdrawal from steroids or from anticonvulsants can be much more dangerous than that from opiates, but that does not prevent the widespread use of those classes of medicines.

Addiction is a pattern of behavior where the need for the stimulus comes to dominate other aspects of life. (See Chap. 14, Disorders of Conduct.) Addiction to opiates appears to be a rare sequel to medical prescription of opiates. One widely quoted estimate is one case in several thousand patients treated. Others have reported higher incidences. The difference depends in part on how addiction is defined, and the extent to which treatable physiological dependence is classified as addiction.

> Before methadone programs were available, a psychiatrist at a New York medical school discussed at Grand Rounds a patient who had been weaned from heroin but needed maintenance Thorazine. A brash medical student asked him, "You have converted the patient from heroin, a physiologically rather safe drug, to Thorazine, a legally available drug with severe and sometimes fatal side effects. Have you helped the patient?" The psychiatrist answered, "Doctor, neither the patient nor I make America's drug laws. We just try to live within them."

After the Vietnam war, many feared an epidemic of opiate addiction among returning veterans who had used opiates, which were readily available in Southeast Asia. The epidemic did not develop. The bulk of the veterans who had been using opiates in Vietnam stopped using them by themselves when they returned to the United States. That amounts to an uncontrolled but epidemiological observation that opiate addiction is not necessarily harder to break than other addictions. As discussed in Chap. 14 (Disorders of Conduct), the word *addiction* is now used in relation to many stimuli. The hardest addiction to break appears to be to nicotine (tobacco). Perhaps the addiction that is the greatest threat to public health is overeating with resulting obesity. A profound emotional drive to obtain and use opiates can be life-destroying and even fatal when these drugs must be obtained illegally. When opiates are available legally, as in methadone programs, their use has frequently been integrated into a reasonable and productive life, even among former opiate addicts.

The success of legal opiate maintenance programs, notably methadone clinics, raises a theoretical question. Are there patients with central endorphin deficiency, who are appropriately treated with opiates? An analogy would be patients with central serotonin deficiency who are appropriately treated with serotonergic agonists such as SSRIs for their "depression". Another analogy would be diabetics with absolute or relative insulin deficiency who are treated with insulin. A functional deficiency in opiates would not have to result from low endogenous levels of endorphins. It could result from receptor or cellular abnormalities in responding to the endorphin signal. In technical terms, it could be a *pharmacodynamic* than a *pharmacokinetic* deficiency. Again, diabetes is an example. Patients with Type II diabetes often benefit from and may require additional exogenous insulin even though this form of diabetes is typically associated with elevated levels of endogenous insulin.

The decision about when and how to use opiates to benefit patients is inevitably influenced by societal concerns. For instance, heroin is available for medical use in Britain but not in the United States. Clinicians must act within the law, but within those limits patient care does not need to be subservient to moralistic political pandering to technically inaccurate convictions within the broader society. Perhaps it is preachy to reiterate that the primary duty of clinicians is to their patients.

Respiratory Depression: Physiologically, the most dangerous side effect of opiates is depression of respiration. This can cause severe brain damage. It is the most common cause of death from opiate overdose. All opiates can depress respiration. They do so by acting directly on the respiratory center in the brain stem. They reduce all aspects of respiration, but their action is most notable on the rate of breathing. That can fall to 2–4 per minute. Respiratory depression from opiates reaches a peak in about 10 minutes after an intravenous dose and within a half an hour to an hour and a half after an intramuscular or subcutaneous injection.

Therapeutic doses of morphine rarely induce clinically significant respiratory depression, but the risk is magnified in at least five situations. One is in patients with pulmonary disease, who already have compromised control of respiration. A second is in patients who have also taken other central nervous system depressants, including alcohol. A third is the use of fat-soluble (lipid-soluble) derivatives of morphine such as *fentanyl.* These can concentrate rapidly in the brain. A fourth is with the application of morphine directly to the spinal cord, to cause a local diminution of pain reception. The opiate can diffuse upward through the spinal fluid until a damaging and potentially fatal amount reaches the respiratory center just above the upper (*rostral*) end of the spinal cord. This is a particular danger with lipid-soluble opiate derivatives, which are often used for this purpose. Patients who have received opiates directly into their spine need close monitoring. A fifth situation is the use of "patient controlled devices" for delivering opiates. The fail-safe mechanisms limiting dosage from these devices can themselves fail. That they sometimes will fail is an inevitable consequence of the fundamental properties of the universe, enshrined in the Second Law of Thermodynamics, which can be stated in a familiar form as Murphy's Law: "That which can go wrong will go wrong." When that happens, the results can be disastrous.

> An 80-year-old farmer had an elective knee repair, which he hoped would allow him to take better care of his disabled wife. The surgery was uneventful, and he was given a partially self-controlled intravenous morphine drip to control his pain. The ward was short-staffed that night, and a number of post-surgical emergencies kept the nurses from checking on him and on the device as meticulously as they would otherwise have done. When the shifts changed in the morning, he was found comatose with very shallow and infrequent respirations. He was promptly intubated and placed on a respirator, given naloxone (see below), and of course the morphine drip immediately stopped. Unfortunately, he was left with such severe brain damage and specifically with so much cognitive impairment that he ended up more disabled than his wife.

As mentioned above, extensive data documents that putting patients in control of their own pain medication usually results not only in better pain control but also in the use of lower amounts of pain medication. (That includes opiates. It is, of course, another piece of evidence that the danger of medically induced opiate addiction has been wildly overstated.) However, the optimal mode of self-administration of pain medication is less well-documented. Patients can become confused and take too much of a liquid like the "Brompton cocktail"[17] left at their bedside. Machines can also fail, as in the case described above. Nurses and other staff can make mistakes setting the machines. As noted above, thermodynamics teaches that a certain number of such failures and mistakes will occur. In the course of preparing this chapter, I could find no documentation of the relative risks of oral versus intravenous or intrathecal opiates, or of self-administered rather than nurse-administered opiates.

My prejudice is to rely on people rather than machines. Machines may make fewer errors, but when they do, the consequences of their errors are often dreadful. Unless programmed to do so, machines do not recognize their errors and stop when what they are doing is obviously harmful to human eyes.

Other Side Effects of Opiates: Opiates have a number of other side effects. They typically induce a feeling of calm and pleasure—of being "mellow." Whether that is a harmful side effect or not is a matter of individual judgment. The ability of codeine and other opiates to suppress the cough reflex can be therapeutically useful, for instance in cough medicines that contain codeine. The opiates tend to cause small pupils (pupillary constriction). Pinpoint pupils in a patient with confusion or in coma and with a depressed respiratory rate almost make the diagnosis (are *pathognomonic*) of opiate overdose. Opiates tend to slow movement of the large gut and can cause chronic constipation. Some clinicians regularly give a stool softener or other weak laxative when they prescribe opiates. Both the pupillary constriction and the constipation are commonly seen and do not tend to diminish with chronic opiate use. Opiates are said to reduce sexual drive, perhaps in part by depressing the secretion of pituitary sex hormones.[18] Opiates can precipitate gall bladder spasm, and are contraindicated in patients with symptomatic gall bladder disease. Similarly, opiates can reduce the ability to urinate, in part by increasing the tone of the *external sphincter* of the *ureter*. Sometimes this side effect necessitates catheterization of the bladder. Opiates sometimes induce nausea and vomiting; some patients tend to vomit after every dose of morphine, while others do not develop this side effect at all. These drugs can have complex effects on immune function, sometimes leading to clinically relevant immunosuppression—for instance in heroin abusers. However, pain itself can depress the immune system. In that case, effective pain medication can enhance immune functions. Opiates can lead to flushing and itching, in part due to release of histamine. Like other chemicals, they can cause rashes in people sensitive to them. Side effects vary somewhat with the opiate used. For instance, as discussed below, the synthetic mixed agonists-antagonists are prone to induce psychotic manifestations.

Types of Opiates: A large number of opium derivatives are available including synthetic and semisynthetic derivatives (Table 7-4). Many of these have been developed in the attempt to find a "nonaddicting form of morphine." Many of them have more undesirable side effects than the natural derivatives. This panoply of opiates can be very useful for specialists in pain management, including anesthesiologists as well as neurologists who specialize in this area. For the general clinician, it is probably better practice to get to know a couple of these medicines well and stick to them. That is why Table 7-4 does not include information about conventional dosages and routes of administration for the wide array of opium derivatives. However, essentially all clinicians will have to become familiar with morphine and codeine.

TABLE 7–4
Opiate medications

I. Morphine
   1. normal release
   2. sustained release (MS Contin, Oramorph, and Kadian)

II. Codeine

III. Heroin (not available legally in the United States)

IV. Methadone

V. Fentanyl
   1. transdermal (Duragesic)
   2. transmucosal (Actiq)

V. Meperidine (Demerol)

VI. Hydromorphone (Dilaudid)

VII. Oxycodone
   1. normal release (Percodan, Percocet, Tylox)
   2. sustained release (OxyContin)

VIII. Hydrocodone (Vicodin, Lortab)

IX. Propoxyphene (Darvon-N, Darvocet-N)

X. Pentazocine (Talwin)

XII. Buprenorphine (Buprenex)

XIII. Butorphanol (Stadol)

XIV. Nalbuphine (Nubain)

Morphine Morphine is the major, pharmaceutically active principle in the juice of the opium poppy. It was isolated in pure form in the beginning of the nineteenth century and had largely replaced cruder extracts for medical use by the middle of that century. Morphine is readily absorbed after being taken by mouth and can also be injected intramuscularly or intravenously. The standard starting dose of morphine is 30 mg by mouth or 10 mg intramuscularly, to be repeated as needed every 4 hours. Doses can be increased, so long as respiratory depression or other side effects do not occur. The side effects discussed above are relatively common with morphine use but are usually relatively minor with therapeutic doses. Oral absorption is rapid and effective, and injectable forms are also available. Morphine is converted by the body to chemical forms that contain glucuronic acid; morphine-6-glucuronide may be responsible for most of the pain-relieving actions of morphine. The morphine glucuronides are efficiently excreted by the kidney. Only small amounts of morphine remain in the body at 24 hours after a single dose. However, small amounts of morphine derivatives can be found for several days in the stool (i.e., in the *enterohepatic* circulation).

Codeine Codeine is a derivative of morphine that also occurs naturally in the juice of the poppy. It is weaker for relieving pain than morphine but more powerful at suppressing coughing. Codeine is so well-absorbed after oral administration that it is only rarely injected. Standard doses are 15–30 mg every 4 hours. If significantly larger doses are needed, it is probably wise to give morphine itself instead. Codeine is converted to morphine in the body by the cytochrome P-450 system—specifically by CYP2D6. Genetic variations (*polymorphisms*) of this cytochrome that occur in about 10% of the Caucasian population can prevent codeine from being effective against pain in those individuals. Codeine also tends to be less effective in people of Chinese extraction than in those of European extraction. As discussed above, combinations of codeine with an anti-inflammatory medication are widely available. The anti-inflammatory and the opiate appear to interact synergistically in relieving pain.

Other Opiates: *Tramadol* (Ultram) is a weak opiate that acts on μ-receptors and also inhibits the uptake of serotonin and norepinephrine. The literature on this medicine concentrates on its use for general surgical patients or in dentistry. It should not be used by people who are at risk for seizures (see Chap. 10, Disorders of Awareness) or who are taking MAO inhibitors (see Chap. 3, Mood Disorders). Heroin is diacetyl morphine. The chemical addition of acetate groups (*acetylation*) leads to it being more rapidly absorbed; that rapid absorption may underline the "heroin rush" described by addicts. Heroin is not available legally in the United States but sees medical use in a number of other countries including Britain. *Meperidine* (Demerol) and its derivatives have a fundamentally different chemical structure than morphine and its analogs. (The meperidines are phenylpiperidines.) They can overexcite the nervous system and lead to convulsions or to other manifestations such as tremors, muscle twitches, hallucinations, and dilated pupils. They are just as "addicting" as morphine and medicines that resemble it in chemical structure (*congeners*). Meperidines now tend to be little used because of side effects. Several lipid-soluble derivatives related to meperidines are popular among anesthesiologists. They include *fentanyl*, as well as *sufentanil*, *alfentanil*, and *remifentanil*. These can be absorbed from skin patches as well as by other routes. As discussed above, the rapid absorption of these agents makes them relatively tricky to use. It is easy to give too much. The use of these powerful, fat-soluble pain medications is best left to specialists.

Methadone Methadone (Dolophine, etc.) has actions like morphine, specifically on μ-receptors, but is more long-lasting. Its chemical structure differs from that of morphine. It undergoes extensive biotransformation in the liver. Methadone and its derivatives bind strongly to plasma and tissue proteins, from which it is released relatively slowly. Its half-life is 15–40 hours, much longer than that of morphine or codeine. Methadone can be used for pain control, except in certain situations such as labor. It is best known, however, for its use in programs to control opiate addiction. Because of its relatively long half-life and resulting persistence in tissues, withdrawal from chronic methadone use tends to be milder than from other opiates. Methadone maintenance programs provide a legal way for individuals psychically dependent on opiates to obtain drug. These programs appear to work well for people whose real problem is a craving or physiological need for exogenous stimulation of opioid receptors. (See discussion of side effects, above.) They typically do not work as well for people in whom the addiction to opiates is primarily an expression of another, underlying and more incapacitating psychiatric disease. These programs have been castigated as "legal horse" (horse being a street word for heroin). A reasonable response to that criticism is, "So what? If they work?"

Other long-acting forms of morphine are now available. *MS Contin*, *Oramorph SR*, and *Kadian* are all forms of morphine. *Oxycodone is* derived from an opium analogue, *thebain*. *Percocet* is a combination with acetaminophen. Different dosage forms of this combination are available, in tablets containing 5, 7.5, or 10 mg of oxycodone and 250 or 500 mg of acetaminophen. These other longer-acting forms of opiates tend to be more expensive than methadone. They can all induce habituation and even addiction. However, they do not have the social stigma that is often attached to methadone use by the general public, who know this medication primarily as a treatment for opiate addiction.

Opioids with Mixed Agonist-Antagonist Properties These have been developed in the attempt to find morphine derivatives with no "addictive potential." Examples include *pentazocine* (Talwin), *nalbuphine* (Nubain), *buprenorphine* (Buprenex), *butorphanol* (Stadol), and *dezocine* (Dalgan) among others. In general, their side effect profiles are not attractive. Among other things, they can induce extremely unpleasant psychological reactions including depersonalization and other reactions, which resemble aspects of psychoses (*psychotomimetic* reactions). People given these drugs can go quite crazy. Patients who have been on opiates and are switched to one of these semisynthetic drugs can go into withdrawal. The use of these medications is best left to specialists in pain management.

Opiate Antagonists This group of semisynthetic morphine derivatives is likely to be useful for the general clinician. *Naloxone* (Narcan) is a well-known opiate antagonist widely used to treat narcotic overdoses. Other drugs in this class have also been developed, including antagonists specific for μ, κ, and δ receptors. *Naltrexone* has been approved for treatment of alcoholism. (See Chap. 5, Cognitive Disorders and Chap. 14, Disorders of Conduct). As normally used, the opiate antagonists have few if any clinical effects in people unexposed to opiates. These medications can, however, rapidly reverse the dangerous side effects of opiate overdoses. Injection of 0.4–0.8 mg of naloxone, either intramuscularly or intravenously, rapidly reverses the dangerous respiratory depression of opiate overdose, typically within 2 minutes. Depressions of blood pressure and of consciousness are also reversed. For heroin overdose, more naloxone may be needed—1 mg of naloxone for 25 mg of heroin. Naloxone can also reverse the psychotomimetic effects of the semisynthetic opiates, but doses as high as 10–15 mg may be required. Naloxone is ineffective if taken by mouth, since it is effectively destroyed by passage through the liver, and must be injected. Its duration of action is relatively short, so repeated injections or an intravenous drip can be necessary.

Optimal use of naloxone or other opiate antagonist involves giving enough to get and keep the patient out of danger but not so much as to cause withdrawal. The patient should regain the capacity to breathe but does not have to wake up fully right away. Too vigorous use of an opiate antagonist can be harmful for the heart.

Antidepressants

Medications that act as agonists on serotonin systems tend to relieve pain as well. (These drugs are discussed in more detail in Chap. 3, Mood Disorders). Sometimes drugs that act on serotonin systems are more effective than other medications in relieving pain—even more effective than opiates. The effectiveness of the older tricyclic antidepressants for pain relief is established. Whether SSRIs and other newer antidepressants are as useful for treating pain as the older medications is still controversial. A number of clinicians think not, but more and larger studies in both humans and experimental animals will be necessary to allow firm conclusions.

The mechanism of action of the serotonergic agonists probably involves stimulation of serotonin-mediated pathways in the spinal cord and probably also elsewhere in the central nervous system. Functional deficiency of serotonin transmission at one site in the nervous system is often accompanied by effective deficiency at others. Thus, patients with a functional serotonergic deficiency in neural systems mediating mood are often frequently also functionally deficient at serotonergic synapses that mediate sleep, appetite, and sexuality. (That is the supposed basis for the "somatic signs of depression.") There is no reason to be surprised if patients with a functional deficiency of serotonin in the spinal cord also have a functional deficiency in central serotonergic synapses and therefore suffer from symptoms or signs associated with "depression." As mentioned above, whether or not one chooses to call the pain in these patients a "manifestation of an underlying depression" or a "depressive equivalent" is a semantic rather than a neurobiological question.

The tricyclic antidepressants reported to be effective against pain include amitriptyline (≤150 mg/day), imipramine (≤200 mg/day), and doxepin (≤200 mg/day). In general, the lowest doses that provide appropriate relief are the optimal doses. The lower ends of these dose ranges are certainly preferable in frail or debilitated people. The side effects of tricyclic antidepressants include unpleasant anticholinergic effects, orthostatic hypotension and cardiac arrhythmias. (See Chap. 3, Mood Disorders.).

Tricyclics have provided effective treatment for pain in a variety of conditions, including persistent pain after infection with the herpes virus (*postherpetic neuralgias* following shingles). Pain syndromes in which tricyclic serotonergic agonists may be particularly effective are fibromyositis and repetitive headaches. These and related syndromes have been called *central pain syndromes*, because they may result from inadequate central modification of central processing of information from peripheral pain receptors. The tricyclic doxepin (Sinequan) has been reported to be effective against itching, which can be quite as great a source of discomfort as pain. Another antidepressant, *mirtazapine* (Remeron; 15 mg/day), appeared even more effective than doxepin in a small series. Both these agents have antihistaminic activities, and appear to be more effective against itch than the antihistaminics that have been used for this purpose (such as *cetirizine* [Zyrtec] or *loratadine* [Claritin]). *Duloxetine* is a putative antidepressant recently approved by the FDA for use in pain, specifically due to diabetic damage to peripheral nerves (*diabetic neuropathy*). This medication has a number of potential side effects including raising blood pressure; it should not be given to patients with narrow angle glaucoma.

Anticonvulsants

These are more useful in relieving pain of central origin than pain arising from peripheral injuries, including injuries to peripheral nerves. Presumably, these drugs modify aberrant electrical activity in the brain that manifests itself as pain. Anticonvulsants used to treat central pain syndromes include *carbamazepine* (Tegretol), *phenytoin* (Dilantin), and *gabapentin* (Neurontin) among others. (See Chap. 10, Disorders of Awareness, for discussion of anticonvulsants.) Carbamazepine (Tegretol, 600–1200 mg/day) is the treatment of choice for tic douloureux. Other anticonvulsants useful for this condition include phenytoin (300–400 mg/day), *valproic acid* (800–1200 mg/day), *clonazepam* (2–6 mg/day), and gabapentin (300–900 mg/day).

A recent review discusses the use of newer antiepileptic medications to treat pain.[19] All tend to cause dizziness and sleepiness that usually gets better with time. Other side effects also tend to be relatively minor. When it occurs, rash indicates that the medicine must be stopped. Controlled clinical trials have shown gabapentin (Neurontin) to be effective for post-herpetic pain, diabetic neuropathy, and in preventing migraine headaches. *Lamotrigine* (Lamictal) was also useful for diabetic neuropathy, as well as AIDS neuropathy and sometimes pain after strokes. This drug slows the removal of the anticonvulsant valproic acid, and caution is necessary in patients taking both those drugs at the same time. Uncontrolled observations suggest that this antiepileptic may also have use in preventing migraines. Controlled studies have shown that *topiramate* (Topamax, 100 mg/day by mouth) is useful for preventing migraines. It has also been also useful for diabetic neuropathy, and also for neuritic pain in the rib area. It should be used with care in patients taking oral contraceptives, because of interactions of these medications at the level of the cytochrome P 450 system. It requires utmost care in patients also taking *acetazolamide* (Diamox) or other drugs that also inhibit the enzyme carbonic anhydrase; the combination can cause metabolic acidosis. Uncontrolled observations suggest that *oxcarbazepine* (Trileptal) can sometimes relieve pain where other antiepileptic drugs have failed, sometimes including the pain of tic douloureux (*trigeminal neuralgia*). This drug can also interact with oral contraceptives. Small, open label studies have suggested that *zonisamide* (Zonegran) may be useful for nerve root pain from back problems, from both the low back and the neck. It has also been claimed to be effective against some cases of diabetic neuropathy, fibromyalgia, and unspecified pelvic pain. It, too, can cause medically significant metabolic acidosis if taken at the same time as acetazolamide or other carbonic anhydrase inhibitors.

Local Anesthetics

Blocking nerves with local anesthetics can sometimes relieve pain. This procedure is particularly useful in pain from damage to peripheral nerves and some types of pain from problems with joints and muscles and other parts of the musculoskeletal system. The application of local anesthetic can be done by injection into the appropriate region to deaden the pain. That is best done by an anesthetist or other specially trained physician. Less invasive alternatives are patches on the skin containing a local anesthetic or other anti-nocioceptive substance (e.g., *lidocaine* patch 5%).[20] They are sometimes gratifyingly effective.

Steroids

These can be specific for pain due to certain kinds of inflammation. In temporal arteritis, their prompt use amounts to a medical emergency because of the risk of blindness. Steroids can, of course, be useful for rheumatic disorders with prominent pain, including polymyalgia rheumatica and polymyositis. General physicians are at least as familiar as neurologists with the use of steroids and the serious side effects of these medications.

Salves and Ointments

A variety of salves and ointments are available to treat local pain. Some of those available contain *methylsalicylate*, *capsain*, or other NSAIDS. Some available over-the-counter are mild vasodilators and may be advertised as providing heat relief. In some patients, these provide significant relief when used in reasonable amount that does not lead to skin rashes or other side effects.[20] There is then no reason not to use them.

Other Forms of Treatment

A variety of non-drug approaches are available to help with the relief of chronic pain. Essentially every society has developed some form of massage, usually justified by the belief system of that society. In the United States, where we believe in science, the most widely used system is Chiropractic. Unskilled chiropractors can seriously injure patients. On the other hand, controlled studies suggest that chiropractic treatment significantly helps some patients with back or head pain. A neurosurgeon in New York who specializes in back problems strongly encourages his patients to try chiropractic treatments first. He says doing that leads to fewer patient complaints after surgery. Other forms of massage including European and Asian types are increasingly available in the United States, at least in the larger cities. Some chronic sufferers get great relief from their use. Acupuncture is sometimes very effective, and is available in most university medical centers as well as from private practitioners.[21] Sterility of the needles used is obviously necessary. Exercise can be useful, particularly in back pain and fibromyositis. A number of other practices are known including herbal treatments. If something helps a patient without incurring undue risks, it makes sense for the patient to use it even if the treatment "doesn't make sense scientifically," according to available scientific knowledge. Harmless mumbo-jumbo that relieves a central pain syndrome is, by definition, harmless.

Specific Syndromes

Treatment of the common pain syndromes discussed above generally depends on NSAIDs and rarely involves opiates. Specific syndromes can also be helped by certain other modalities.

Headache

The first line of medical treatment of a tension headache is NSAIDs. Most people try aspirin or some other over-the-counter preparation themselves, and only ask for medical help if they do not get adequate relief. Instructing the patient to find the NSAID that most helps him or her can be a good way to identify an over-the-counter medication that the patient finds effective. Chronic overuse of NSAIDs can induce dangerous side effects including kidney failure.

Tension headaches that do not respond to self-treatment with an over-the-counter NSAID may respond to a combination drug. Sometime a combination containing an antihistaminic that induces restful sleep can break a headache cycle; sometimes it needs to be taken for several nights running. In some patients, a headache cycle or even a pattern of daily headaches responds to a "sleep cure," as discussed below under "anecdotal" treatments. The chronic use of NSAIDS combined with codeine can lead to tolerance and dependence, depending on the severity and chronicity of the pain. Most authorities use opiates to treat chronic headaches only when these drugs are clearly necessary.[22] The syndrome of "daily headache" is currently believed to be due in large part to rebound to the chronic use of headache medicines. The currently recommended treatment for headaches of this type is weaning the patient off medication. This approach is difficult and best tried in specialty headache clinics. It is hard to convince patients that to get rid of pain, they must stop taking the medicine that has been making their pain bearable. A recent report suggests that the antidepressant mirtazapine (Remeron) may help control recurrent tension headaches.[23] This agent acts on many different receptors in the nervous system including certain histamine receptors. Further studies to determine its usefulness in this condition are needed. Recurrent headaches can be a very difficult condition to treat, even for specialists, and more effective treatments would save many people from suffering.

Migraine headaches can be treated in a number of ways. Often one-sided headaches respond to an NSAID, even if they are classified as "migrainous" rather than "tension" headaches. Over-the-counter preparations that are "specific" for migraine are available, although from reading the label it can be hard to see how these preparations differ from other NSAIDs without the label. Perhaps the label has a beneficial placebo effect on some migraine sufferers who know no pharmacology. Combinations of NSAIDs with other drugs can be used, as noted above. Patients can often "sleep off" a migraine, making the combination of an NSAID and a sleep medication useful. Combinations of an NSAID and codeine or another narcotic are not a treatment of choice, but can be very useful in certain patients who have relatively rare migraines and therefore are at relatively little risk for developing tolerance and dependence. (The arguments made above about chronic opiate use can, however, also be applied to chronic migraineurs whose lives are otherwise unbearable. That may be particularly true for patients whose heart disease argues against the use of *triptans.*)

The *triptans* are favored drugs for reducing the frequency of migraines that do not respond to milder medications. They include *sumatriptan* (Imitrex), *zolmitriptan* (Zomig), and *rizatriptan* (Maxalt, Maxalt-MLT). These agents act as selective agonists for a specific subtype of receptor (for 5-hydroxytryptamine) that occurs in blood vessels. They are not used to treat migraines but to prevent them. Orally, these medications are typically effective within 2 hours, and their effects can last a full day. The usual oral dose of sumatriptan is 50–100 mg, with repeat dosage after 2 hours until relief is gained or a total dose of 200 mg has been administered over a period of 24 hours. For zolmitriptan, the oral dose is 2.5–5.0 mg, repeated as needed every 2 hours up to a total dose of 10 mg over 24 hours. For rizatriptan, the recommended dose is 5–10 mg with a total of no more than 30 mg over a 24-hour period. Nausea and vomiting associated with a migraine may prevent a patient from taking a medicine by mouth, and sumatriptan is available not only orally but also in injectable forms, including a self-injectable form, and as a nasal spray The usual dose for subcutaneous injection is 6 mg. Pain or burning at the site of the injection is common. Effects of the nasal spray can be rapid, becoming noticeable after 15 minutes. Unfortunately, the triptans can have potentially serious although relatively rare side effects. These drugs act on blood vessels of the heart as well as those involved in migraine pain. They are contraindicated in people who are considered at risk of heart disease or have heart disease, including angina as well as other manifestations of ischemic heart disease. Heart disease affects a significant part of the population—particularly the elderly population. It is often silent clinically until something trips the coronary vessels into spasm. Therefore, prescribing triptans to people with risk factors for ischemic heart disease can be worrisome. The triptans are also contraindicated in people with underlying liver or kidney disease. Despite these side effects, these drugs can be very useful in appropriate patients, particularly younger patients. *Ergotamine* can be an extremely effective treatment of migraine, but its use is again worrisome in people with or at risk for ischemic cardiovascular or other vascular disease. Giving ergotamine for headache is probably best left to specialists.

β-Blockers including propranolol can be useful for prevention of full-blown migraine in appropriate patients. They are best taken during the prodrome or with the "aura." Sometimes regular treatment is necessary to significantly modify headache recurrence and pain. General clinicians are familiar with the dosages and potential side effects of β-blockers, which do not need to be enumerated here.

Calcium channel blockers help some migraineurs, sometimes dramatically. Again, this group of medications is familiar to general clinicians.

SSRIs as well as other antidepressants can be very useful for some patients who suffer from migraines. Indeed, some specialists in treating headaches have suggested that intractable headaches are often a manifestation of "depression." (i.e., of central serotonin deficiency; see Chap. 3, Mood Disorders.) Sometimes headaches respond to other psychiatric medications, including benzodiazepines (see Chap. 6, Anxiety) or dopamine blockers (see Chap. 4, Thought Disorders). Dopamine blockers have, in my admittedly anecdotal experience, been useful in treating some patients whose headaches appear to be triggered by foods containing tyramine. One might speculate that in the tyramine-sensitive patients who respond to this treatment, the dopamine blocker cross-reacts with and more or less blocks the responsible tyramine receptor as well as acting on dopamine receptors.

Anticonvulsants can be effective prophylactic treatment for migraine in appropriate patients. The data is best for topiramate (Topamax), but head-to-head trials of different anticonvulsants for prevention of migraine are lacking. (Anticonvulsants are discussed in Chap. 10, Disorders of Awareness.)

Cluster Headaches: No single medication is a specific for cluster headaches. The clinician must, as usual, work with the individual patient to find what helps him (or, for cluster headache, less often her). To simplify, the same medications are used as for tension headaches and migraines. The first line is over-the-counter NSAIDs, including particularly combinations of NSAIDs that help with sleep. In my own anecdotal experience, the combination of an NSAID and an antihistaminic is particularly useful in patients whose headaches are associated with runny nose, watering eyes, and flushed face, that is, with "cold" symptoms that also respond to antihistaminics. Indomethacin (75–200 mg/day) relieves cluster headache so specifically in a number of patients that its use can be indicated in them, despite its serious potential side effects. A course of a few days of prednisone or other steroids, starting with a high dose and then tapering down rapidly, gives dramatic relief to some patients. Triptans and ergotamine can also be useful in cluster headache, particularly if taken to abort the expected headaches, but they have the potentially dangerous side effects discussed earlier. Some patients with frequent or chronic cluster headaches respond to a calcium channel blocker such as *verapamil* (Calan, Isoptin), as do some patients with migraines. Lithium has a confirmed role in the management of chronic cluster headache. Blood lithium levels should be maintained between 0.7 and 1.2 meq/L. The mechanism of action of lithium in cluster headaches is understood as poorly as its role in mania. (See Chap. 3, Mood Disorders.) Verapamil and lithium can safely be given together.

Anecdotal Suggestions: One of the "old-fashioned" ways of treating chronic headaches is with an "elimination diet." This technique is based less on objective studies than on clinical experience. The full form of this approach is for the patient to go on a diet of white rice, water, and vitamin pills. This diet is admittedly deficient in fat and essential amino acids, but the patient usually does not need to stay on it for more than a few days to a week or two or three. If headaches do not clear by that time, another approach can be undertaken. If the headaches do clear, then other foods are added one by one. When headache follows the ingestion of a foodstuff or beverage, the patient goes back on the rice diet until the headaches clear again. (That specifically includes alcoholic beverages, including not only red wine but also beer and white wine and whiskies.) Eventually the patient develops a list of foods and drinks that appear to trigger headaches in him or her. If avoiding those foods significantly helps the patient avoid headaches—for whatever reason, including placebo effects—the treatment has been useful.

Another technique that sometimes breaks a headache cycle is for the patient to sleep for most of a couple of days or more. The easiest way to induce such long sleep is with a relatively mild, over-the-counter sleep medication. That can be in combination with an NSAID, such as Tylenol PM or Excedrin PM. It can also be a benzodiazepine that also has "anti-tension" and "muscle relaxant" actions. (See Chap. 6, Anxiety and Chap. 8, Sleep.) The patient can take a repeat dose when the sleepiness from a previous dose wears off. Patients should not be so doped up that they fail to move in bed, to get up to drink and perhaps to eat, and to relieve themselves. Sleeping over a long weekend—Friday night to Monday morning—is often enough to break a headache cycle or a pattern of chronic headaches. Headaches that persist despite this treatment should increase suspicion of a new, organic cause of headaches even in patients who say that their type of headache has not changed. Unfortunately, the effects of "sleeping off" one's headaches are rarely permanent or even excessively long-lasting.

Back Pain: NSAIDs are the first line of pharmacological treatment for the pain of back pain, as they are for headaches and other types of pain including arthritis. The use of NSAIDs for back strain/sprain is particularly rational, since the mechanisms of these conditions typically involve inflammation. Local heat or ice can provide useful adjunct treatment. Different patients and different practitioners argue strongly for heat, others for ice packs. Whether to use heat or cold in wet or dry form depends, as always, on what helps the specific patient being treated. As the back pain gets better, appropriate exercises can be very helpful. Again, the best exercise for any patient is what helps that patient and what the patient enjoys enough to keep doing. Moderate swimming can be very good for Americans or Australians who swim the crawl or side-stroke; it is not likely to help Europeans and others who do the breast-stroke. Push-ups can strengthen the back muscles for those willing to do them regularly. For the more troublesome types of back pain, consultation with a Physical Therapist is advisable.

Opiates including medications containing codeine are not widely recommended for back pain. However, they can be very useful in brief regimens to break the cycle of pain → spasm → more pain → more spasm → and so on.

Muscle relaxants help some patients and do not help others. A high enough proportion of patients are helped that controlled studies have found these agents effective, particularly in acute back strain/sprain. Some clinicians are convinced that the "muscle relaxants" act primarily by their effects on mood and anxiety and their ability to induce sleep. How they act is, of course, less important clinically than whether they act in the particular patient being treated and do so safely. Benzodiazepines are widely used for this purpose. (See Chap. 6, Anxiety.) Other more putatively specific muscle relaxants include *carisoprodol* (Soma), which is metabolized in the body to the anti-anxiety agent meprobamate. Soma can be a drug of abuse. Alcohol is a muscle relaxant in addition to its effects on mood. Some patients with chronic back pain benefit greatly from having the equivalent of a couple of glasses of wine with dinner. Obviously, drinking oneself into a stupor night after night is not good for back pain or any other aspect of health. The possibility of being given money for having continuing back pain is obviously a motivation to continue to complain of back pain. That mechanism can work unconsciously or consciously. People may be more or less aware that they are exaggerating pain that they would otherwise just live with in order to get money, but they may not admit that even to themselves. Prompt settlement of workman's compensation claims or other litigation can work wonders for chronic back pain.[24]

Fibromyositis/Fibromyalgia

There is no specific treatment for fibromyositis that has been well-documented to be effective in most patients. Empiric trials of the usual panoply of NSAIDs, antidepressants, anti-anxiety agents, and non-pharmacological interventions can often uncover something that the patient feels benefits her. Whether a particular medicine or other intervention appears to work because it was coincidently given at a time when the patient was feeling better anyway or by a specific biological effect is often unclear. As discussed above, even if the improvement on the medicine or other intervention is "coincidental," that experience may set up a (visceral) conditioned response that can be used to help the patient in future attacks.

Opiates are not recommended for the treatment of this chronic pain syndrome, because of the problems of tolerance, dependence, and possible addiction. This is standard American practice and the wise practitioner will respect it. On the other hand, the biology behind this decision is hardly obvious. A rational, "scientific" argument can be made that if fibromyositis results from excessive sensitivity to pain, it may involve a functional deficiency of endorphins and analogous endogenous forms of the "body's own opium." In that case, replacement therapy with opiates would be the rational treatment. Patients treated in this way would, however, probably become habituated and perhaps medically addicted to opiates. The concerns about opiate use in the United States are such that a physician who chooses to treat fibromyositis with opiates puts himself or herself at risk.

A recent paper describes a small series of patients with fibromyositis who had evidence of sleep apnea. They reportedly improved with treatment for the upper airways resistance syndrome (UARS; *sleep apnea*) with the standard treatment for this condition, namely continuous positive airway pressure.[25] UARS (sleep apnea) is discussed in more detail in Chap. 8 (Sleep). If these preliminary observations hold up in further work, there will be something more to offer patients with fibromyositis.

Summary

Pain is one of the most common reasons patients see physicians. A simple approach to this complex problem can be formulated as follows. Treat any underlying disease to which the pain can be attributed as effectively as possible. Try NSAIDs first, unless they are contraindicated by gastrointestinal or other problems. Let the patient find the NSAID that works best for him or her. Move on to an NSAID-codeine combination when necessary. If that fails, do not let fear of medical addiction prevent the use of morphine, usually in combination with an NSAID. Where indicated, use other medications for specific indications, for example, triptans for migraine headaches. If problems persist, do not hesitate to get a consultation with a pain specialist.

Our duty as physicians is not only to treat effectively when possible but also and always to try to relieve suffering. Happily, the array of medications available to treat pain usually allows us to treat physical pain relatively effectively.

REFERENCES

1. A clear and concise discussion of the neurobiology of pain is Jessel TM, Kelly DD. Pain and Analgesia, In. *Principles of Neural Science*. EM Kandel, JH Schwartz, TM Jessel, eds, 3d edition, Elsevier, NY, pp. 385.
2. During the late 1960s, a resident physician at a well-known Boston teaching hospital was using large doses of morphine to treat an older man, who was wracked with pain and cough from the lung cancer that was rapidly killing him. A government office called to complain to the resident that the doses of morphine fell outside of Federal guidelines. The government official pointed out that the patient might even have become addicted to morphine. (The phrasing he should have used was "become dependent on morphine.") The resident—who was very tired—responded that the patient probably was habituated to the drug, but that was not a long-term problem since he was rapidly dying anyway. The drug was being given to lessen his pain and cough. The resident requested to be allowed to go back to trying to take care of patients, while the government official went back to doing whatever he took taxpayer money to do. The resident suggested that if there was a problem, the government official should complain to the director of the hospital. He did. The hospital director, a crusty old Yankee, asked how the young doctor had responded to the charges. The government official told him. The hospital director said, "Sounds like good advice. See you!" and hung up.
3. In accord with the intellectual traditions of the specialty of Neurology, erudite Latinate or Greek names are available for other types of visual prodromes for classic (neurological) migraine.
4. Kruit MC, van Buchem MA, Hofman PA, et al. Migraine as a risk factor for subclinical brain lesions. *JAMA*. 2004;291:427–434.
5. Estevez M, Gardner KL. Update on the genetics of migraine. *Hum Genet*. 2004;114:225–235.
6. This entirely descriptive term can appear erudite, since it uses the Greek word *cephalalgia* instead of the English word *headache*.
7. Carragee EJ, Kim DH. A prospective analysis of magnetic resonance imaging findings in patients with sciatica and lumbar disc herniation: correlation of outcomes with disc fragment and canal morphology. *Spine*. 1997;22:1650–1660.

8. Jarvik JG, Deyo RA. Diagnostic evaluation of low back pain with emphasis on imaging. *Ann Intern Med.* 2002;137:586–597.
9. Staud R. Fibromyalgia pain: do we know the source? *Curr Opin Rheumatol.* 2004;16:157–163.
10. Yunus MB, Young CS, Saeed SA, et al. Positron emission tomography in patients with fibromyalgia syndrome and healthy controls. *Arthritis Rheum.* 2004;51:513–518.
11. The lack of pain sensors in the brain has allowed the mapping of functions of the human brain in "awake" patients undergoing neurosurgery for other therapeutic indications.
12. This technique works. I learned it when a physician who had been in the Navy gave me an injection. I have used it successfully when giving injections myself. (Patients have been surprised and pleased at getting an injection that "did not hurt.")
13. Enright E. Goodbye Pain. AARP The Magazine 2004; September–October, pp. 52–56, 97–99.
14. To oversimplify, this is the ready association of an ingested substance with the feeling of being sick. The classic example is of people who eat a dessert on an ocean liner and then become seasick, and who thereafter become sick when eating that dessert. See Garcia J, Holder MD. Time, space and value. *Hum Neurobiol.* 1985;4:81–89.
15. It has been used for centuries, although the chemically pure principle was not isolated until about 150 years ago. The medicinal properties of willow bark against fever (ague) were justified by the *Doctrine of Signatures*, as was the use of digitalis for heart failure ("dropsy"). This doctrine held that a munificent Deity had put a clue ("signature") on every plant to indicate its use for humans. It is up to the reader to decide whether the success of this theory with willow bark and foxglove proves the theory is correct or rather proves the risks of theorizing.
16. For a recent review of mainstream American practice with opiates, see Ballantyne JC, Mao J. Opioid therapy for chronic pain. *N Eng J Med.* 2003;349:1943–1953.
17. The *Brompton cocktail* is a mixture of medicines against pain and anxiety. Hospices often provide it at the bedside for the patient to use as needed.
18. A city hospital patient who was a pimp told me that addicting prostitutes to heroin made sex an entirely mechanical act for them, allowing them to turn more tricks a night.
19. Pappagallo M. Newer antiepileptic drugs: possible uses in the treatment of neuropathic pain and migraines. *Clin Ther.* 2003;25:2506–2538.
20. Mason L, Moore RA, Derry S, et al. Systematic review of topical capsaicin for the treatment of chronic pain. *BMJ.* 2004;328:991–994.
21. A successful trial of acupuncture for recurrent headache is described in Vickers AJ, Rees RW, Zollman CE, et al. Acupuncture for chronic headache in primary

care: a large, pragmatic, randomized trial. *BMJ*. 2004;328:744–747. Melchart D, Streng A, Hoppe A, et al. (The acupuncture randomised trial (ART) for tension-type headache—details of the treatment. Acup Med 2005;23:157-165) confirmed that result, but found that sham acupuncture and correct acupuncture were equally effective, and both were more effective than placebo.

22. Saper JR, Hamel RL, Lutz TE, et al. Daily scheduled opioids for intractable head pain: long-term observations of a treatment program. *Neurology*. 2004;62:1687–1694.
23. Bendtsen I, Jensen R. Mirtazapine is effective in the prophylactic treatment of chronic tension-type headache. *Neurology*. 2004;62:1706–1711.
24. Deyo RA, Weinstein JN. Low back pain. *New Eng J Med*. 2001;344:363–370.
25. Gold AR, Dipalo F, Gold MS, et al. Inspiratory airflow dynamics during sleep in women with fibromyalgia. *Sleep*. 2004;27:459–466.

CHAPTER EIGHT

Sleep

One of the commonest requests physicians get from patients is for "something to help me sleep." Many more patients worry about how much or little they sleep than have biologically significant disorders of sleep. The notion that a healthy life requires 7–9 hours of unbroken, "restful" sleep is based in part on studies that indicate that mortality and morbidity in the United States is greater in populations that do not conform to that pattern.[1,2] Whether the altered sleep patterns are the result of underlying illness or contribute to it is, however, not clear. There are documented individuals who appear otherwise healthy who sleep no more than 4 hours out of 24. There is at least one well-documented, otherwise healthy lady who needed no more than 45 minutes of sleep each 24 hours. Other individuals who appear equally healthy routinely sleep 10–12 hours out of 24, or even more. In an environment without time cues, most people entrain to a cycle of 25 hours and some to much longer cycles. A nap during the noon break and less sleep at night is the socially accepted pattern in many countries with warm climates, including Mediterranean countries of undoubted civilization and with relatively long average life spans. The "natural" sleep pattern of pre-agricultural Homo sapiens may have been two periods of sleep a day, each of about 4 hours. Despite these biological caveats, many patients are upset if they do not conform to the sleep patterns that their family and friends expect of them. In order to do so, they want sleep medication. These people will typically find a practitioner who will prescribe "something" to help them sleep according to the pattern that they want. In addition to the "worried well" who want to "normalize" their sleep cycle, there are also people who have medical disorders of the sleep-wake cycle that need treatment by physicians.

CLASSIFICATION AND DIAGNOSIS

Table 8-1 presents a classification of disorders of sleep adapted from that of Kelly.[3]

Disorders of sleep are usually but certainly not always associated with variations from normal in the EEG patterns of sleep, as discussed below under Neurobiology. In some patients, discrete organic causes for these disabilities related to sleep can be found; in others, not.

The first question about a putative "sleep disorder" is whether or not it needs treatment. Variations in sleeping time are wide among otherwise healthy human beings.[4] They can vary within a single individual over time as well as among different individuals. The Zen Buddhist teaching, "sleep when tired," can be excellent medical advice for healthy people who need more or less sleep than the U.S. average. On the other hand, sleeping too little (*insomnia*) or too much (*hypersomnia*) can be a sign of depression or other serious and even life-threatening disease, as can certain other disorders of sleep.

Insomnia

Insomnia—too little sleep—is a common complaint among patients seen in general clinical practice. Insomnia can be a disorder of expectation. The patients believe that they should sleep according to a pattern. When their perceived sleep pattern differs from their expectations, they want the doctor to fix that discrepancy even if there is no other evidence that it harms them.

TABLE 8–1

Classification of disorders of sleep (Dyssomnias)

Insomnia
Hypersomnia
Parasomnias
Sleep apnea
Narcolepsy
Other dyssomnias

The following anecdotal experience describes an instance where prescribing a sleep medication could easily have interfered with psychic healing.

> The daughter of a 53-year-old man died unexpectedly in an auto accident. The father was utterly grief stricken. He was a disciplined and controlled man with no ready emotional outlet for his grief. A month after his daughter's death, he found he could sleep no more than 2 hours a night. He became worried and asked his doctor for a sleep medication. The doctor explained that the sleeplessness was part of necessary and healthy grief work, which the father was doing in his own way. The man began to use the time when he couldn't sleep to do work he had not gotten done during the day. That was the best way he found to distract himself from brooding about his dead daughter. As time passed, he became able to sleep longer during the night. A year and a half after the child's death he was back to 7–9 hours a night of unbroken, restful sleep.

The current American psychiatric definition of primary insomnia (in DSM-IV-R, the Diagnostic and Statistical Manual of Mental Disorders) requires that the condition lasts for at least a month, impairs life in some significant way, and is not attributable to any other medical condition including a medication. As many as half or more of patients who complain of insomnia and are studied in a sleep laboratory turn out to have normally long periods of sleep with normal sleep patterns on EEG recording. (See discussion of sleep architecture below.) These patients tend not to drop their body temperatures as much as others do during deep sleep, and they may have more episodes of very brief wakening during sleep. Such "microwakes" last no more than a few seconds. Apparently these relatively minor physiological variations can interfere with the perception of having had restful sleep.

The first cause to look for in insomnia is poor sleep hygiene. That can result from many factors, including ingestion of inappropriate materials, often too much coffee or tea or over-the-counter or prescription medications that interfere with sleep. The key to sleeping better may just be relaxing for a little while before going to sleep.

Insomnia can be a sign of so many different medical and neurological illnesses that it has to be approached as a non-specific manifestation of disease, that taxes the full diagnostic capability of the general clinician. A stuffy nose (*allergic rhinitis*) is a classic cause of troubled sleep. Pain can keep people awake. Headaches that wake a person during sleep should raise a suspicion of organic disease of the brain, possibly a brain tumor, although that is certainly not always true. (See Chap. 7, Pain.) Endocrine disorders can also interfere with sleep.

Trouble with sleep is a classical somatic sign of depression. The trouble can take many forms. A typical pattern is falling asleep easily but trouble staying asleep through the night. When a patient describes such "early morning wakening," further questioning is in order even if the patient attributes the wakening to an external cause such as a need to urinate. It pays to find out how much trouble the patient has going back to sleep, and what he or she thinks about if they lie awake. If they brood (have "bad thoughts"), the insomnia may be the give-away sign of a depression that needs treatment. Other types of sleep impairment can also accompany depression. Some patients with depression sleep abnormally long. As discussed in Chap. 3 (Mood Disorders), depression is a life-threatening disease. The general clinician should dig for other evidence of depression or anxiety disorder in patients who complain of insomnia. As discussed elsewhere in this monograph, both depression and anxiety disorders can usually be treated effectively. (See Chap. 3, Mood Disorders, and Chap. 6, Anxiety).

Changes in sleep patterns often accompany aging. The "classic" change in sleep pattern in elderly people is more naps during the day and shorter periods of sleep at night. This can become their "natural" pattern. It may be harmless and even convenient in people who adapt to it—for instance, retired people who do not need to meet the demands of employment or other rigidly scheduled activities. If it does not bother anyone or interfere with anyone's health, why treat it? On the other hand, if this alteration in sleep pattern destabilizes a living arrangement—for instance, an elderly parent living with adult children and grandchildren—then it can be considered a disability. Recent studies suggest that falls in elderly patients during the night tend to result from grogginess due to sleep medications more often than they do from the fact of getting up itself (for instance, to urinate). However, more data is needed before that conclusion is accepted.

It is common practice to prescribe sleep medication as needed (p.r.n.) as part of admission orders in hospitals. Hospitals can be noisy and distracting places. They can be weird environments at night as well as during the day, for staff and certainly for patients. Some patients will want a sleeping pill. Some, particularly patients in pain, may benefit from that treatment. However, all sleep medications are to some extent central nervous depressants, and their use to treat harmless wakefulness is not optimal medical care.

Hypersomnia

Hypersomnia—too much sleep—is a rarer complaint than insomnia among patients who are not medically ill. The diagnosis of *Primary Hypersomnia*, by *DSM-IV-R* criteria, requires symptoms to recur over at least a month or last at least 3 days several times a year for 2 years. The symptoms must also interfere with life and not be attributable to insomnia or other known cause, including drugs or other specific types of sleep disorder. Patients who are somnolent from too much of a medication or other toxin or are in stupor or coma are not correctly described as having hypersomnia, since those states differ in important ways from normal sleep.

Detailed evaluation usually uncovers a cause for excessive sleeping. Obtaining all the medications in the home of a person who is "always sleepy" will often uncover an over-the-counter medication or other sedative that the patient failed to mention. Sleeping is a common response to many illnesses including the common cold and flu. An increasingly recognized cause of daytime sleepiness is *sleep apnea*, which is discussed below. Diseases affecting the mesencephalon, a part of the brain associated with sleep regulation, can characteristically cause excessive sleep. The brain disease can be a small tumor or a vascular or other insult. These patients classically can be roused easily, but fall asleep promptly when a stimulus is withdrawn. *Narcolepsy*, discussed below, can cause daytime sleepiness. The classical example of a disease that causes excessive sleep is *von Economo encephalitis*, which occurred as an epidemic after World War I. Hypersomnia is a typical manifestation of *trypanosomiasis*, a disease caused by a parasite. It is fortunately seldom seen in the United States.

If a patient begins to sleep much more than his or her previous pattern, a work-up is indicated. If medical examination does not turn up a disease that provides a reasonable explanation for the increased sleeping, referral to a specialist is indicated. In fact, work-up by a specialist is a wise precaution even if an adequate medical cause seems to have been uncovered. Mistakes in diagnosis are likely to be too expensive.

Parasomnias

Parasomnias are disorders of sleep more complex than simply sleeping less or more than one wants to, or not sleeping on a schedule approved of by others. They arise by a number of different mechanisms, more or less specific for the type of parasomnia. Many of these have been described in terms of the alterations in sleep architecture. (See discussion of Neurobiology, below.) Many involve loss of the smooth, "normal" relationship between sleep state and muscle tone. Some parasomnias are also understood on a more molecular and cellular level. These conditions are diagnosed by their characteristic clinical patterns and by other examinations including electroencephalography (EEG) during sleep. The diagnosis and treatment of these disorders is an area for specialists. Ideally, these are neurologists with a special interest in sleep disorders and access to a sleep laboratory. The continuing treatment of these disorders optimally involves collaboration between the sleep specialist and the patient's general physician.

Nocturnal Enuresis (Bed-Wetting): This is largely a problem of children but has been observed in young adults, including military recruits. Sometimes the cause is a problem with the urinary tract that is best treated by a urologist. In other cases, urinating during sleep tends to be associated with rapid waking from stage 4 of slow-wave sleep. It is not associated with REM sleep. (See discussion of sleep architecture below.) This condition is usually not of itself a significant threat to health, except for the patient's or others' reaction to this unappetizing behavioral variant. Bed-wetting can be associated with sleepwalking.

REM Sleep Disorder: This occurs in unfortunate individuals in whom REM sleep is not associated with loss of muscle tone. This disorder is dangerous. People with it tend to act out their dreams, including violent dreams. They frequently harm themselves and not rarely harm their bed partners as well. Confusion of REM sleep disorder with simple sleep walking (*somnambulism*) may have contributed to the idea that sleepwalkers are acting out dreams. As noted below, patients with REM sleep disorder tend to respond to anticonvulsants. This condition is often associated with manifestations of *Parkinson disease*.

Hypnic Starts (Somnolescent Starts): They are movements of the legs or trunk and more uncommonly the arms that occur while a person is falling asleep. The movements tend to wake the patient. If they happen regularly, they often bother the patient. They do not have pathological implications apart from their inconvenience. They are not a sign of underlying epilepsy or related condition.

Sensory Paroxysms: These are related to hypnic starts but affect the sensory system. Sometimes they lead to the sensation of one's head exploding—a “thunderclap sensation.” They are unpleasant but not otherwise harmful.

Restless Legs Syndrome and Related Conditions: Some people tend to move more actively in sleep than others, including movements of their legs. Some patients develop a very strong urge amounting to a compulsion to move their legs while falling asleep or in the early stages of sleep. The urge tends to be associated with abnormal “drawing” sensations in the legs. This can disturb a bed partner and lead to disarray of the bedclothes by morning, but is otherwise without pathological implications. Rare patients develop true *myoclonic jerking* during sleep; in some, this is part of a movement disorder that carries on into the day and typically responds to opiates. (See Chap. 11, Disorders of Motility.)

Nocturnal Paroxysmal Dystonia: This consists of abnormal movements that occur during sleep. The movements may include writhing (*choreoathetotic*) movements, spasmodic movements (*dystonia*), or flinging of an arm or leg (*ballismus*). They typically occur during deep (slow wave) sleep.

Sleep Paralyses (Pre- and Postdormital Paralyses; Hypnagogic Paralyses): These often unpleasant episodes are periods of loss of tone of the voluntary muscles while falling asleep or waking up. These spells tend to be brief and transient. Patients can often be “snapped out” of that state if their bed partner or other person touches them. Sleep paralysis has no particular medical significance unless the attacks continue to bother the patient even after their nature and lack of medical implications have been explained. Happily, bothersome sleep paralyses usually respond to treatment with tricyclic antidepressants.

Kleine-Levin Syndrome: This rare disorder is seen most often in adolescent boys. Perhaps four times a year, these patients go through periods of a few days or a few weeks of sleeping too much, eating too much, usually becoming hypersexual, and typically showing other behavioral abnormalities including cognitive disturbances and social withdrawal (above the level normally associated with adolescence in males). Happily, this condition tends to go away with time. Neither its cause nor a treatment for it is known.

Sleepwalking (Somnambulism): Sleepwalking tends not to lead to medical complications unless people become upset by it. It typically occurs during deep sleep. Sleepwalking is more common in children than in adults. Sleepwalking in an adult who does not have childhood history of this activity requires a reasonably extensive work-up, particularly new onset sleepwalking. A sleepwalker (somnambulist) may perform apparently purposive actions such as dusting a table. Sometimes sleepwalkers mumble incoherently. Generally the somnambulist returns to bed with no visible side effects and no memory of the activities he or she carried out while asleep. Antisocial and even violent acts are rare during sleepwalking but have been recorded. A psychoanalytic interpretation of sleepwalking has been the acting out of dreams, which are themselves ways to deal with ideas and emotions unacceptable to the conscious mind. (See below.) However, sleepwalking is not associated with the REM stage in which formed dreams are most likely. Sleepwalkers can be hard to wake, but do not appear to be harmed by being awakened while engaged in their nighttime activities. Bed-wetting and sleepwalking both tend to occur in the same families.

Sleep Automatisms (Half-Waking Somnambulism): Sleep automatisms are stereotyped activities in people who are half-awake and typically do not remember the activity when fully awake. Waking up from deep sleep can be difficult, particularly after being sleep-deprived and getting very tired. Many of us have occasionally been surprised by what others tell us we did or said while half awake. On the other hand, if sleep automatisms occur frequently enough to bother the patient or if the automatisms put someone at risk, they can become a medical problem. Fortunately, they tend to respond to treatment with a benzodiazepine such as flurazepam.

Narcolepsy: People with this serious condition fall asleep during the day, typically two to six times a day. They develop an irresistible urge to sleep, sometimes in very inappropriate settings such as while driving a car. Attacks typically last no more than a quarter of an hour, although if left alone narcoleptics can sleep for an hour during an episode. This condition affects perhaps 0.05% of both men and women. It is usually fully established by age 25.

People who suffer from narcolepsy may also have episodes of automatic behavior that they do not remember, without obviously falling asleep. In these episodes, patients often feel drowsy and fight off sleeping but then lose track of what they are doing. These spells can obviously be dangerous, depending on what the person is doing when they go onto automatic. Narcoleptics tend to have more automobile accidents than do epileptics.

Many narcoleptics also suffer from episodes of loss of skeletal muscle tone, that is, from *cataplexy*. Cataplexy can be brought on by laughter or by emotional activity. The phrase "I laughed until I dropped" describes a form of cataplexy. Simply slipping to the ground because of loss of skeletal muscle tone is usually not harmful of itself. However, this can be a dangerous event, depending on where the victim is and what he or she is doing when the attack occurs.

The combination of narcolepsy, cataplexy, sleep paralysis, and hallucinations make up a clinical entity.

Nightmares: Dreams occur regularly during sleep (They are more vividly and better remembered in REM sleep than in slow-wave sleep.) Unfortunately, about two-thirds or more of dreams are unpleasant. Nightmares are unpleasant dreams that we remember, often because they occurred during episodes of REM sleep shortly before awakening. Dreams at that time tend to be rich in emotional content. Nightmares are part of the human condition in the imperfect world in which we exist. They become a medical problem only if they clearly interfere with a person's life. During psychoanalysis, the contents of recurrent dreams are sometimes clues to problems of which people are not consciously aware.

Sleep Terrors (Night Terrors): Night terrors are generally worse than nightmares and are associated with other symptoms. These are most frequent in children, but can occur in adults as well. In adults they tend to be associated with a feeling of pressure on the chest that impairs breathing. Formed dreams beyond the abnormal sensation are rare. Associated signs of anxiety occur, including perspiration, dilated pupils, and partial paralysis. Night terrors in adults tend to be accompanied by increased anxiety during waking hours. They occur during deep (slow wave) sleep, not typically during periods when dreams are common (REM sleep). The idea that a devil is sitting on the chest of the sufferer has been incorporated into words for a frightening sleep disturbance in several European languages. The Latin term for such an attack is *incubus* (from *incubare*, to lie upon). An old Teutonic root for devil, namely, *mar*, is incorporated into the English word nightmare, the French word *cauchemar*, and the German word *nachtmar*.

Hypnagogic Hallucinations: These are auditory or visual hallucinations that occur when a person is falling asleep or waking up. They are particularly common in patients who suffer from narcolepsy, as discussed above. They are associated with paralysis of the muscles of the limbs, so that the sufferer is not only hallucinating but can have the often frightening sense of being unable to do anything about the events in the hallucination. The word "sufferer" is chosen carefully. Hypnagogic hallucinations can be extraordinarily unpleasant. However, they are not by themselves a sign of mental illness.

Sleep Apneas

Well-recognized disorders that affect breathing during sleep sometimes cause insomnia but more often—in perhaps 90% of cases—cause too much sleep (hypersomnia). By definition, sleep apnea involves at least five episodes a night in which breathing stops for at least 10 seconds. In severe cases, there are hundreds of episodes a night. Sleep apnea is broadly divided into central, obstructive, or mixed. In central sleep apnea, breathing stops including the movement of the chest muscles of breathing. An extreme example is "*Ondine's curse*," in which conscious control is required to maintain adequate breathing. These patients can die while they are asleep because they literally forget to breathe. Appropriate protective machinery for them is available. In obstructive sleep apnea, an obstruction in the nose or mouth blocks breathing even though the motion of chest muscles is intact; it often involves increased effort to get air past the obstruction. Patients who have obstructive sleep apnea tend to be obese and to snore. The combination of obesity and daytime sleepiness has a literary name, *Pickwickian syndrome*, after a boy described in Dickens' *Pickwick Papers* who epitomized this combination. Mixed sleep apnea is a mixture of both types.

Sleep apnea is not now thought to be a benign condition. The periodic episodes of low oxygen (*hypoxia*) and too much carbon dioxide (*hypercarbia*) due to inadequate breathing often have longer-term effects on health. These disorders have been proposed to be a cause of cognitive impairment, at least in severe cases.[5–7] "Vigilance" and "executive functions" are often affected. In other words, people with sleep apnea tend to have trouble paying attention and organizing themselves during the day. They also tend to have high blood pressure and a number of other disorders, even if they are not obese.

Disorders of Circadian Rhythm of Sleep

These are broadly of three types. Some people fall asleep earlier and wake up earlier than most other people; this can be medicalized as

Advanced Sleep Phase Disorder. Some other people fall asleep later and wake up later than other people. People with this *Delayed Sleep Phase Disorder* function perfectly well if they can work at night—for instance, as entertainers or chefs. There are situations where they are at a major disadvantage, such as Marine Corps basic training. Shift workers have a societaly-induced condition that sometimes deserves medical intervention. They have jobs that require them to switch the time of their sleep cycle. Many of us are familiar with this syndrome in the form of "jet lag," when we have traveled through time zones and our inner clock is not in tune with the light-dark cycle of the place where we have arrived. This can be a very difficult problem for airline personnel who fly long distances, such as pilots and cabin staff on international routes. It can also be a problem for nurses and other medical personnel whose duty assignments vary between daytime and night shifts.

Having interns and residents on duty for 36 hours on with 12 hours off is a practice hallowed by American medical traditions. It is supported by many aging members of the medical profession because of their recollections of how energetic and virile they were when they were interns and residents. The known physiology of sleep and the known effects of sleep deprivation argue that this practice is unlikely to optimize the quality of care for patients for whom the house staff is responsible.

Other Dyssomnias

A number of other types of disorders of sleep have been described in the literature. They include seizures revealed during sleep. (The increased evidence of seizures during sleep is the justification for doing sleep EEGs. See Chap. 10, Disorders of Awareness.) *Carpal tunnel syndrome* manifesting itself during sleep has a special scholarly name, *acroparesthesias*. This and other disorders are discussed in textbooks of Neurology and Psychiatry and in the large and rapidly expanding literature on sleep and sleep disorders.

NEUROBIOLOGY

Studies of sleep and disorders of sleep have been extensive. There are four stages of progressively deeper slow-wave sleep, characterized by progressively slower frequencies and higher voltages on the EEG. They are numbered stage 1 through to stage 4. In these stages, heart rate, blood pressure, and usually body temperature decline but stay within healthy physiological limits. Muscle tone is maintained in slow-wave sleep. Another sleep stage that contrasts with slow-wave sleep is REM (Rapid Eye Movement) sleep. In this stage, the cortical EEG has high frequency, desynchronized, low voltage pattern but the hippocampal EEG remains synchronized (*theta waves*). Muscle tone is lost, and rapid eye movements occur. Patients awakened from REM sleep are more likely to remember relatively detailed dreams than those awakened from slow-wave sleep. The belief that REM sleep is necessary to maintain sanity is demonstrably wrong. For instance, MAO inhibitors tend to abolish REM sleep without inducing psychosis.

Why sleep is necessary is still not clear in neurobiological terms. On the other hand, sleep deprivation if prolonged and extensive enough wreaks havoc with the personality. Evidence is available from the experiences of those of us who did our internships and residencies where the standard schedule was to be on duty every other night and every other weekend. Our spouses can provide even more evidence of the bizarre effects of severe sleep deprivation on the behavior of previously healthy and reasonably sane young people.

Sleep is driven actively by centers in the brain stem. Current theories propose a balance between serotonergic activity of the raphe nuclei and cholinergic activities that involve the nucleus tractus solitarius. REM sleep has been related to periods of lower activity of the serotonergic raphe nuclei. The preoptic area and the suprachiasmatic nucleus in the hypothalamus and basal forebrain have a critical role in controlling circadian rhythms including the sleep-wake cycle. Light appears to be an important trigger for these rhythms, that is, light acts as a "*zeitgeber*" (time-giver). Other parts of the brain also appear to be involved in sleep as well. The complexity of the mechanisms involved in sleep allow for a variety of neurobiological and behavioral causes of aberrations of sleep that are brought to the attention of physicians. Substances that induce sleep have been isolated and characterized from brain or spinal fluid of sleep-deprived experimental animals or humans. They are generally peptides. Lack of a hypothalamic peptide, *hypocretin*, is responsible for most cases of narcolepsy. (See discussion above.)

Why we dream is even less clear than why we sleep. Freud provided a mechanistic explanation of dreaming in terms of brain function. He proposed that dreams are ways of releasing ideas or drives that are—for a variety of reasons—unacceptable to the conscious, verbal mind. One can express this in language that is more neurobiological than psychoanalytic. *Engrams* can be laid down, particularly in the hippocampus, which can influence behavior and be powerful but are not acceptable to conscious, socialized life. For instance, the thought that "I want to kill that son-of-a-bitch" or "that son-of-a-bitch" wants to kill me" can be powerful ideas, but are better not acted on except in unusual situations. Gazzaniga among others has shown that we can have potent, behavior-altering ideas in our non-dominant hemisphere that do not normally make it through the filter in our dominant hemisphere. Freud may have intuited correctly that sleep and dreaming provide a physiological state in which the brain can organize biologically encoded memories (engrams) into a more or less harmoniously functioning whole. That statement is more or less in accord with a suggestion by Jouvet, that REM sleep is a chance for the brain to "practice" the neural part of complex activities before they are carried out in the real world while awake.

Insomnia

Insomnia is not a single entity. It is a syndrome rather than a disease. As discussed above, many illnesses can keep people awake, particularly painful illnesses. People can also be kept awake by habits that do not promote sleep, such as drinking too much coffee late in the day. Recent studies suggest that cigarette smoking can impair sleep—yet another reason to give up smoking. Often, however, insomnia is a complaint without clear biological correlates. Not rarely it is the avowed complaint of people who turn out to have a psychiatric disease, especially a mood disorder. ("Schizophrenics" appear to sleep relatively normally, despite their many other problems.) The differential diagnosis of insomnia is discussed above. As already noted, some patients who complain of insomnia sleep as long as most other people and have normal sleep electrophysiologically. Their perception that they "sleep badly" may be related to their failure to drop body temperature during slow-wave sleep as well as to excessive numbers of "microwakenings." Fortunately, modern medication can help these people greatly.

Hypersomnia

Hypersomnia is also a syndrome not a disease. Some apparently healthy people just need more sleep than others.[7] Sometimes sleepiness is a side effect of the perception of not sleeping well at night even in people in whom the duration and architecture of sleep were normal. Wanting to go to bed and sleep is a standard response to feeling sick. Medical causes of increased sleepiness and sleep time include infections, heart failure or failure of a number of other organ systems, endocrine disorders such as *hypothyroidism*, and other illnesses. "Sleepiness" can be an effect of a drug or other condition that impairs cognition and consciousness—for instance a metabolic encephalopathy due to alcohol, other drugs, or endogenous conditions such as liver failure. Occasionally hypersomnia is a manifestation of a local lesion in one or more brain areas modulating sleep. A pathologically important cause of hypersomnia is impaired breathing during sleep, due to sleep apnea and *alveolar hypoventilation*. The extent to which *idiopathic hypersomnia* is associated with increased production or slowed removal of sleep-inducing substances or with abnormalities of other systems modulating sleep is not clear at this time.

Parasomnias

Parasomnias have different causes, depending on the condition.

Bed-Wetting and Sleepwalking: These conditions have a genetic component revealed by family studies. Some of the same genes may be involved, since these conditions tend to occur together in the same families. Specific genes for these conditions have not yet been identified.

REM Sleep Disorder, Hypnic Starts and Sensory Paroxysms: These appear to involve aberrations in the normal mechanisms by which sleep modifies the actions of motor or sensory systems.

Restless Legs Syndrome and Related Condition: These are occasionally the first manifestations of a disease of peripheral nerve (*neuropathy*), particularly due to kidney failure (*uremic neuropathy*). Myoclonic jerking during sleep may be released by the electrophysiological mechanisms involved in sleep. Not rarely it is associated with *myoclonus* and other evidence of a movement disorder during waking times as well. (See Chap. 11, Disorders of Motility.)

Nocturnal Paroxysmal Dystonia: The common form of this problem is a seizure disorder, primarily frontal. Attacks typically last only minutes and respond to anti-seizure medication. A rarer form, with attacks that can last up to 40 minutes, is not associated with seizure activity on the EEG and generally does not respond to anticonvulsants.

Sleep increases seizure susceptibility, as discussed in Chap. 10 (Disorders of Awareness). EEG recordings during sleep are often requested when searching for evidence for a subtle predisposition to seizures.

Sleep Apnea

Sleep apnea (*upper airways resistance syndrome*, UARS) This common cause of daytime sleepiness is frequently associated with obesity, snoring, and high blood pressure.[5–7] Effective treatment, as discussed below, tends to benefit blood pressure as well as other signs and symptoms. There are at least two distinct forms of this syndrome.

Central sleep apnea is a manifestation of damage to the brain stem and specifically to the structures in the brain stem that modulate sleep. This damage can arise from a variety of sources, including stroke, trauma, infection, or degenerative disease. When of unknown cause (idiopathic), the syndrome is referred to as *Ondine's curse.*

Obstructive sleep apnea is more common than the central form. As its name implies, it involves some kind of mechanical limitation on breathing when asleep. The immediate cause is inadequate contraction of the upper respiratory muscles, allowing the pharynx to be relatively closed when the diaphragm contracts. Obesity is a major risk factor, as are a variety of diseases including hypothyroidism as well as neuromuscular syndromes such as *motor neuron disease*. As discussed below, these patients typically snore.As noted in Chap. 7 (Pain), a recent paper reports a small series in whom the pain syndrome, *fibromyalgia*, was associated with sleep apnea (*UARS*)[8]. If *fibromyositis* were to turn out to be the result of sleep apnea, then sleep apnea is even more common than has been thought.

Narcolepsy and Related Conditions

These include sleep paralyses. Narcolepsy and related disorders are associated with a generalized disorder of sleep architecture, frequently with REM sleep preceding slow-wave sleep. This condition tends to cluster in families, and a genetic susceptibility seems likely. A specific genetic defect has been described in narcolepsy in dogs, affecting the receptor for the sleep peptide *hypocretin* (*orexin*). In humans, narcolepsy can be secondary to a variety of types of damage to the brain stem or to structures surrounding the third ventricle. Multiple sclerosis can cause this syndrome.

Other Dyssomnias

These have various causes that are discussed in medical literature on sleep and sleep disorders. Nightmares can be precipitated by drugs, notably by the cholinesterase inhibitor *donepezil.* They can be so unpleasant as to prevent use of that medicine, including in people who are too demented to understand the explanation of why they are having bad dreams.

TREATMENTS

The first-line of treatment of clinically significant sleep disorders is what is formally called good sleep hygiene. That amounts to informed common sense. Patients should test whether drinking coffee or tea in the evening or even afternoon interferes with their sleep. If so, they should drink coffee and tea only at breakfast or not at all. Patients should be advised not to be overexcited before trying to go to sleep. If working in bed before they go to sleep keys them up too much to sleep well, then they should not work in bed before going to sleep. On the other hand, for some of us working in bed until we get too sleepy is a wonderful way to get a restful night's sleep. We should not be discouraged from doing what works for us. If the need to urinate awakens a person during the night, he or she should try to drink less fluid in the evening and even with supper. Smokers who have trouble sleeping have another good reason to stop smoking. Such "common sense" interventions can often obviate the need for drugs to induce sleep, or to provide a good enough night's sleep so that a person is not drowsy during the day. The extensive literature on sleep hygiene is beyond the scope of this monograph, which focuses on pharmacological agents. As noted above, there are also more specific disorders of sleep that fortunately tend to respond to specific treatments.

Insomnia (Inadequate Sleep)

A wide variety of medications are available for sleep, over-the-counter as well as by prescription. The discussion below attempts to go from the mildest to pharmacologically more powerful interventions. The group of medications that can induce sleep are variously called sedatives, hypnotics, or drugs that induce somnolence.

Old-Wives Potions: Warm Milk and Honey: There are many safe "old wives" potions for aiding sleep. When one of these home remedies works for a person, that person should use it. Neurochemistry supports the use of at least one of these, namely warm milk and honey. The major protein in milk, *casein*, is rich in the amino acid tryptophan. This amino acid is the precursor of the brain neurotransmitter *serotonin*. (Chemically, serotonin is 5-hydroxtryptamine.) Stimulation of serotonin receptors is one of the mechanisms involved in sleep, as discussed above. Transport of tryptophan into the brain is favored by sugar, including sugar from honey. Warm milk and honey is pleasant and safe and often comforting to people who prefer "natural" interventions to pills. People who want "scientific medicine" may be convinced to try milk and honey if the neurochemistry summarized in this paragraph is recited to them.

Alcohol: Alcohol has been used as a sedative in medicine for thousands of years. Its older name in the medical literature is *spiritus fermenti*, the Latin for "fermented spirit." Although relatively small amounts of alcohol can seem to be a stimulant by loosening inhibitions, large amounts of alcohol put people to sleep (e.g., a man "sleeping off his drunk"). For some people, an excellent and entirely adequate aid to relaxation and sleep is a glass of something alcoholic and nice when going to bed or even after climbing under the covers. However, if the equivalent of one shot of whiskey or one glass of wine is not enough to help a person sleep, then that person should probably try something else. Drinking oneself into a stupor with toxic amounts of alcohol is not to be recommended, even though enough booze will put anyone out. (Before the discovery of ether, alcohol was the conventional way to render patients coming to surgery semi-conscious [stuporous] or unconscious. In fact, enough booze can kill you promptly from *acute alcoholic toxicity*.) In many people, alcohol is a poor way to induce sleep because it also induces a sympathetic response that wakes them up later in the night. The pharmacology of alcohol is discussed in Chap. 5 (Cognitive Disorders) and in more detail in Chap. 14 (Disorders of Conduct).

Tryptophan: As discussed above, this amino acid is a precursor of serotonin, and ingesting it tends to increase serotonin functions in the brain. Tryptophan is an essential amino acid. It must be included in the diet, since the body can not manufacture (i.e. *synthesize*) it. Foods rich in tryptophan include turkey and milk. Serotonin function contributes to sleep. Ingesting tryptophan can favor sleep, i.e. tryptophan can be an effective hypnotic.[9] Formal trials have indicated that as little as 2 g of L-tryptophan can induce sleepiness in healthy young volunteers. That dose is much lower than the amount recommended by many purveyors of natural remedies. Commercial preparations of tryptophan have in the past been reported to induce significant side effects, perhaps because of contaminants in poorly manufactured lots. It seems unlikely that 2 g of uncontaminated tryptophan are likely to harm ordinary people. Theory suggests, of course, that there may be people with rare genetic variations that make them tolerate ingestion of tryptophan poorly. Tryptophan is contraindicated in people taking serotonergic antidepressants including SSRIs, tricyclics, and MAO inhibitors. (See Chap. 3, Mood Disorders.)

Melatonin: This natural hormone is produced by the pineal gland. It can help induce sleep in susceptible individuals. The proportion of such individuals is high enough in the general population that the effect of melatonin has been demonstrated in formal clinical trials. This compound acts via high affinity G protein-coupled membrane receptors, three of which have been identified. Melatonin has been described as a "chronobiological agent," that helps the body restore circadian rhythms that have been interfered with. Some academic physicians claim that this compound is the best agent to help them sleep when they cross time zones in the extensive travel our profession now requires.

The optimal dose of melatonin to induce sleep in most people is 0.3 mg by mouth about a half hour before bedtime.[10] Larger doses, up to 3 mg, sometimes help people whom the lower dose does not, but also increase the risk of side effects. These include daytime sleepiness ("hangover effects"), impairment of sexual responses in men, increased chance of seizures in those with epilepsy, and occasionally psychotic reactions in people also taking the SSRI fluoxetine. (See Chap 3, Mood Disorders.) Melatonin, particularly in larger doses, can have additive effects with other drugs that may cause grogginess, including benzodiazepines, antihistamines, some antidepressants, alcohol, herbal preparations such as valerian or kava kava, and other sedating preparations. Melatonin may decrease the effectiveness of anti-inflammatory medicines including aspirin and corticosteroids. This drug should be avoided by people taking MAO inhibitors (Chap. 3, Mood Disorders), people with autoimmune diseases such as lupus, and women trying to get pregnant.

Tablets of melatonin are available in a wide range of doses, from 0.2 mg to 5 mg. A melatonin solution that is also available contains 0.05 mg/drop (50 μg/drop) and therefore allows very low doses. Lozenges containing 0.5 mg are available, but other forms such as capsules contain a minimum of 0.2 mg.

Benzodiazepines: These drugs are discussed in more detail in Chap. 6 (Anxiety). Essentially all drugs in this class can help to induce sleep if taken at bedtime. Indeed, somnolence can be one of their unfortunate side effects if taken during the day. Certain benzodiazepines have been marketed specifically for helping people sleep, in part on the basis of their pharmacological properties and in part to enlarge the market for those medications. Table 8-2 lists benzodiazepines recommended particularly for this purpose. Triazolam is not included in this table, because of its side effects. (See Chap. 6, Anxiety.) If triazolam is used to induce sleep, that use should not exceed a week or 10 days. This medication is now banned in Britain.

Benzodiazepines are so successful as to be almost a specific remedy for people who complain of insomnia despite normal duration and architecture of their sleep. Whether these medications work by altering temperature in slow-wave sleep, by diminishing "microwakenings," or just by calming these worried individuals is not clear. Nor is it particularly important for the clinical use of these drugs for these patients.

Chronic benzodiazepine use, whether for sleep or for anxiety, typically leads to habituation. Whether the benefits to a specific patient outweigh the risks entailed by this physiological effect is a matter of clinical judgment. People who have become used to taking a benzodiazepine in

TABLE 8–2

Benzodiazepines marketed as sleep medications

Drug name	Common name	Half-life (hours)	Usual dose (h.s.)
Flurazepam	Dalmane	<6	15–30 mg
Temazepam	Restoril	6–20	7.5–15.0 mg
Estazolam	Prosom	6–20	1–2 mg
Quazepam	Doral	>20	7.5–15.0 mg
Zolpidem	Ambien	<6	5–10 mg
Zaleplon	-	1	5–10 mg

order to sleep should taper these medications rather than stopping them suddenly. Patients who are reducing their use of benzodiazepines often need continuing counseling as well. *Cognitive-behavioral therapy* has been reported to be useful.

Benzodiazepines used for sleep typically also have anti-anxiety effects that continue through the day. The obverse is also true. Benzodiazepines given during the day to alleviate anxiety may also allow the patient to sleep better. The rule is, as always, to do what helps the patient. Theory including the way a drug company chooses to market a particular benzodiazepine matters much less.

Antihistaminics: Antihistaminics as a group have sedative properties. Stimulation of histamine (H_1) receptors in the brain favors wakefulness, so blocking them favors sleep. Antihistaminics as a group tend to be antagonists at these receptors. In appropriate doses, this group of medications can be extremely useful sleep medications.

In addition to antihistaminics available by prescription, there are over-the counter preparations that also aid sleep. Combination of a non-steroidal, anti-inflammatory, and antihistaminic are marketed in several forms, often with "PM" in their label. Examples are Tylenol PM and Excedrin PM. The author's anecdotal experience suggests that these over-the-counter preparations can be very well tolerated and gratifyingly effective, although there is effectively no published evidence that the NSAIDs themselves help sleep, except perhaps by relieving pain.[11] Doses of powerful over-the-counter preparations of antihistaminics (such as Contac) can induce prolonged sleep, particularly in people who are pharmacologically naïve to these medications. Excessively large doses of any antihistaminic can put anyone into a long and deep sleep, and can even cause confusion, coma, and death. Table 8-3 lists antihistaminics that are typically prescribed to aid sleep.

TABLE 8–3

Antihistamines commonly used as sedatives

Name of drug	Common name	Sedative dose
Diphenhydramine	Benadryl	25–50 mg
Hydroxyzine	Atarax, Vistaril	50–100 mg
Promethazine	Phenergan	25–50 mg

The most common and dangerous side effect of antihistaminics is excessive sleepiness. Patients taking these medications should be warned about driving or operating machinery if they get sleepy. They should also be warned about additive and synergistic effects of these agents with other central nervous system depressants, specifically including alcohol. The sedative effects of antihistaminics can be a very annoying side effect when these medications are used to treat colds or allergies. Television advertisements for these agents often emphasize a relative lack of drowsiness with the sponsor's allergy remedy compared to the antihistaminics marketed by others.

Antihistaminic drugs can induce anticholinergic side effects in susceptible people. These can include relatively mild effects such as gastrointestinal (GI) distress, dry mouth, urinary retention, and blurring of vision. Both the sedative effect and the anticholinergic effects of antihistaminics can interfere with memory and other aspects of cognition in people with Alzheimer disease or other dementia, including those with mild, "subclinical" disease. They can even induce psychotic delirium. Chapter 5 (Cognitive Disorders) describes an instance of antihistaminic-induced delirium in an elderly man that was originally mistaken for dementia. That has been seen particularly with *diphenhydramine* (Benadryl) and *cyproheptadine* (Periactin). Other antihistaminics reported to have such side effects include both agents that block H_1 histamine receptors (*H_1 antagonists*) as well as those that are marketed as more or less specific blockers of H_2 receptors (*H_2 antagonists*). The former include *loratadine* (Claritin), *cetirizine* (Zyrtec), and *fexofenadine* (Allegra), and the latter *cimetidine* (Tagamet), *Ranitidine* (Zantac), *famotidine* (Pepcid), and *nizatidine* (Axid). If a patient taking one of these medications presents clinically with confusion, other signs of delirium, or other altered states of consciousness, the antihistaminic should be stopped.

Other Sleep Medications: *Zolpidem* (Ambien) is widely advertised. Dosage is 5 or 10 mg a night by mouth. As always, the lower dose is safer as a starting dose or for use in debilitated people, elderly people, or people taking other medications that can depress the central nervous system. It is usually reasonably well tolerated. However, its side effects include drowsiness and nausea and vomiting in mentally healthy people and exacerbation of symptoms in people with a mood disorder. *Zaleplon* (Sonata) is another non-benzodiazepine hypnotic. Doses vary from 5 mg a night by mouth to a maximum of 20 mg a night for people who are not helped by 5 or 10 mg doses. Elderly and debilitated people typically do not tolerate the higher doses. Zaleplon, like zolpidem, can have "hangover effects" and has been associated with "strange thoughts" in some people taking it. Animal studies suggest it is not safe for the fetus during pregnancy. Also, it interacts with a variety of other drugs and conditions. Both of these drugs are recommended only for short term use—perhaps 2 weeks.

The FDA recently approved *Esopiclone* (Lunesta) for sustained treatment of difficulty sleeping. Dosage is 2 mg a night orally in adults, rising to 3 mg a night if needed. In the elderly, the dosage is 1 mg and 2 mg. This drug significantly reduces anxiety as well as accelerating the onset of sleep. Its drawbacks include "hangover" effects such as drowsiness. It appears to impair attention and memory more than zolpidem and zaleplon do. Headache is the most prominent side effect, and patients may complain of the taste.

Another drug recently approved for sleep is *ramelteon* (Rozerem). This agent acts on melatonin receptors (i.e., is a melatonin receptor agonist). The standard dose is 8 mg by mouth about half an hour before going to sleep. Taking it after a fatty meal slows its absorption and therefore its action. Patients with liver disease should avoid it. Known side effects are mild and reversible. As yet, there are no reports of withdrawal, rebound insomnia, or utilization as a drug of abuse.

Chloral Hydrate: Chloral hydrate is no longer a drug of choice for aiding sleep in adults or the elderly, but in occasional patients is the only effective medication that is also reasonably convenient to use. It has a simple chemical structure, part of which is an ethanol moiety. Its mechanism of action may be to facilitate the release in the brain of the neurotransmitter GABA, whose action is mimicked by benzodiazepines. (The benzodiazepines are of course effective sleep medications, as discussed above.) Chloral hydrate is effective orally in doses of 0.5–1 gram, although higher doses have sometimes been used. Sleep usually comes in half an hour or so.

The side effects of chloral hydrate sharply limit its use. It causes tolerance, requiring increasing doses. It can cause dependence similar to dependence on alcohol, including a withdrawal syndrome. The lethal dose of chloral hydrate is only about 10–20 times the therapeutic dose, and this drug acts additively or synergistically with other central nervous system depressants. The combination of alcohol and chloral hydrate, known as a "Mickey Finn," was classically used to quiet rambunctious drunks in bars in the slums of New York. Not rarely, they got too much and quieted down permanently (died).

The risk of fatal overdose of chloral hydrate is high even when it is used medically. This risk is high not only in people who are actively suicidal but also in those who are too confused or agitated to monitor their medications accurately. Chloral hydrate, like other central nervous system depressants, can induce delirium, and sometimes does so even when given in "standard, recommended" doses. The delirium can be either apathetic or agitated. (See Chap. 5, Cognitive Disorders.) Depressant effects of chloral hydrate can last after a person wakes up, that is, "sleep hangover" can occur. As noted, confusion can be dangerous in a person who becomes unclear about how much chloral hydrate he or she has taken or should take.

Among other problems with this drug is that it is irritating to the stomach and other parts of the gastrointestinal tract. It should be taken with milk or antacids. Chronic use has been associated with stomach problems including ulcers. Chloral hydrate can cause severe skin rashes that are sometimes accompanied by fever, including *erythema multiforme*. It should be avoided in nursing mothers and people with significant kidney, heart, or liver disease or with porphyria.

With all these disadvantages, why mention chloral hydrate here? The reason is that it sometimes remains the best available medicine despite its drawbacks. A number of brain disorders damage the systems in the brain that modulate sleep. Alzheimer disease is one common example. Patients with these disorders may show little response to other sleep medications but still respond to appropriate doses of chloral hydrate. The inability of these people to sleep through the night can be a serious complication, not so much for their physical health as for the stability of their social situation. The patient's sleeplessness can exhaust the caregivers by keeping them awake, and thus precipitate placement of the patient in a nursing home or other custodial facility. The combination of sleeplessness with the other strains of caring for a brain-damaged person may add up to more than the caregiver can bear. *Judicious* use of chloral hydrate can sometimes solve these problems for long enough to stabilize a care situation that has been falling apart. When chloral hydrate is used, the reasons for prescribing it rather than some other hypnotic should be well documented in the medical records.

Barbiturates: These are another group of central nervous system depressants that were once widely used to induce sleep but have been largely superceded by newer medications. In the short run, the clinical effects of the barbiturates are similar to those of the benzodiazepines, but the latter drugs are much safer. In the longer run, barbiturates become relatively ineffective in inducing sleep. Tolerance can occur within several weeks. Several mechanisms are involved, including more rapid metabolism of barbiturates due to induction of the cytochrome P-450 system in the liver.

A major problem with the barbiturates is the relatively small margins between the doses that are therapeutic and the doses that are toxic. In other words, these drugs as a group have a low therapeutic index—much lower than the benzodiazepines. The barbiturates depress respiration, and their effects are additive with those of other respiratory depressants including morphine. Death from respiratory failure is a significant risk in patients on barbiturates. These are effective agents for committing suicide. The barbiturates are also addicting, and their abuse can lead to a variety of unpleasant complications including withdrawal syndromes.

Barbiturates are often still used in the induction of anesthesia, in the treatment of some kinds of seizures sometimes including status epilepticus, and in psychiatry in *narcoanalysis*, that is, sodium amytal interviews. A general clinician might want to prescribe a barbiturate in a special case—for instance, for a patient who has not responded to newer and safer medications, or for a patient who has been using a barbiturate for so long that he or she is unwilling to change to a more up-to-date drug. When barbiturates are prescribed for sleep, the medical records should document the reasons for choosing to prescribe one of these relatively toxic drugs rather than a newer and safer hypnotic.

Antidepressants: As discussed in Chap. 3 (Mood Disorders), sleeplessness can be a manifestation of depression or mania. Medication that effectively treats the mood disorder usually remedies the sleep disorder as well. These medications are discussed in Chap. 3 (Mood Disorders). Sometimes, when sleeplessness is a particularly annoying manifestation of a mood disorder, a sleeping medication can be added to a more specific agent for the underlying psychiatric disease, particularly in the early stages of treatment. Most often this is a benzodiazepine. The risk of suicidal and even accidental overdoses in these patients should, however, not be forgotten. It is wise never to prescribe central nervous system depressants to these patients in amounts great enough to be fatal if taken all at once, or if taken with large amounts of alcohol. It is also wise to try to check that patients with mood disorders have taken previously prescribed medicine before giving them more. These cautions are presented with full awareness of how effectively some patients lie to their doctors, including specifically patients bent on committing suicide.

Trazodone (Desyrel) is an antidepressant with particularly useful sleep-inducing ("hypnotic") properties. When used alone, it is not a particularly powerful antidepressant. It is however a reasonably powerful medication for inducing sleep. It works well in the elderly, and can be very useful in mildly depressed older people. It can be used in combination with SSRIs in depressed people troubled by lack of sleep. Doses of trazodone as high as 400 mg/day have been recommended for the treatment of depression. Doses as low as 50 mg/day have often been effective for sleep in somewhat sad older people (at least in the author's experience). Where necessary, of course, that low dose can be titrated up. Increasing doses, of course, increase the risk of side effects. Trazodone can cause "sleep hangover." Chapter 3 (Mood Disorders) describes the less common but unpleasant and sometimes dangerous side effects that trazodone can have.

Other Medications for Sleep: Many other medications depress the central nervous system enough to facilitate sleep. A number of drugs are rarely used any more because their side effect profile is even less attractive than that of chloral hydrate or the barbiturates. Examples include *paraldehyde* and *glutethimide*. The general clinician who is driven to prescribing one of these relatively toxic drugs should probably do so in collaboration with an anesthetist, psychiatrist, or other specialist, both for the safety of the patient and for medicolegal reasons.

Hypersomnia

In treating patients who complain of sleeping too much, it is important to determine whether their increased sleep results from a medical or neurological condition that needs treatment. As discussed above, sick people respond to many illnesses by sleeping more. Classic examples include hypercarbia due to lung disease and endocrine disorders such as hypothyroidism. Specific lesions of the brain can also lead to excessive sleepiness. For instance, multiple sclerosis is well known to sometimes do so. For such patients, the basic treatment for the hypersomnia is treatment of the underlying illness.

Another group of patients who complain of sleeping too much are not harmed by spending more time sleeping than other people. For such patients, encouragement and counseling on adjusting their life style to their sleeping pattern can be the best help the physician can offer. That can often involve patients finding jobs where their sleep patterns are acceptable.

A variety of stimulants are available for people who truly need pharmacological aids to stay awake an adequate amount of the time. One of the most commonly used is, of course, coffee[12]—or in England, tea. Prescription medications for staying awake are best prescribed in collaboration with a sleep specialist, including modafinil (Provigil). None of these drugs is entirely safe, and many of them can be addicting.

Other Disorders of Sleep

Other drugs are used for specific and rarer types of sleep disorder. These conditions, like sleeping "too much" (hypersomnia), are best treated by a specialist in sleep disorders or by collaboration between the patient's personal physician and a specialist consultant.

REM Sleep Disorder: This usually responds to treatment with an appropriate anticonvulsant. (See Chap. 10, Disorders of Awareness.) It is a potentially dangerous condition, and treatment should not be delayed. This disorder is highly associated with Parkinson disease. (See Chap. 11, Disorders of Motility.)

Nocturnal Paroxysmal Dystonia: This is a seizure disorder whose clinical manifestations are prominent during sleep. It also responds to appropriate anticonvulsant medication.

Narcolepsy: For narcolepsy, *modafinil* (Provigil) is an FDA-approved treatment. Doses of 200 mg by mouth are usually effective, although some patients require 400 mg. As noted above, the FDA has recently extended approved uses for this medication to shift work disorder and obstructive sleep apnea/hypopnea syndrome.

Sleep Automatisms: Sleep automatisms that cause enough problems to deserve medical treatment can be treated with benzodiazepines. (See Chap. 6, Anxiety.) Again, consultation with a sleep specialist is wise when caring for the patients with these unusual disorders.

Disturbances of Circadian Rhythms: Disturbances of circadian rhythms including those occurring in shift workers are often treated with melatonin if the affected people need to sleep and with modafinil (200 mg) if they need to stay awake. Both medications are used in standard doses. The FDA approval of modafinil for shift workers points out the lack of long term studies in of the use of this potentially habituating medication for this indication.

Sleep Paralyses: These conditions often do not need treatment. If they do, antidepressants are often effective.

Sleep Apnea: Sleep apnea is treated in different ways depending on the cause of the apnea. Obstructive sleep apnea is typically treated by continuous positive airway pressure (CPAP). Central sleep apnea, which is potentially fatal, can sometimes be effectively treated with one of a number of drugs, particularly the tricyclic antidepressant clomipramine. Other medications that have proven effective in some patients include *acetazolamide*, *medroxyprogesterone*, and *protriptyline*. Monitoring devices are available to ensure that if the pharmacological treatment fails, the patient does not die in his or her sleep. Modafinil has been approved to treat the daytime sleepiness that night time sleep apnea can cause. As noted above, sleep apnea is a serious and potentially life-threatening condition. It should be treated promptly and appropriately, if at all possible, in consultation with a physician with special expertise in sleep disorders including sleep disorders of this type.

Benign Sleep Disorders: Conditions such as restless legs syndrome or slow wakening are appropriately treated by a mixture of encouragement and advice on how to adapt one's life style to the problem. For instance, people who have trouble waking up should arrange their sleeping schedules and alarm clocks so that they can wake up slowly. An automatic coffee maker (or tea maker) by the bedside can allow a person to awaken slowly without getting out of bed. So can a spouse or other bed partner who is willing to help. Drug therapy can have unforeseen complications. For instance, drugs that activate receptors for dopamine can often relieve restless legs syndrome but have been reported to induce compulsive behavior—notably gambling—in a minority of patients. (See Chap. 11, Disorders of Motility). Psychological counseling may help people who have recurrent nightmares or night terrors. Even if the night time problems persist, counseling may help the affected people to live with their disability more comfortably.[13]

Odd and Unusual Sleep Disorders

These deserve to be referred to specialists. Often the specialist will be able to do no more than the general clinician, but at least the patient and family will know that everything possible is being done. So will a lawyer who tries to make a case out of the disorder.

REFERENCES

1. Patel SR, Ayas NT, Malhotra MR, et al. A prospective study of sleep duration and mortality risk in women. *Sleep*. 2004;27:440–444.
2. Kripke DF, Garfinkel L, Wingard DL, et al. Mortality associated with sleep duration and insomnia. *Arch Gen Psychiatry*. 2002;59:131–136.
3. Kelly DD. Disorders of Sleep and Consciousness. In: ER Kandel, JH Schwartz, TM Jessel, eds. *Principles of Neural Science*. 3d edition, Elsevier, NY, 1991, pp. 805–819.
4. The author of this monograph has slept for 24–48 hours at a stretch every few months or so since early puberty. He awakens refreshed and happy. While these prolonged bouts of sleep are as weird as much of his other behavior, there is no obvious reason to classify them as a sleep disorder.
5. Gale SD, Hopkins RO. Effects of hypoxia on the brain: neuroimaging and neuropsychological findings following carbon monoxide poisoning and obstructive sleep apnea. *J Int Neuropsychol Soc*. 2004;10:60–71.
6. Beebe DW, Groesz L, Wells C, et al. The neuropsychological effects of obstructive sleep apnea: a meta-analysis of norm-referenced and case-controlled data. *Sleep*. 2003;26:298–307.
7. Sateia MJ. Neuropsychological impairment and quality of life in obstructive sleep apnea. *Clin Chest Med*. 2003;24:249–59.
8. Gold AR, Dipalo F, Gold MS, et al. Inspiratory airflow dynamics during sleep in women with fibromyalgia. *Sleep*. 2004;27:459–466.
9. Although turkey meat is rich in tryptophan, eating turkey is not recognized to aid sleep. People do often enjoy napping after a big Thanksgiving meal, however.
10. Zhdanova IV, Tucci V. Melatonin, circadian rhythms, and sleep. *Curr Treat Options Neurol*. 2003, May 5;3:225–229.
11. Some of my patients have said to me things like, "Doc, you won't believe this, but aspirin helps me sleep." Obviously, if aspirin or other NSAID works for them and has no untoward side effects, there is no medical reason to discourage them from using it.

12. In my office there is a mug on which is written, "I can't start my day without c-c-c-c- coffee."
13. Many wry jokes by and about psychoanalysts point out that learning to live with a disability more comfortably can be as important and gratifying outcome of psychiatric care as doing away with the disability completely. Psychoanalysis can not do away with traumas that have already happened. When successful, it can make such traumas less troublesome in current life. There is a Buddhist teaching that in this world one can not eliminate pain but one can largely eliminate suffering.

CHAPTER NINE

Cerebrovascular Disorders

The treatment of vascular diseases including attempts to prevent them is part of the armamentarium of the general clinician. This chapter does not dwell at any length on such issues as the mechanisms or treatment of hypertension, or atheroma formation, or autoimmune vasculitis, or bleeding diatheses. It is assumed that the readers of this volume are already familiar with these topics.[1]

The effects of strokes are so revealing for understanding the functions of the different parts of the human brain that neurologists are said to learn their specialty "stroke by stroke." A reasonably complete discussion of cerebrovascular disorders including specific stroke syndromes would involve so much of Neurology as to be out of place in this monograph. The focus here is on information directly relevant to pharmacological treatment of these patients by general clinicians. More extensive discussions of cerebrovascular disease are available in textbooks of Neurology[2,3] and in review articles.[4]

Cerebrovascular disease is common. General clinicians can expect to see and care for patients with disease of the brain circulation, even in areas where neurologists have the primary responsibility for such care. In the United States, there are about half a million strokes a year, and between 150,000 and 200,000 people die of stroke annually. The costs of caring for these patients are high. In the widely admired French health care system, costs are estimated at between 15,000 and 20,000 Euros per patient during the first year post stroke.

CLASSIFICATION AND DIAGNOSIS

Cerebrovascular diseases can be divided by etiology into five groups: clots (thrombi); bleeds; vasculitides (inflammatory diseases of blood vessels); general disorders of the circulation; and other. The discussion below is organized according to this classification by etiology. The "other" category includes strokes secondary to a variety of medical illnesses, such as disorders of coagulation. These categories are not mutually exclusive. For instance, bleeds can cause clots, and clots can cause bleeds. Medical disorders of coagulation can cause both.

Strokes can, however, also be classified in a number of other ways. Examples are: by size; by location; by duration; by the artery affected; and by the clinical syndrome. The latter two classifications relate closely to each other. Textbooks of general Neurology[2] and texts and review articles on stroke[3,4] describe in detail stroke syndromes associated with particular arteries or damage to particular parts of the brain. Neurologists are trained to recognize these "classical"stroke syndromes.

Vascular disease often involves more than one organ system. Having symptoms due to atherosclerosis in the heart, the head, or the legs makes it likely that the other two organ systems are or will also become affected. As discussed below, atherosclerosis leading to heart disease is so often associated with strokes that part of the work-up of stroke is examination for heart disease.

The first and in some ways most important step in the diagnosis of cerebrovascular disease is to recognize when a person has it. In major strokes, this is relatively easy. Even there, traps exist for the unwary clinician. Recognizing minor strokes or incipient strokes can be more challenging but therapeutically more gratifying. While it is now recognized that the brain does have a capacity to form new neurons, that capacity is limited. Better that brain cells not die from vascular insufficiency to begin with.

Modern brain imaging techniques have revolutionized the diagnosis of strokes and other forms of cerebrovascular disease, as discussed below.

Major Strokes

These tend to be relatively easy to recognize. The clinical picture is that of a rapid onset of clear cut neurological impairment with no other obvious cause. Often the patient has risk factors for cardiovascular disease or a history of such disease. Strokes are far and away the major cause of this

TABLE 9–1 Causes of sudden neurological deficits other than strokes
Trauma (unrecognized, poor history, and so on)
Migraine
Seizure
Cardiac arrhythmia or other failure leading to inadequate brain perfusion (Stokes-Adams attacks)
Temporal arteritis associated with blindness (see Chap. 7, Pain)
Rapidly expanding tumor, for example, some glioblastomas
Sudden onset of weakness of cranial nerve VII (Bell palsy)
Severe attacks of dizziness (vertigo) due to labyrinthine disease
Ophthalmoplegia due to diabetes
Acute peripheral nerve disease

syndrome. However, other conditions can also lead to sudden neurological impairment and more or less mimic this syndrome. Table 9-1 lists some of the more important.

Seizures can cause sudden neurological impairment that can last for hours or up to 2 days (*Todd's paralysis*). It is uncommon for the first manifestation of a stroke to be a seizure, but the differential diagnosis is not always easy.

Certain neurological syndromes are typically associated with blockage of specific vessels. Learning these syndromes is an important part of specialized training in Neurology. Only a few generalizations are worth mentioning here. A stroke arising from blockage of a carotid artery or the middle cerebral artery leads to weakness and sensory loss on the opposite side. Strokes of the left (dominant) cortex often lead to aphasia as well. Those of right (nondominant) cortex can lead to neglect of the left side of the body. Strokes that involve the brain stem typically lead to loss of consciousness. A particularly nasty form of brain stem (typically basilar artery) stroke leaves the patient in a "locked-in" syndrome, in which consciousness is maintained but movement is absent or nearly absent, except perhaps of the eyes. The course of major stroke syndromes tends to vary with the cause and type of stroke.

Clots

Clots in vessels supplying the brain account for about 80% of strokes. They can be divided conveniently into three groups: emboli; cerebral thromboses, usually atheromatous; and obstructions of veins.

Emboli: Emboli into arteries supplying the brain are the most common cause of clinically significant strokes in most series. (Emboli are, of course, clots or other materials that move in the circulation and get caught in and stop up specific blood vessels.) The most common source of embolism is the heart, emphasizing again the close relationship of general medicine to the prevention of strokes. Strokes are common in patients with *atrial fibrillation*, particularly in those who are not on anticoagulants. Cerebral emboli secondary to other kinds of clots accumulating in damaged hearts are not rare, however. Emboli that break off from clots (*thrombi*) in the carotids or other blood vessels are less common. Emboli can also arise from vegetations on the heart valves, from medical or surgical manipulations (e.g., trauma to blood vessels during catheterization), and from a variety of other sources. Emboli from traumatized fat or other tissue are rare, except in special situations such as after auto accidents or other major trauma. In principle, metastatic cancers get to the brain as emboli, but they rarely lead to stroke-like syndromes in their early stages.

Embolic strokes are typically sudden in onset. They usually occur without warning. Often, they are associated with pain, perhaps due to the clot distending the blood vessel it blocks. (Cerebral blood vessels have pain sensors; brain tissue itself does not.) Cardiac ultrasound can identify previously unsuspected clots that have announced their presence by causing a cerebral embolus. Emboli that break off from clots in the carotids or cerebral vessels can have a more stepwise progression, in part as the primary embolus breaks up and gives rise to further emboli in the more distal arterial tree.

Cerebral Thromboses: These develop as primary clots in blood vessels supplying the brain. They usually reflect atherosclerosis of the vessel. These patients often have elevated blood pressures and other risk factors for atheromas. The mechanisms of clot formation are fundamentally similar in the brain to those in other organs. They are well known to general clinicians. As noted above, the processes that lead to formation of atheromas typically although not invariably also affect organs besides the brain, including the heart.

Thromboses in intracranial vessels tend to lead to strokes with a relatively "stuttering" onset. They are often preceded by minor strokes or *transient ischemic attacks* (TIAs), often in the same vascular distribution as the eventual major thrombotic stroke. (See discussion of TIAs below.) Primary thromboses in cerebral vessels are not typically associated with headaches, unless there is massive brain swelling.

Venous Thromboses: Patients with obstructions of veins or of venous sinuses have as high a death rate as do those with obstructions to cerebral arteries.Venous thromboses or clotting off of venous sinuses can be difficult to diagnose. They tend to be associated with conditions in which blood has a dangerously increased tendency to clot. Examples include *post-partum* state, *thrombocytosis* with or without accompanying *polycythemia*, sickle cell disease, *antiphospholipid antibody syndrome*, mutations in the genes encoding clotting factors such as factor V Leiden mutation, and a variety of other states that favor clotting and are well known to general clinicians. Clinically, venous thromboses tend to have a slower clinical onset than arterial blockages. They tend to be associated with lesions outside a typical arterial vascular distribution, with hemorrhages, and with a tendency to seizures. Brain imaging can be the key to the diagnosis.

Bleeds

Bleeds that affect the brain can be not only into the brain substance but also into the *ventricles* (the areas in the brain normally filled with cerebrospinal fluid) or into the *meningeal spaces* (the spaces formed by the membranes that surround the brain). The latter include *subarachnoid* hemorrhages or bleeds causing *subdural* or the less common *epidural* hematomas.

Bleeding into the brain is less common than clots. Hemorrhages account for about 20% of strokes. They can arise from a variety of sources—essentially, whenever blood vessel walls are not strong enough to contain the blood pressures to which they are exposed. That can occur even in undamaged vessels, but is more likely in vessels that are damaged from atherosclerosis or from a variety of congenital or acquired disorders that compromise the integrity of arteries. *Hyalinization* of blood vessels due to high blood pressure can damage blood vessels enough to increase the chance of bleeds. Table 9-2 gives a list of risk factors for bleeding into the brain or meninges.

Bleeds into the brain lead to different clinical pictures depending on the location and size of the bleed. Massive hemorrhages into the brain typically present with a sudden attack of "apoplexy." A person who seemed intact moments before falls down unconscious, can not be roused, and soon dies (unless treated; see below). Smaller bleeds into brain substance can present clinically like other strokes, with increasing symptoms as the bleed expands. Very small bleeds can lead to *lacunar* strokes, which are asymptomatic or lead to only minor symptoms and signs. (See below.)

TABLE 9–2
Common causes of cerebral hemorrhages

Hypertension
Aneurysms
  Congenital
  Acquired
Vascular Malformations
  Arteriovenous
  Cavernous
Amyloidosis/Hyalinosis of cerebral vessels
Impairments of blood clotting
  Iatrogenic (e.g., anticoagulant therapy)
  Spontaneous (e.g., in blood dyscrasias such as leukemia)

Arteriovenous malformations manifest themselves clinically as hemorrhage in about half the patients, seizure in about a quarter, headache in about 15%, and other signs and symptoms in the remaining 10%. Large arteriovenous malformations can cause signs and symptoms due to local expansion before they bleed. Subarachnoid bleeding is associated with variable combinations of severe headache, vomiting, and loss of consciousness. (The arachnoid is one of the membranes that line the brain, the *meninges.)* Intermittent minor bleeding—"oozing"—often but not necessarily precedes the onset of a major bleed from an arteriovenous malformation or an aneurysm.[5]

Subdural and epidural bleeding is often associated with trauma. (The dura is another of the meningeal membranes.) Sometimes the history of trauma is hard to obtain, particularly if the patient is too impaired to give a reliable history and no good informant is available. Subdural or epidural bleeding can also result from other causes such as a disorder of blood clotting (natural or due to excessive anticoagulation therapy). Acutely, subdural bleeding is often associated with coma. The milder forms of subdural bleeding into the *posterior fossa* are associated with dysfunction of the brain structures there, and therefore with incoordination and other signs of cerebellar damage and/or of cranial nerve malfunction. Chronic subdural hematomas tend to be associated with disturbances of mentation and consciousness rather than with localizing (focal) neurological abnormalities. Chronic subdural hematoma is classified as a treatable cause of dementia. (See Chap. 5, Cognitive Disorders.) Often the patient or other informant does not volunteer or even remember a history of head trauma. Headaches sometimes occur.

TABLE 9–3
Medical conditions predisposing to strokes

Primary disorders
Atherosclerosis of blood vessels
Blood dyscrasias
Leukemias
Polycythemias (to a lesser extent)
Platelet disorders
Thrombotic thrombocytopenic purpura
Other thrombocytopenias
Aplastic anemia
Anticoagulants (inappropriate doses)
Lymphomas
Liver disease (advanced)
Renal dialysis
Cancers (including brain metastases)
Infection (including mycotic aneurysms of cerebral vessels)
Oral contraceptives
Pregnancy and postpartum state
Hereditary diseases (e.g., CADASIL)

Abbreviations: CADASIL, cerebral autosomal dominant arteriopathy with subcortical infarcts and leukoencephalopathy.

Table 9-3 gives a partial list of the systemic illnesses that can be important contributing causes to bleeding that affects the brain. Systemic illnesses or medical treatments that compromise blood clotting can be major contributors to cerebral hemorrhages, whether or not there is prior damage to blood vessels supplying the brain. So can trauma. Cancers of the brain can lead to stroke-like syndromes if a bleed complicates the cancer. That includes rapid enlargement of a cancer from a bleed into it, as well as bleeding from an eroded blood vessel

Vasculitis

Vasculitis affecting the brain is rarely limited to that organ, with the exception of some forms of giant cell arteritis (temporal arteritis; see Chap. 7, Pain). Other tissues besides blood vessels of the brain are also involved in the inflammatory/autoimmune process. For instance, *Disseminated Lupus* can present clinically with abnormalities in thinking or behavior that indicate brain disease and turn out to be due to cerebral vasculitis, but systematic work-up usually reveals other systemic manifestations as well that aid in the diagnosis. That generalization also holds true for most other vasculitides. For instances, patients with brain disease as well as dry mouth and dry eyes deserve a work-up for Sjögren syndrome and possible treatment with steroids. These "*collagen-vascular*" diseases are well known to general clinicians. There is no need to belabor their mechanisms or clinical characteristics or even to list them here.

Vasculitides affecting the brain typically lead to variable neurological signs and symptoms that cannot be attributed to a single vascular distribution. They are often multifocal but can appear clinically to be unifocal. The neurological picture can resemble multiple sclerosis. (See Chap. 13, Disorders of Both Sensation and Motility.) The first important clinical manifestation of cerebral vasculitis can mimic a major psychiatric disorder—for instance, in women with Lupus. Usually the tip-off to the diagnosis is the peripheral manifestations of the disease, but finding those manifestations may require a focused work-up.

General Disorders of the Circulation

These are often due to primary disease of the heart, but can be due to blood loss (shock) or other forms of volume depletion. For cardiac disease to compromise the supply of blood to the brain significantly, cardiac output must fall enough that the "autoregulation" of the cerebral circulation fails. Arrhythmias can do that, if they are severe enough, frequent enough, and prolonged enough. So can cardiac arrest (which is of course a very bad disturbance of cardiac rhythm). The latter often leads to stupor and/or coma and/or death, despite attempts at prompt resuscitation. However, quantitatively milder forms of "global" hypoxia/ischemia can give rise to relatively selective brain damage, depending on the extent and duration of the compromise of circulation. Brain regions that can be relatively selectively damaged by global hypoxia/ischemia include the hippocampi (which are involved among other things in memory) and the basal ganglia (which are involved among other things in control of involuntary movements) .

Circulatory insufficiency that leads to clinically important brain damage is usually obvious from history, e.g. of cardiac arrest, fainting spells (including *Stokes-Adams* attacks), or prolonged shock.

Other Conditions

Other causes of strokes include other types of damage to blood vessels or to the mechanisms of coagulation. The former include, for instance, dissections of the carotids or cerebral vessels. The proportion of strokes caused by dissections is greater in those under forty years than in older patients—as much as one-third of patients in some series. Disorders of coagulation are usually well known to general clinicians. Table 9-3 gives a partial list of some of the most important of these conditions. As with vasculitis, the first manifestation of these systemic diseases may be referable to the brain. Systemic diseases that lead to bleeds or other cerebrovascular brain damage can usually be identified by their peripheral manifestations. Recognizing them is part of a good general medical work-up, which should always be done in patients with strokes.

Minor Strokes

Minor strokes—small strokes—can be harder to differentiate from other conditions affecting the brain than are larger strokes. Minor strokes can be of a number of types.

Transient Ischemic Attacks (TIAs): These are stroke-like episodes that by definition leave no neurological sequelae. The criterion of lasting neurological sequelae is *clinical.* Whether vascular disease of the brain can lead to symptoms without causing even minor permanent damage to the brain is now debated. With diffusion-weighted MRI imaging (DWI), detectable abnormalities persisted in the brains of patients who had more severe TIAs in terms of duration (>30 minutes) or disturbance of higher brain function (e.g., aphasia).[6,7] The speculation has been advanced that even more sensitive ways of detecting damage would detect persistent abnormalities even in the brains of people with milder TIAs. Presumably, meticulous neurological examinations including extensive neuropsychological testing might find residua in patients in whom a more cursory, practical exam had found none. Whether it would be worthwhile clinically to call these minor residual disabilities to the attention of the patients and their families is another question.

Unfortunately, there is as yet no way to know confidently in advance which TIAs will be followed by major strokes and which will not. Emboli can cause single attacks without sequelae. Repeated TIAs leading to the same symptoms and signs can be a warning of an impending (often thrombotic) stroke in the affected vascular area. Recently, a group at Oxford has crafted a simple clinical scoring system to help predict which "TIAs" will go on to "completed strokes."[8] Larger, independent, prospective studies are needed to evaluate whether this simple checklist is useful in general clinical practice.

When short-lived signs and symptoms like those of a TIA lead to permanent clinical evidence of a stroke, then the event is called a stroke. The permanent evidence may be limited to abnormalities on brain imaging, or it may lead to minor abnormalities that are evident on a careful neurological examination but do not bother the patient. Sometimes the patient or family will state that the patient has "never been the same" since the event, even if neurological and imaging examinations are unrevealing. Sometimes the reason may be that the "minor" event has tipped the patient into a depression. (See Chap. 3, Mood Disorders.) Sometimes the patient and family are sensitive to changes that are not demonstrable to others in the professional setting. Analogously, a famous ballerina once said, "If I do not practice, after one day I know. After two days my teacher knows. After three days the audience knows."

Accumulated damage from small strokes can lead to detectable neurological deficits. The accumulation of small strokes in white matter has been called by various names: *leukoaraiosis*, *lacunar state*, *état criblé*, and *Binswanger disease*. The neurological disabilities can take a variety of forms, varying with the functions of the nerve cells that the damaged axons were connected to. Gait abnormalities, abnormal eye movements, cognitive impairment, and probably depression are relatively common clinical expressions of "lacunar state." A recent unconfirmed report claims that small strokes in white matter often lead to "executive dysfunction" associated with frontal lobe damage, independent of where in the white matter they occur. High grade (>70%) carotid stenosis is also associated with impaired mental function, probably because of its association with strokes and perhaps because of an association with periods of underperfusion of the brain on the side of the stenosis.[9] However, it is important not to over diagnose "vascular dementia" on the basis of small strokes, clinically or on an imaging study. Small strokes in patients with dementia not only do not rule out but do not even argue against the concomitant presence of Alzheimer disease or other degenerative disease of the nervous system. (See Chap. 5, Cognitive Disorders.)

Small strokes can be asymptomatic—"silent." That may be because they occur during sleep or in areas of the brain where small decrements in tissue do not lead to obvious disabilities. Silent strokes are, however, a manifestation of vascular disease of the brain. Their presence increases the risk for both symptomatic strokes and cognitive disability. The diagnosis of silent strokes is normally made by imaging.

Depression and other psychiatric manifestations can be a result of both small and large strokes, as discussed later and in Chap. 3 (Mood Disorders). One or more small strokes knocking out regions of the brain involved in the mediation of emotion can lead to depression without clinically significant motor or sensory signs. This syndrome is particularly relevant in patients with first onset depression in later life. It is worth emphasizing again that becoming depressed is not a "normal part of aging." Excessively prolonged grief is not a healthy reaction to the personal losses that accompany reaching a ripe old age. First onset depression in an older person is an indication to look for organic brain disease and specifically for strokes, including small strokes. (See Chap. 3, Mood Disorders.) Depression is a well-recognized complication of larger strokes, perhaps more of vascular disease involving the left (normally dominant) side of the brain than the right. Fortunately, stroke-related depression usually responds eventually to standard treatment for depression, although relatively large doses of medication for relatively long times are sometimes needed.

Other psychiatric disorders can also follow strokes, including hallucinosis. Late onset psychiatric disease raises the possibility of psychiatric manifestations of cerebrovascular disease or other "organic" brain disease. Evaluation of possible stroke should be part of the work-up of such patients, including brain imaging.

Imaging

Imaging studies of the brain have become crucial to the diagnosis of stroke and to the differential diagnosis of the type of stroke. CT (computed tomography) readily detects blood within the brain or elsewhere in the cranial vault except in the posterior fossa (i.e., brainstem and cerebellum), where CT is less effective because of interference from bone. CT frequently does not reveal embolic or thrombotic strokes for several hours. MRI (magnetic resonance imaging) is better than CT for visualizing the posterior fossa and for the immediate visualization of strokes due to blood clots.

For a general clinician evaluating a patient with a clinical picture consistent with a stroke, a prompt imaging study read by a competent neuroradiologist is necessary if at all possible. Such a study is a valuable guide to treatment, as discussed below, in part by detecting bleeding that is a contraindication to *thrombolysis* with tPA and to *anticoagulation*. Treating a patient who appears to have had a cerebrovascular accident without a modern imaging study is like treating a patient with serious shortness of breath without a chest X-ray. It can be done when necessary in relatively primitive settings, but can not be defended as state-of-the-art medicine or even as conventional medical practice in the USA.

NEUROBIOLOGY

In every mammalian species, there is an organ system that is particularly prone to disease, especially in later life. Failure of that organ system becomes the most common cause of death, at least under conditions where animals do not die earlier from such external causes as infections or violence. For Wistar rats raised under laboratory conditions and eating lab chow, that organ system is the kidneys. For humans living in the Western world, it is the blood vessels. The most common cause of death in the United States is vascular disease of the heart, and the third most common is vascular disease of the brain. These together with other disorders of the blood vessels probably account for over 80% of deaths in the United States and other developed countries.

The mechanisms leading to diseases of the blood vessels tend to be relatively independent of the organs in which those blood vessels lie. That is specifically true for atherosclerosis, the most common form of blood vessel disease in the United States and other developed countries. It is also true for hyalinization of blood vessels related to high blood pressure, for infectious (*mycotic*) aneurysms, and for congenital malformations of the vasculature. These mechanisms are well known to general clinicians and well described in textbooks of Internal Medicine and Family Practice.

It is worth emphasizing here that poorly controlled hypertension is the most important single, medically modifiable risk factor for stroke. Systolic blood pressure is even more important than diastolic blood pressure.[10–13]

Since heart disease is a risk factor for stroke, measures to prevent heart disease are not only part of good general medical care but also tend to decrease the likelihood of stroke. A number of risk factors for heart disease other than high blood pressure are also independent risk factors for stroke. These include excessive weight, diabetes, and *metabolic syndrome*. Previous stroke is quantitatively the important risk factor for future stroke. That may be because having a stroke is a marker for having enough vascular disease and/or enough risk factors for stroke. Whatever the basis of the relationship, a previous stroke is not a "reversible risk factor." Once a completed stroke has happened, it can not be reversed. A number of other risk factors for stroke are also not amenable to medical intervention—for instance, advanced age and male sex. As a generalization, maintaining good health, and specifically good cardiovascular health, is good practice for avoiding strokes as well as many other disabilities.

Whether abnormalities in blood lipids are an independent risk factors for stroke is at best controversial.[10–12] Whatever relationship there might be may be mediated by their role as a risk factor for heart disease, which is itself an independent risk factor for stroke. Blood triglyceride levels above 150 mg/dL have even been reported to be associated with a diminished incidence of severe stroke. Documenting an epidemiological association between fat intake and stroke has also been hard, even though elevated fat intake contributes to atherosclerosis and cardiac disease, which are themselves risk factors for strokes.

Genetic factors can predispose to strokes. That is expected, since they can predispose to high blood pressure and other forms of cardiovascular disease. There is also a tendency for congenital aneurysms and arteriovenous malformations to run in families. Genes linked to the formation of arteriovenous malformations include those encoding the cytokine interleukin 6 (the *IL6-174G* polymorphism) and the *CCM1* and *CCM2* genes. Mutations in the endoglin and *ALK1* genes can cause a rare disorder predisposing to stroke, namely *hereditary hemorrhagic telangiectasia.* Linkage of congenital aneurysms to several regions of the human genome has been reported. Possession of the plasminogen activator-inhibitor-1 4G allele in the 4G/5G promoter polymorphism tends to worsen the outcome of subarachnoid hemorrhage. So does possessing the e-4 allele of the *APOE* gene, an allele that tends to be associated with a worse course in a number of diseases including Alzheimer dementia. It is, of course, not surprising that congenital malformations including those of the vascular bed tend to be associated with abnormalities in DNA. Presumably future research will identify links of other specific genes to risk factors for stroke.

TREATMENT

Cerebrovascular disease, like cardiovascular disease with which it is so often associated, is now a treatable condition even though it remains a major cause of death. Advances in the prevention and treatment of strokes are now occurring rapidly and are clinically important. The following discussion attempts to present the state of the art at the time this monograph is being written, but the author confidently predicts that the state of-the-art will continue to change—and to do so relatively rapidly. This discussion does not cover the rapidly developing area of surgical treatment for strokes: *carotid endarterectomy*, surgical removal of clots from the cerebral vasculature, stents, and other techniques. Nor does it cover the rapidly evolving rehabilitative techniques for stroke. It is and will remain a challenge for general clinicians to keep up with what they are obligated to know in this rapidly evolving field of therapy. Fortunately, "state-of-the-art" reviews appear regularly in major medical journals, and neurologists are widely available for consultations.

Pharmacological treatment of cerebrovascular disease is conveniently divided into three topics: prevention, acute treatment, and chronic treatment.

Prevention

Measures to hold off the progression of cerebrovascular disease are in general the same as those to retard cardiovascular disease. Guidelines for the prevention of stroke have been published.[10–14] The available evidence indicates that general clinicians often do not pay attention to these guidelines, either in the United States or in European countries with more centralized health care payment systems. Physicians need to realize that clinically silent or insignificant cerebrovascular disease is quite as important a signal of vascular disease as is clinically silent or insignificant cardiovascular disease. Both require active intervention to try to prevent clinical progression and disability. Fortunately, largely the same measures are used to control the progression of cerebrovascular disease and cardiovascular disease.

Control of high blood pressure plays if possible an even greater role in the prevention of strokes than of heart attacks. Follow-up studies are tending to imply that perhaps everyone who has had a stroke or TIA should be treated with antihypertensive medication, even if their blood pressures are not elevated according to current guidelines. As noted above, the contribution of abnormal levels of blood lipids including cholesterol to ischemic stroke is controversial. Lipid abnormalities nevertheless deserve modification as risk factors for cardiovascular disease, even apart from the role of cardiovascular disease as a risk factor for stroke.[15] Treatment with statins appears to lower the risk of stroke.[16,17] Whether statins do so directly or by their action on cardiac disease is less important than their beneficial effects. Close management of diabetes has been reported to reduce its complications including vascular complications. In essence, good general medical care to reduce cardiovascular risk factors—especially hypertension—is also good care for reducing the risk of strokes.

Anticoagulation to prevent stroke is clearly indicated in three situations: atrial fibrillation; a blood clot in the heart, particularly an anterior wall thrombus; and the presence of a prosthetic valve. Anticoagulation for these conditions is usually with a coumadin anticoagulant. It is maintained long term, unless severe enough bleeding or some other contraindication occurs. The optimal INR (international normalized ratio) is about 2 to 3. At higher INR, the risk of bleeding outweighs the benefits of anticoagulation, in prospective studies. Individualization of the coumadin dose and regular monitoring of anticoagulant status are, of course, necessary. General clinicians are very familiar with these issues. Some neurologists recommend aspirin instead of coumdin for patients with atrial fibrillation who do not have other risk factors for stroke, i.e. patients under 75 years who are free of other evidence of vascular or endocrine disease. In patients with atrial fibrillation who do not tolerate more vigorous measures, appropriate therapy is with aspirin or clopidogrel, or aspirin and clopidogrel, or other newer anticoagulants.[18–20]

Antiplatelet agents are currently the preferred treatment to prevent recurrent strokes, even in patients without atrial fibrillation or mural thrombi (Table 9-4).[18–20] Aspirin is as effective as anticoagulation in preventing recurrent nonembolic strokes and causes fewer side effects. Antiplatelet therapy may also be appropriate in patients with cognitive impairments or other evidence of brain damage from carotid disease, even in the absence of "frank strokes." Doses of aspirin within the range of 50–325 mg/day appear effective. Many clinicians recommend 82 mg/day. Other antiplatelet agents have also been recommended in some studies, notably clopidogrel (75 mg/day). If and when combined therapy with more than one antiplatelet agent is indicated is still under study. Aspirin combined with dipyridamole has been recommended by some workers for prevention of recurrent stroke in people who have already had a stroke. Probably the best course for a general clinician is to find out what is the "local standard of practice" in stroke prevention, from a neurologist or other specialist in stroke working in the same geographic area, and to document in the chart that the current local standard is being used. The "state-of-the-art" according to "expert opinion" is likely to continue being changed—"refined"—as the results of new studies become available

TABLE 9–4
Antiplatelet agents to prevent recurrent stroke

Drug(s)	Dose	Advantage over ASA alone	First-line therapy if:
Aspirin	82 mg/day	-	Cost is a factor, or intoler ance to other agents
Ticlopidine	250 mg 2id	121%	Not recommended; severe, potentially fatal side effects
Clopidogrel	75 mg/day	107%	True aspirin intolerance
Aspirin + extended-release Dipyridamole	200 mg ASA + 25 mg di pyridamole, 2id	122%	Angina: *a contraindication

Abbreviation: ASA, acetylsalicylic acid.
* Specifically unstable angina.
Source: Derived in part from Weinberger J. Managing and preventing ischemic stroke: Part II—Risk assessment and prevention of secondary ischemic stroke. *Clinical Geriatrics.* 2004;12:41–46.

In patients with risk factors for stroke but no cerebrovascular or cardiovascular events and no evidence of clinically significant brain damage, the benefits of anti-platelet or anticoagulant therapy do not outweigh the risks. A recent Cochrane data base study concluded

> Acetylsalicylic acid (ASA) did not reduce stroke or 'all cardiovascular events' compared to placebo in primary prevention patients with elevated blood pressure and no prior cardiovascular disease. Based on one large trial (HOT trial), ASA taken for 5 years reduced myocardial infarction (ARR, 0.5%, NNT 200 for 5 years), increased major hemorrhage (ARI, 0.7%, NNT 154), and did not reduce all cause mortality or cardiovascular mortality. There was no significant difference between ASA and copridogel for the composite endpoint of stroke, myocardial infarction or vascular death in one trial (CAPRIE 1996). In two small trials warfarin alone or in combination with ASA did not reduce stroke or coronary events.[21]

Surgical intervention to reduce the likelihood of stroke in patients with *symptomatic* carotid stenosis is recommended by current guidelines.

Stents are increasingly used. Whether such surgery should be done for high grade occlusions (>75%) that are not symptomatic depends in part on the skill and experience of the available vascular surgeons.[22] Expert consultation is advisable in making this decision. If preventive surgery is contemplated, there is usually enough time for the patient to go to a center where the necessary expertise is available.

Antioxidants such as vitamin E have been used to slow the progress of disease of the blood vessels, but their effects if any are controversial. A recent study reported that concomitant administration of antioxidant vitamins actually impaired the efficacy of treatment with a statin and niacin in preventing the progression of vascular stenoses.[23] Giving folate to reduce homocysteine levels has not proven useful in preventing strokes, in prospective studies.

Treatment of Acute Stroke

The optimal treatment for different types of acute strokes is a rapidly changing area. New data and new techniques are appearing. Consensus conferences lay down new guidelines with some frequency. Specialists in the treatment of stroke are obligated to keep up with this large literature. Where possible, the care of acute stroke should be left to such specialists. This is almost always possible in large medical centers, particularly those that have designated stroke centers and/or stroke teams. The use of telecommunications to make such expertise available to clinicians in other institutions is becoming more frequent. Such consultations not only improve clinical care but also can help protect against future lawsuits by disappointed patients and their families.

An ACCP (American College of Clinical Pharmacy) conference recently put forward a set of consensus guidelines.[24] The key recommendations are:

> For patients with acute ischemic stroke (AIS), we recommend administration of i.v. tissue plasminogen activator (tPA), if treatment is initiated within 3 h of clearly defined symptom onset (Grade 1A). For patients with extensive and clearly identifiable hypodensity on CT, we recommend against thrombolytic therapy (Grade 1B). For unselected patients with AIS of >3 h but <6 h, we suggest clinicians not use i.v. tPA (Grade 2A). For patients with AIS, we recommend against streptokinase (Grade 1A) and suggest clinicians not use

full-dose anticoagulation with i.v. or subcutaneous heparins or heparinoid (Grade 2B). For patients with AIS who are not receiving thrombolysis, we recommend early aspirin therapy, 160 to 325 mg q.d. (Grade 1A). For AIS patients with restricted mobility, we recommend prophylactic low-dose subcutaneous heparin or low molecular weight heparins or heparinoids (Grade 1A); and for patients who have contraindications to anticoagulants, we recommend use of intermittent pneumatic compression devices or elastic stockings (Grade 1C). In patients with acute intracerebral hematoma, we recommend the initial use of intermittent pneumatic compression (Grade 1C+). In patients with noncardioembolic stroke or transient ischemic attack (TIA) [i.e., atherothrombotic, lacunar or cryptogenic], we recommend treatment with an antiplatelet agent (Grade 1A) including aspirin, 50 to 325 mg q.d.; the combination of aspirin and extended-release dipyridamole, 25 mg/200 mg b.i.d.; or clopidogrel, 75 mg q.d. In these patients, we suggest use of the combination of aspirin and extended-release dipyridamole, 25/200 mg b.i.d., over aspirin (Grade 2A) and clopidogrel over aspirin (Grade 2B). For patients who are allergic to aspirin, we recommend clopidogrel (Grade 1C+). In patients with atrial fibrillation and a recent stroke or TIA, we recommend long-term oral anticoagulation (target international normalized ratio, 2.5; range, 2.0 to 3.0) [Grade 1A]. In patients with venous sinus thrombosis, we recommend unfractionated heparin (Grade 1B) or low molecular weight heparin (Grade 1B) over no anticoagulant therapy during the acute phase.

These recommendations require some comments. Those labeled (1A) are supported by solid evidence from structured clinical trials. The other recommendations are supported by less solid evidence. These recommendations are up-to-date for 2005, when this monograph was being written, but some of them will probably be outdated soon thereafter. As noted above, the literature in this area is in flux, is massive, and is hard to keep up with.

The use of recombinant tPA (Alteplase) to dissolve clots causing strokes has been a major advance in the treatment of cerebrovascular disease. Meta-analyses have shown clear cut benefits in properly selected patients treated within 90 minutes of a thrombotic stroke, and some benefit in patients treated for the next 90 minutes.[25] However, dissolving clots is obviously inappropriate in patients who are or have been bleeding into their brains, since the clots are preventing further brain damage in them. Imaging studies and other examinations to rule out significant hemorrhage or predispositions to bleeding (*bleeding diatheses*) are necessary before giving tPA. Major medical centers usually have designated stroke centers with special teams trained in the use of tPA for patients with strokes. The procedure does have definite risks even with experienced teams in place. The most important of these risks is hemorrhage into the brain. At the present time, tPA is the standard thrombolytic therapy for acute ischemic stroke in the United States. *Streptokinase* has proven not to be as safe, and recombinant *urokinase* is not widely used.

Treatment with tPA is spreading from hospitals with designated stroke centers to smaller community hospitals, where this treatment is usually done in consultation by telemedicine with experts in the nearest designated stroke center. The procedure currently recommended for a community hospital without a stroke center is to determine if the onset of symptoms and signs of the stroke occurred less than 3 hours before the patient arrived at the hospital. If so, an emergency brain imaging study is done to rule out bleeding. Simultaneously, blood tests are done to determine platelet count, INR, and blood glucose. The inclusion and exclusion criteria for starting intravenous therapy of tPA are listed in Table 9-5. Following these criteria is critically important. Breaks in protocol have been shown to lead to major increases in bleeding and other complications. Use of tPA in a patient who did not meet protocol is as difficult to defend as not using tPA in a patient who did. The treating physician(s) should if possible consult with the nearest stroke center, reporting the results of the initial brain scan and blood tests. If practical—that is, if it can be done rapidly enough—the consultation should be ongoing before starting the tPA drip. Logistical problems should not, however, be permitted to postpone treatment until a patient has passed beyond the time for optimal outcomes. For patients meeting the consensus for use of tPA, the agent should be given intravenously, at a dose of 0.9 mg/kg (maximum 90 mg). A bolus of 10% of this dose is given initially, and the rest infused by IV drip over the next hour. The patient should then be transported by ambulance to the stroke center. Obviously, clinical records including copies of imaging studies and results of blood tests should be sent with the patient, and the stroke center should be warned that the patient is on the way. A jargon term for this protocol is "drip and ship".

Anticoagulation for acute stroke when tPA is not suitable remains an area of controversy. Disagreements among experienced, well-informed practitioners exist despite extensive clinical research, extensive data analyses, and consensus conferences. Anticoagulation clearly benefits patients with atrial fibrillation or other cardiac sources for emboli, but anticoagulation for other stroke patients is more "iffy." Decades ago, a distinguished

TABLE 9–5

Inclusion and exclusion criteria for tPA treatment of acute ischemic stroke

Inclusion criteria

Age >18 years

Clinical diagnosis of stroke, including

- Meaningful neurological deficit
- Defined time of onset less than 3 hours previously
- No evidence of hemorrhage on CT scan

Exclusion criteria

Physical examination

- Minor impairments and/or rapidly improving clinical picture
- BP >185 systolic or >110 diastolic
- Aggressive treatment required to lower BP
- Subarachnoid hemorrhage (clinically or by imaging)
- Pericarditis complicating myocardial infarction
- Pregnancy
- Lactation

Bleeding

- Intracranially (e.g., by CT)
- History of intracranial bleeding
- GI bleeding within the previous 3 weeks
- Urinary tract bleeding within the previous 3 weeks

Bleeding diathesis

- Platelet count < 100,000 per μl
- INR >1.7
- Prothrombin time >15 seconds
- Current use of anticoagulants (including heparin with 48 hours of the stroke)

Other blood tests

- Blood glucose >400 mg/dL or <50 mg/dL

Other aspects of history

- Arterial puncture at a noncompressible site within 1 week
- Lumbar puncture within 1 week
- Seizure at stroke onset
- Head injury or stroke within the previous 3 months
- Major surgery within 2 weeks
- Major trauma within 2 weeks

Abbreviations: CT scan, computerized tomography; BP, blood pressure; GI, gastrointestinal; INR, international normalized ratio.

Source: See references 24,25 for details.

Canadian neurologist was an eloquent supporter of anticoagulation in acute stroke. When a controlled study appeared in the late 1960s that claimed that anticoagulation provided no benefits to victims of stroke, his response was "I didn't anticoagulate those people." Despite the many large studies and massive literature on this topic that have accumulated over the last 40 years, the decisions on whether or not to anticoagulate stroke victims and if so how to do so remain more or less where they were then.

The guidelines formulated by a recent conference are summarized earlier.[24] Those guidelines differentiate clearly between situations where there are solid data and other situations where the members of the consensus conference are expressing their opinions. Again, a safe practice for the general clinician is to find out what the accepted standard of practice is in the geographical region in which he or she is practicing and then to follow that standard. It is important to keep informed as changes in accepted practice occur.[25] A straightforward way to do that is to collaborate with a consultant neurologist or other clinician with special expertise in stroke care and prevention. If such an expert is not available locally, it is wise to keep in touch with the changing standards of the nearest designated stroke center.

Recently, encouraging but still preliminary results have been presented for a new treatment of hemorrhagic strokes, the injection of (recombinant) clotting factor VII to stop the bleeding.[26,27] If borne out by future studies, this would be a major advance in the treatment of this often devastating and even fatal form of cerebrovascular accident.

Surgical treatment of strokes is a burgeoning and controversial field.[28,29] Enthusiastic initial reports of successes of surgical removal of clots from arteries sometimes giving gratifyingly good results, even with surprising delays after the stroke before the patient came to surgery,[28] require extensive confirmation before this controversial technique is adopted.[30] Surgical treatment of acute stroke is beyond the scope of this monograph, which focuses on pharmacological treatments.

One of the complications of severe strokes—of bleeds even more than clots—is brain swelling, often leading to compression of the brain stem and death (coning). The recognition and treatment of this set of complications is discussed in Chap. 10 (Disorders of Awareness) of this monograph. Treatment includes both medical and surgical interventions. It can sometimes be life-saving. In patients who are suspected of having this complication, *immediate* treatment and consultation with a neurosurgeon are indicated.

The process of recovery from stroke usually follows a more or less logarithmic curve. Recovery of function is most rapid at early times, as brain swelling decreases and blood supply increases to areas where it was compromised by swelling. Progress then becomes slower over the coming weeks and months. Clinically significant progress is less likely after 6 months. Rarely, it can occur even years later, particularly with newer rehabilitation techniques.

Good general medical care is critically important in the acute treatment of stroke. Blood pressure should be maintained in a high normal or slightly above normal range. Both excessively high and excessively low blood pressures have bad prognostic implications in this population. The occurrence of a stroke does not change the guidelines for age appropriate blood pressure levels. In stroke, as in many other disabling neurological diseases, infection is often the immediate cause of death. Infections including pneumonia typically require active treatment. That specifically includes *aspiration pneumonia*. Prevention of bed-sores is important. As usual, *incontinence* can contribute to severe local infections. Other aspects of good medical care are also important, including nutrition and maintaining salt and water balance (*hydration, electrolyte balance*). The association between stroke and heart attack is close and requires monitoring of cardiac health in stroke patients, including diagnostic ECGs (electrocardiograms) as part of the stroke work-up. If cardiac arrhythmia is suspected, longer term (Holter) monitoring can be in order. The indications for heart medications are well known to general clinicians and do not need to be discussed here. That includes the principle that even appropriate anti-arrhythmics have an inherent potential to become pro-arrhythmics as cardiac status changes.

Rehabilitation

Patients who have had a stroke tend to fall into three groups in regard to prognosis. In perhaps 30% of patients who have had a first stroke, the clinical sequelae are so mild that rehabilitation has not been found to improve clinical outcome significantly. In another group—perhaps 50%—rehabilitation in a specialized, expert setting improves not only short term recovery but also the extent of recovery after 2 years. The remaining patients are typically so severely brain damaged that there is little hope for significant rehabilitation. This group tends to need chronic nursing care for as long as they live, most often in nursing homes. As strokes recur and damage more and more brain, the prognosis and the utility of rehabilitation worsen. How long intensive medical care is justified in patients who are very severely disabled by strokes is a contentious topic that goes far beyond the scope of this monograph.

Rehabilitation for stroke is a highly specialized area with its own body of knowledge and its own continuously growing literature. Non-pharmacological care involves splints, exercises, teaching the patient to use optimally what brain he or she has left, and modifications of the patient's environment to allow maximal independence. Medications are available for complications such as pain, spasticity, urinary or fecal incontinence or retention, and so on. These medicines are the same as for these problems in other settings. It is probably wise for the general clinician to provide such medical treatment in consultation with an expert in stroke rehabilitation.

Recent studies at both the laboratory and clinical level show unexpected and gratifying plasticity in the brains of adult humans and other mammals. Newer techniques including robotics have led to surprising benefits even in patients who had their strokes as much as 2 years ago and appeared clinically stable.[31] Studies in experimental animals suggest that innovative techniques such as stem cell transplantation and the use of growth factors may eventually reach the point of being clinically useful. As yet, they have no clinical relevance beyond hope.

Chronic Care after Strokes

A number of problems common in people who have had strokes can respond gratifyingly to medications. Prominent among these problems are psychiatric issues. A degree of coarsening of behavior (*disinhibition*) is common. Strokes also predispose to dementia and to depression. Sometimes they lead to frank hallucinations or delusions that may require treatment. As always, the principle is to treat disability not statistical abnormality. Training the people who will provide care for stroke survivors at home improves outcome and is economically valuable, at least in England.[32] That can include training in when and how to use medication, including not using medication too much or too often.

Disinhibition is a common and often difficult consequence of a stroke. Loss of brain substance can lead to loss of socialization skills and other inhibitions that we have hopefully learned while growing up. That generalization clearly applies to people who have had strokes. Stroke survivors sometimes say that having been close to death makes them care less what they say and do. That may be a conscious reaction to a life-threatening event, a rationalization of a change in behavior due to brain damage, or both.

Whether or not "coarsening" of behavior needs treatment depends on circumstances. It can be fatal if an unarmed stroke survivor in a wheel chair insults terrorists so bluntly that they throw him in the ocean to drown. Disinhibited behavior can be very unpleasant and lead to placement if it disrupts a family or threatens a paid caregiver. Treatment is symptomatic, with anti-anxiety drugs discussed in Chap. 6 (Anxiety) or when necessary with antipsychotics discussed in Chap. 4 (Thought Disorders). As always, clinical judgment is required. Behavior that doesn't bother anyone doesn't need treatment.

Dementia occurs in as many as one-third of patients studied a few months after having had a stroke. Also, a stroke at least doubles the likelihood of developing dementia.[33] That appears true even allowing for the inability of patients with aphasia to perform on tests that require language. Chapter 5 (Cognitive Disorders) discusses at some length the complex relationship between cerebrovascular disease and degenerative disease in causing dementia—specifically the relationship between "Alzheimer disease" and "multi-infarct dementia." As pointed out there, dementia as now defined neuropsychologically is not a frequent result of cerebrovascular disease alone without concomitant neurodegenerative disease.

Depression is a frequent and treatable complication of cerebrovascular disease. Using a strict definition, depression may occur in as many as a third or more of patients with strokes. The suggestion has been made that depression is more common in people with left-sided (dominant) rather than right-sided (non-dominant) brain damage, and frontal brain damage rather than primarily posterior damage. As discussed in Chap. 3 (Mood Disorders), depression can be the presenting clinical problem in a patient whose stroke-affected part of the brain is involved in the modulation of affect. Post-stroke depression can occur without motor or sensory signs, if the stroke did not cause enough damage to areas involved in movement or sensation to lead to clinically detectable abnormalities. Patients with stroke who also suffer from depression have a poorer functional outcome.[34] That correlation does not indicate whether poor functional outcome leads to depression or depression to poor functional outcome. As discussed in Chap. 3 (Mood Disorders), the biology of depression involves impaired central serotonin and sometimes noradrenaline function. Both the serotonergic cells of the raphe nuclei and the noradrenergic cells of the nucleus cereolus project widely in the brain, so that strokes are likely to damage their nerve endings. Extensive enough damage to the projections of these cells may damage the bodies of these cells as well. An attractive, simple explanation of the correlation between depression and poor outcome from stroke is that the worse the stroke, the more likely there is to be a biological basis for concomitant depression.

Happily, stroke-related depression typically responds well to standard treatments discussed in Chap. 3 (Mood Disorders). These specifically include SSRIs. Poorly responsive stroke-related depression may require more vigorous treatment, up to and including electric shock. Depression after stroke is common but is *not* a "normal," "reasonable" reaction. These patients are suffering. They deserve treatment that is as vigorous as necessary.

Medical problems requiring good general medical care are common in patients who survive stroke. This is in general an elderly population with proven atherosclerotic vascular disease. Stroke survivors are at risk for hip fractures, particularly on the side of a paretic leg. Guidelines for caring for stroke survivors have been put forward.[35] These are, of course, guidelines. As always, individualization of care and good clinical judgment about which treatments are appropriate are necessary.

REFERENCES

1. Indeed, more familiar than the author of this monograph.
2. Victor M, Roper AH. *Principles of Neurology*. 7th ed. McGraw-Hill, New York, pp. 821–924.
3. Adams HP, Hachinski V, Norris JW. *Ischemic Cerebrovascular Disease (Contemporary Neurology Series)*. Oxford, NY, 2001.
4. Witt BJ, Brown RD Jr, Jacobsen SJ, et al. A community-based study of stroke incidence after myocardial infarction. *Ann Intern Med*. 2005;143:785–92.
5. A tragic misdiagnosis is attributing intermittent neck pain to tension headache or psychosomatic causes instead of to an aneurysm that is potentially curable by surgery. By the time the aneurysm calls attention to itself by bleeding massively, it may be too late.
6. Inatomi Y, Kimura K, Yonehara T, et al. DWI abnormalities and clinical characteristics in TIA patients. *Neurology*. 2004;62:376–80.
7. Warrach S, Kidwell, CS. The redefinition of TIA: the uses and limitations of DWI in acute ischemic cerebrovascular syndromes. *Neurology*. 2004; 62:359–360.
8. Rothwell PM, Giles MF, Flossmann E, et al. A simple score (ABCD) to identify individuals at high early risk of stroke after transient ischaemic attack. *Lancet*. 2005;366:29–36.
9. Johnston SC, O'Meara ES, Manolio TA, et al. Cognitive impairment and decline are associated with carotid artery disease in patients without clinically evident cerebrovascular disease. *Ann Int Med*. 2004;140:237–247.

10. Smaha LA, American Heart Association. The American Heart Association Get with the Guidelines Program. *Am Heart J*. 2004;148(suppl 5):S46–48.
11. Akopov S, Cohen SN. Preventing stroke: a review of current guidelines. *J Am Med Dir Assoc*. 2003;(suppl 5):S127–132.
12. Chapman N, Huxley R, Anderson C, et al. Writing Committee for the PROGRESS Collaborative Group. Effects of a perindopril-based blood pressure-lowering regimen on the risk of recurrent stroke according to stroke subtype and medical history: the PROGRESS trial. *Stroke*. 2004:35: 116–121.
13. Chobanian AV Chobanian AV, Bakris GL, et al. Joint National Committee on Prevention, Detection, Evaluation, and Treatment of High Blood Pressure. National Heart, Lung, and Blood Institute; National High Blood Pressure Education Program Coordinating Committee. The seventh Report of the Joint National Committee on Prevention, Detection, Evaluation, and Treatment of High Blood Pressure: The JNC 7 report. *J Amer Med Assoc*. 2003;289:2560–2572.
14. Bowman TS, Sesso HD, Ma J, et al. Cholesterol and the risk of ischemic stroke. *Stroke*. 2003;34:2930–2934.
15. He K, Merchant A, Rimm EB, et al. Dietary fat intake and risk of stroke in male US healthcare professionals: 14-year prospective cohort study. *BMJ*. 2003:327:777–781.
16. Heart Protection Study Collaborative Group. Effects of cholesterol lowering with simvastatin on stroke and other major vascular events in 20,356 people with cerebrovascular disease or other high-risk conditions. *Lancet*. 2004;363:757–767.
17. Trubelja N, Vaughan C, Coplan NL. The role of statins in preventing stroke. *Prev Cardiol*. 2005 Spring;8(2):98–101.
18. Rockson SG, Albers GW. Comparing the guidelines: anticoagulation therapy to optimize stroke prevention in patients with atrial fibrillation. *J Am Coll Cardiol*. 2004 March 17;43(6):929–935.
19. Waldo AL. New possibilities in anticoagulant management of atrial fibrillation. *Rev Cardiovasc Med*. 2004;(suppl 5)5:S30–38.
20. Tran H, Anand SS. Oral antiplatelet therapy in cerebrovascular disease, coronary artery disease, and peripheral arterial disease. *JAMA*. 2004;292: 1867–1874.
21. Lip GY, Felmeden DC. Antiplatelet agents and anticoagulants for hypertension. *Cochrane Database Syst Rev*. 2004;(3):CD003186.
22. Bond DR, Rerkasem K, Shearman CP, et al. Time trends in the published risks of stroke and death due to endarterectomy for symptomatic carotid stenosis. *Cerebrovasc Dis*. 2004:18:37–46.
23. Brown BG, Zhao XQ, Chait A, et al. Simvastatin and niacin, antioxidant vitamins, or the combination for the prevention of coronary disease. *N Eng J Med*. 2001;345:1583–1592.

24. Albers GW, Amarenco P, Easton JD, et al. Antithrombotic and thrombolytic therapy for ischemic stroke: the Seventh ACCP Conference on Antithrombotic and Thrombolytic Therapy. *Chest.* 2004;(suppl 3):483S–512.
25. Hacke W, Donnan G, Fieschi C, et al. ATLANTIS Trials Investigators; ECASS Trials Investigators; NINDS rt-PA Study Group Investigators. Association of outcome with early stroke treatment: pooled analysis of ATLANTIS, ECASS, and NINDS rt-PA stroke trials. *Lancet.* 2004;363:768–774.
26. Mayer SA, Brun NC, Begtrup K, et al. Recombinant Activated Factor VII Intracerebral Hemorrhage Trial Investigators. Recombinant activated factor VII for acute intracerebral hemorrhage. *N Eng J Med.* 2005;352:777–785.
27. Brown DL, Morgenstern LB. Stopping the bleeding in intracerebral hemorrhage. *N Eng J Med.* 2005;352:828–830.
28. Alexandrov AV. Ultrasound identification and lysis of clots. *Stroke.* 2004;35(11 suppl 1):2722–2725.
29. Gobin YP Starkman S, Duckwiler GR, et al. A Phase I study of mechanical embolus removal in cerebral ischemia. *Stroke.* 2004;35:2848–2854.
30. Nakano T, Ohkuma H. Surgery versus conservative therapy for intracerebral haemorage: is there an end to the long controversy? *Lancet.* 2005;365:361–362.
31. Lynch D, Ferrar M, Krol J, et al. Continuous passive motion improves shoulder joint integrity following stroke. *Clin Rehab.* 2005;19:1–6.
32. Patel A, Knapp M, Evans A, et al. Training caregivers of stroke patients: economic evaluation. *BMJ.* 2004;328:1102–1104.
33. Ivan CS, Seshadri S, Beiser A, et al. Dementia after stroke: the Framingham study. *Stroke.* 2004;35:1264–1268.
34. Apprelos P, Viitanen M. Prevalence and prediction of depression at one year in a Swedish population-based cohort with first ever stroke. *J Stroke Cerebrovasc Dis.* 2004;13:52–57.
35. Gordon NF, Gulanick M, Costa F, et al. American Heart Association Council on Clinical Cardiology, Subcommittee on Exercise, Cardiac Rehabilitation, and Prevention; the Council on Cardiovascular Nursing; the Council on Nutrition, Physical Activity, and Metabolism; and the Stroke Council. Physical activity and exercise recommendations for stroke survivors: an American Heart Association scientific statement from the Council on Clinical Cardiology, Subcommittee on Exercise, Cardiac Rehabilitation, and Prevention; the Council on Cardiovascular Nursing; the Council on Nutrition, Physical Activity, and Metabolism; and the Stroke Council. *Circulation.* 2004;109: 2031–2041.

CHAPTER TEN

Disorders of Awareness: Dizziness, Fainting, Fits, Stupor, and Coma and Related Conditions

This chapter groups together a number of conditions that impair awareness and eventually consciousness. General clinicians frequently see patients with these problems. Effective treatments are available for some of these disorders. Even where treatment is primarily in the hands of neurologists—such as for seizures—general clinicians need to be sensitive to the side effects of the medications used, since generalists are very likely to have patients who need to take these medicines.

The terms *awareness* and *consciousness* are widely used but hard to define. Psychologists and philosophers have proposed definitions and even developed formal procedures to measure these capacities as they have defined them. Detailed discussion of these ideas and their philosophical and theological underpinnings is beyond the scope of this monograph. Here the terms are used in their widely understood, "common sense" meanings.

DIZZINESS

Classification and Diagnosis

Many patients complain to their general physicians of having suffered episodes of "dizziness." That same term is used colloquially both for "light-headedness" or "feeling faint" and for true vertigo.

Light-Headedness: *Light-headedness* can refer to a number of conditions, varying from trivial to serious. Fortunately, this sensation most often turns out not to be associated with major disease. Feelings of being "light-headed" or "not quite there" are often a physical expression of a psychological disability. They are often physical expressions (*somatizations*) of anxiety, and are frequently mediated by excessively rapid breathing (*hyperventilation*). (See Chap. 6, Anxiety, and Chap. 14, Disorders of Conduct.) These feelings can disappear as external stress lessens. When hyperventilation is the mechanism for light-headedness, breathing into the proverbial paper bag or similar container can "cure" the sensation by preventing loss of CO_2 (hypocarbia). If it does, the successful treatment more or less establishes the diagnosis. When light-headedness is associated with specific situations it can be a manifestation of a phobia, for example, "supermarket syndrome" or "movie-theatre syndrome." (See Chap. 6, Anxiety.) Medications can cause light-headedness, including many psychiatric medications.

Light-headedness can have a medical cause, sometimes serious. Current American textbooks of psychiatry discuss dizziness in the context of drug side effects. Lightheadedness can also be the presenting complaint of *postural hypotension*, *hypoglycemia*, reasonably severe *anemia*, *aortic stenosis*, and *cardiac arrhythmias* with episodes of inadequate perfusion of the brain. Occasionally, this relatively non-specific complaint is a clinical manifestation of significant brain disease—for instance, seizures (see below) or an impending stroke. (See Chap. 9, Cerebrovascular Disorders.). Extensive biological work-up of all patients with this complaint is not feasible practically nor is it good clinical practice. Medical tests can encourage somatization in a suggestible person and thereby tend to perpetuate what could have been a self-limited problem. On the other hand, no one wants to pooh-pooh a complaint that turns out to be the signal of a serious illness. The differential diagnosis of light-headedness challenges a physician's clinical acumen. As usual, physicians must exercise clinical judgment and continually reevaluate that judgment in the light of the patient's clinical course.

Vertigo: *Vertigo*, in contrast to light-headedness, is generally a sign of organic disease, involving the labyrinth, the vestibular nerve, or the vestibular nuclei in the brain stem. The exceptions to that generalization are uncommon to rare. Patients with vertigo complain of their surroundings moving around them, or of feeling that their body is rotating or whirling, or of sensing an up-and-down or to-and-from movement. Sometimes they say the feel like they are on a ship in a rough sea. Nausea, vomiting, ringing in the ears (*tinnitus*) or deafness frequently accompany episodes of vertigo. Lying still in an appropriate position usually stops true vertigo. Vertigo that occurs only on lying down, standing up, or turning is typically harmless (the benign positional vertigo of Bárány). Vertigo can constitute the aura of a seizure (*vertiginous epilepsy*), but the balance problem is typically rapidly overwhelmed by other manifestations of the fit. A variety of diseases can affect the labyrinth and lead to vertigo. The common, self-limited diseases of the labyrinth are often attributed to viral infections. Streptomycin and other aminoglycoside antibiotics are potentially toxic to the ear. They can damage both hearing and balance, sometimes permanently. Vertigo typically diminishes or goes away entirely if patients lie down. Sometimes they must lie down in a specific position. *Vestibular rehabilitation* consists of a series of exercises that stimulate the vestibular system and often benefit patients by leading to better central nervous system compensation for vestibular input. Medications used to treat vertigo are similar to those used to treat Ménière disease, as discussed in the next paragraph.

Ménière Disease: This is a relatively common form of recurrent vertigo associated with deafness and tinnitus, and attributed to abnormalities of fluid within the labyrinth. Treatment is a combination of bed rest, oral antihistaminic agents such as *meclizine* (Bonine, Antivert), or the cholinergic blocker *scopolamine* transdermally. Conventional attempts at reducing recurrences include a low salt diet and/or diuretics or other dehydrating agents such as glycerol, but these interventions have not been tested in rigorous clinical trials. Often Ménière disease can be controlled by standard doses of antihistaminic medications such as meclizine (Antivert, Bonine) or *cyclizine* (Marezine). Sometimes transdermal scopolamine is necessary, and sometimes suppositories against vomiting are helpful, such as *promethazine* (Phenergan, 200 mg) or *trimethobenzamide* (Tigan). Not rarely, medication needs to be combined with bed rest. Severe Ménière disease should be treated by—or at a minimum in consultation with—a specialist. Surgery can become the best treatment in severely disabled patients. Surgery risks accidentally cutting the auditory portion of cranial nerve VIII in the course of transecting the vestibular portion of that nerve However, for people who are already deaf in that ear, that does them no further practical harm.

FAINTING

People who faint not only "feel faint" but actually lose consciousness and with it postural tone and therefore the ability to stand. Typically, such episodes of *syncope* have a sudden onset, are short, and finish with complete recovery without medical intervention. The difference between syncope and a number of other disorders such as catalepsy is that people with syncope characteristically lose consciousness, at least transiently. In practice, the relationship between light-headedness and fainting—between presyncope and syncope—is often close. Furthermore, there are some patients—primarily elderly women—who have "drop attacks" in which they fall without losing consciousness. The evaluation and care of patients with drop attacks is similar enough to that for patients with syncope that most the following discussion applies to both. In some series, careful medical investigation can yield a specific cause for the attacks in a high proportion of patients.[1]

The cause of fainting is almost always inadequate blood flow to the brain. A variety of conditions can cause transiently inadequate cerebral blood flow, most of them extrinsic to the nervous system (Table 10-1). Primary diseases of the heart that can cause fainting are well known to general clinicians. Failure of control of blood pressure by the blood vessels can cause faints. These *vasogenic* attacks could also be classified as *neurogenic*, since they typically involve failures of neural control of the reactivity of blood vessels. The term *neurocardiac syncope* has therefore replaced the older term *vasovagal attack*. These episodes typically involve the release of a pulse of adrenalin in response to a frightening episode, followed by increased activity of the cholinergic vagus nerve. Different people are susceptible to different stimuli—sometimes something as mild as the sight of blood. A painful illness can also precipitate such an attack, particularly pain in the abdominal or sexual organs. Excessive dilation of the peripheral blood vessels can prevent the return of adequate blood to the heart—for instance, people can faint on a very hot day when their peripheral vessels dilate to help themselves cool off. Drinking too much alcohol increases that risk.

TABLE 10–1
Causes of fainting

Cardiac
Arrhythmias
Myocardial infarction
Heart failure with low cardiac output
Aortic stenosis (including hypertrophic subaortic stenosis)
Tamponade (pericarditis)
Pulmonary embolism
Vasogenic
Vasovagal (vasodepressor)
Vasodilatation (exposure to heat, alcohol, etc.)
Orthostatic hypotension
Postprandial failure of vasogenic regulation
Carotid sinus sensitivity
Other causes of impaired venous return (urination, coughing, Valsalva)
Autonomic failure
Other
Psychogenic (hysteria)
Hypoxia
Hypoglycemia
Small strokes

(That of course includes drinking lots of beer on a holiday spent on the beach or in a park.) In some people too much exercise can precipitate a faint, perhaps because of dilatation of the blood vessels in their muscles. Inappropriate sensitivity of the *carotid sinus* can cause fainting, which can be mimicked by massaging the carotid sinus. Often these faints are benign, but they can be the signal of serious disease including atherosclerosis of the opposite carotid artery or tumor pressing on a carotid artery. Carotid massage should not be done if there is a bruit or other evidence of atherosclerosis of either carotid artery.

Several types of fainting occur much more often in older than in younger people. *Orthostatic hypotension* occurs when the peripheral blood vessels do not contract quickly enough on standing up, resulting in pooling of blood in the legs and sometimes abdomen. As general clinicians know, the diagnosis is made by history, by measuring blood pressure when the patient is lying down and then standing up, and by observing the patient for symptoms when he or she stands up quickly. Tilt-table testing is another useful diagnostic maneuver. Medicines that can contribute to orthostasis include

β-blockers, diuretics, some antidepressants, and some drugs against high blood pressure (particularly antihypertensives that act on the sympathetic nervous system). *Post-prandial hypotension* is a special form of orthostatic hypotension in which blood pools in the abdominal vessels after meals, without adequate compensatory constriction of other vessels. Post-prandial hypotension can cause falls in older people, particularly in nursing homes. Fainting after urinating (*micturition syncope*), after coughing (tussive syncope), or after straining that causes a Valsalva maneuver are also well known. Fainting incurs the risk of falling, and falls can be dangerous in older people with brittle bones and a tendency to heal slowly. A faint that leads to a hip fracture can start a train of events that kills an older person.

The diseases of the brain associated with neurological failure to regulate blood vessels are discussed elsewhere in this monograph. Peripheral neuropathies including diabetic neuropathy can cause orthostatic hypotension by interfering with the transmission of information to the blood vessels to constrict. Other examples include diseases such as *Combined Systems Disease* that impair autonomic function in the brain. (See Chap. 11, Disorders of Motility.) Postural hypotension and failure to control cardiac rate in response to activity can be major problems in these syndromes. People with transient ischemic attacks or minor strokes can have brief episodes of unconsciousness that can be mistaken for faints. Fainting can be the first manifestation of a bleed, either into the brain or into a meningeal space. This is typically associated with headache. An imaging study can help with this diagnosis. (See Chap. 9, Cerebrovascular Disorders.) Seizures, which are a classic cause of transient loss of consciousness, are discussed below.

Fainting can be a manifestation of "hysteria," but that is a risky diagnosis to make. A famous study in the 1960s from the National Hospital for Neurological Diseases in Queen Square, London, described follow-up studies of women who had received that diagnosis. Within 15 years, half were dead of the disease that had been misdiagnosed as hysteria. More recent studies have claimed much higher accuracy in diagnosis, but follow-up periods were also shorter.[2] The frequent "fainting" among proper Victorian women may have been due in part to their very tight corsets, which interfered with their taking a deep breath. Cultural expectations also played a role, although even at that time Rudyard Kipling pointed out that "the colonel's lady and Suzy O'Grady are sisters under the skin." The current edition of the DSM-IV-RT (Diagnostic and Statistical Manual of the American Psychiatric Association) does not include the word "hysteria" in the index.

Acute treatment of fainting involves keeping the patients lying flat until their head clears. The prone position counteracts the pooling of blood in the periphery and thereby tends to restore circulation to the brain. Positioning the patient with legs higher than the head makes sense. The patient's tongue should not be allowed to slip into the throat, and the patient should be watched for a few minutes after getting up. Obviously, if the faint is due to blood loss or cardiac arrhythmia or other concomitant condition, appropriate medical care needs to be given promptly. More chronic interventions to prevent fainting depend on the cause of the faints. Treatment of primary disease of the heart is part of the mainstream of general medicine. There is neither space nor reason to discuss it in any detail here, including the potential difficulties with diagnosing and treating episodic cardiac arrhythmias, and the principle that all anti-arrhythmics are potentially pro-arrhythmics. Common sense measures well known to general clinicians can frequently reduce the frequency of fainting. A reasonable treatment is avoiding the situation that induces the faint or, where necessary, desensitizing the patient to that situation. Treatment with anti-anxiety agents may be useful. (See Chap. 6, Anxiety). People with orthostatic hypotension should get up slowly and hold on to something until their head clears. Where necessary, they can wear support stockings (Supp-Hose) to prevent blood pooling in their legs. In younger patients with relatively severe orthostatic hypotension, it is sometimes appropriate to institute high salt diets or treatment with salt-retaining steroids (e.g., fludrocortisone acetate (Florinef), 2.5 mg PO q. 4 hours, slowly titrated up to 5 mg PO q. 4–6 hrs). These are, however, risky interventions in older people at risk of heart failure. Drugs that are associated with orthostasis should be replaced where possible by drugs that are not. Patients with post-prandial hypotension should sit still after eating rather than getting up promptly to engage in activities. Men with micturitional syncope should pee sitting down. People in whom straining causes fainting should avoid straining. People with hypersensitive carotid sinuses should wear loose shirts and learn to turn their heads without putting pressure on the carotid sinus.

FITS (SEIZURES)

Fits (seizures, epilepsy) are a common cause of transient loss of awareness. Their cause is disordered electrical activity in the brain. Generally but not invariably this leads to abnormal activities of muscles. The common term *epilepsy* tends to have a bad connotation in the minds of many non-professionals. It is often wise to avoid it when talking to patients and their families. One reason for this fear is the association of epilepsy with a number of disorders that slow mental development in children, including certain inborn errors of metabolism and other conditions which shorten a child's life. Seizures can also be the first manifestation of unpleasant and life-threatening diseases of the brain in adults including elderly people—for instance, of cancers in the brain.

Fits are common. About 1% of the United States population suffer from epilepsy. Perhaps 20% will have a seizure at some time in their lives. General clinicians are very likely to have patients who suffer from fits. Although the seizure disorder is best treated primarily by a neurologist, general clinicians need to be familiar with the common anti-seizure medications and particularly with their side effects.

Classification and Diagnosis

Fits take many forms. How a fit manifests itself in an individual patient depends on the nature of the disturbance in the brain of that person and on the detailed characteristics of his or her brain. Classifying seizures into groups is useful, however, for convenience and as a guide to treatment. Nomenclature has changed over the last 40 years and continues to be modified. Table 10-2 presents the international classification of seizure disorders at the time this monograph is being written. A number of patterns of generalized seizures occur primarily in children and are therefore beyond the scope of this monograph. They include classical *Petit Mal* epilepsy (absence spells lasting some seconds, which may interfere with schoolwork), variants associated with slow mental development including the *Lennox-Gastaut syndrome* and *West syndrome,* and *atonic* and *myoclonic* epilepsy including juvenile myoclonic epilepsy.

Recognizing seizures requires differentiating them from other types of transient loss of consciousness. Table 10-3 lists some diagnostic clues that the cause of transient unconsciousness is a fit rather than a simple faint. As noted in the legend to that table, these differences are rough statistical impressions. They are *not* absolute distinctions. Classic generalized tonic-clonic (*Grand Mal*) seizures or typical focal seizures that progress to generalized seizures require little diagnostic acumen, but more subtle manifestations can be hard to recognize, as in many *complex partial* seizures involving the temporal or frontal lobes. EEG can be a valuable tool, although it is important to recognize that seizures can occur

TABLE 10–2
International classification of seizures

Generalized seizures

(Symmetrical, without focal onset)
1. Tonic, clonic, tonic-clonic (*grand mal*)
2. Absence (*petit mal*)
   >With loss of consciousness only
   >Complex—with brief tonic, clonic, or automatic movements
3. Lennox-Gastaut syndrome
4. Juvenile myoclonic epilepsy
5. Infantile spasms (West syndrome)
6. Atonic (astatic, akinetic), sometimes with myoclonic jerks.

Partial (Focal) seizures

(With focal onset)
1. Simple (consciousness not impaired)
   >Motor (frontal lobe origin; tonic, clonic, tonic-clonic; Jacksonian; epilepsia partiala continualis
   >Somatosensory or special sensory (visual, auditory, olfactory, gustatory, vertiginous)
   >Autonomic
   >Pure psychic
2. Complex (consciousness impaired)
   >Beginning as simple partial seizures, going on to impairment of consciousness
   >Impairment of consciousness at outset

Special epileptic syndromes

1. Myoclonus and myoclonic seizures
2. Reflex epilepsy
3. Acquired aphasia with convulsive disorder
4. Febrile and other seizures of infancy and childhood
5. Hysterical seizures

in people with normal EEGs, and that all people with abnormal EEGs do not have clinically significant seizures. (Some of the childhood epilepsies are associated with characteristic EEG findings.)

The basic tool for diagnosing seizures is history. Seldom do patients make life easy for the diagnostician by having a seizure in the examining room.

Generalized Fits: These can, as noted above, be relatively easy to recognize, particularly in adults. In classical *Grand Mal* epilepsy, a prodrome ("aura") often occurs immediately before the attack. It is followed

TABLE 10–3
Clues to distinguishing seizures and faints

Seizures	Faints
Occur sitting, standing, or lying down	Occur while standing*
Color in face normal	Face pale
More sudden onset†	Often preceded by faintness
Tongue often bitten	Tongue rarely bitten
Slower return of consciousness	Relatively rapid return of consciousness
Sequelae largely mental or headache	Sequela largely physical weakness
Relatively frequent recurrence	Less-frequent recurrence††

* Except unconsciousness due to heart block, that is, Stokes-Adams attacks
† Not counting prodrome and aura
†† Does not hold in older people

by patients falling unconscious and then having *tonic* (tense) and then *clonic* (shaking) movements. The patients often wet themselves and often bite their tongues, and generally end up limp in a deep coma from which they awake spontaneously with no memory of the event. Often they have a pulsating headache after they regain consciousness. Sometimes there is weakness for hours or more (*Todd's paralysis*), which may involve only a single limb. Characteristic abnormalities are usually present on the electroencephalogram (EEG) during the seizures and even between seizures (e.g., an *epileptogenic focus*).

Focal Fits: These begin with abnormal electric activity in a particular part of the brain, which can be recognized by the initial manifestations of the seizure. Focal epilepsy beginning in the motor area leads to motor manifestations, for instance of the eyes (*versive seizures*), of the hand (Jacksonian seizures), of the toes, or more rarely of other parts of the body. If the epileptic focus is primarily in the motor areas involved in speech, the seizures can cause brief loss of the ability to speak (*ictal aphasia*), which does not always generalize and is not always associated with loss of consciousness. These fits can thus manifest themselves as brief episodes of *productive aphasia.* Seizures beginning in the somatosensory cortex lead to unusual sensations as their earliest manifestation—most commonly "pins and needles," sometimes visual, sometimes auditory, and sometimes a sense of vertigo. Odd smells, tastes, or vague and indefinable sensations are often associated with seizures beginning in a temporal lobe.

Complex Partial Seizures: Fits involving the temporal lobe require special discussion. These can take many forms, some of which are difficult to distinguish from a number of other diseases including "psychiatric" diseases. The initial event of the seizure may be a hallucination or perceptual illusion including "undescribable" and often unpleasant smells, tastes, or sensations. These seizures can lead primarily to altered intrapsychic experiences. Intense joy, sadness, sexual arousal, or other intense emotions may occur without motor manifestations or loss of consciousness. Intense religious experiences can occur, and the patient can be convinced that these were revelations from a Deity.[3] Sometimes these patients have a sense that they have previously experienced something going on currently (*déjà vu*) or a sense of depersonalization and not experiencing a current event (*jamais vu*). Rarely brief attacks of loss of memory are the only clinical manifestation of temporal lobe epilepsy (*transient epileptic amnesia*). Combinations of subjective experiences can occur. Sometimes complex partial seizures involving the temporal lobe progress to a period of unresponsiveness.

Patients may exhibit altered behavior of which they are typically not consciously aware—"automatisms." These can be simple behaviors such as smacking of the lips but can also take the form of apparently purposive complex behavior such as undressing in public. Patients can strike out at people whom they perceive as threatening or otherwise disturbing them. Whether temporal lobe disease can lead to planned violent or criminal behavior is controversial. Some neurologists are sure that it can; many others strongly doubt that. In patients with temporal lobe epilepsy, about a quarter have primarily psychic manifestations, about a third automatic behavior, and between 40% and 50% have motor abnormalities. As noted, all three can occur in the same patient.

A difficult and unsettled question is how often "psychiatric" disease is a manifestation of aberrant electrical activity in a temporal lobe. After seizures affecting this part of the brain, some patients become psychotic for weeks, often with paranoid delusions. In epilepsy referral centers, where particularly difficult patients tend to be seen, perhaps two-thirds of patients with temporal lobe seizures have also carried a psychiatric diagnosis at some time during their lives, and 10% are psychotic when first seen. Behavioral problems can be so characteristic in epileptics, even between seizures, that an "epileptic personality disorder" has been described. Characteristics include a tendency to speak and particularly to write at length, relatively slow and rigid thinking, a tendency to religious mysticism,[3] often bad temper and aggressiveness, emotionality including mood swings, and a tendency to paranoia. Temporal lobe disease can mimic classical psychiatric syndromes, including not only schizophrenia and schizoid personality disorders but also anxiety and mood disorders. The author has seen temporal lobe disease manifest itself as typical manic-depressive illness, as diagnosed by an expert psychiatrist.[4]

EEG can often help with the diagnosis. Sometimes *nasopharyngeal* leads reveal aberrant temporal lobe activity undetected by scalp electrodes. Sometimes studies with implanted electrodes reveal a previously undocumented seizure disorder. Other less invasive techniques are in development, and are available through consultations with neurologists in specialized centers.

Patients who do not respond to classic psychiatric medications sometimes respond well to antiseizure medications. (See Chap. 4, Thought Disorders.) It does not require imagination to wonder if these patients may actually have a seizure disorder presenting clinically with psychiatric symptoms, as a portion of partial seizures involving the temporal lobe are known to do.

Status epilepticus occurs when seizures continue to recur so rapidly that the patient does not regain consciousness between them. This is a dangerous condition that requires immediate treatment, even if a neurologist is not available. Death rates as high as 20% or more have been reported. It can also cause permanent brain damage, as discussed later.

Neurobiology of Fits

Seizures occur when a part or parts of the brain becomes overactive electrically. Generalized seizures occur when this over activity triggers analogous over activity in other parts of the brain.

The over activity may result from hypersensitivity to stimulation resulting from loss of connections to the affected neurons (*deafferentation*), including loss of inhibitory as well as excitatory input. Deafferentation can occur with a number of types of injury to the brain. If the injury is unknown, the seizures are considered *primary* (idiopathic). If the site of damage is known, they are considered *secondary*. Typical causes of secondary epilepsy include tumors, strokes, congenital malformations such as *hamartomas*, and other brain lesions such as abscesses. Withdrawal from alcohol or other brain depressants can lead to seizures, particularly if there is a potentially irritable site—even if that "potential focus" has not previously revealed itself clinically. Some have hypothesized that the differences between primary and secondary epilepsy result from the limits of our ability to detect subtle brain damage. In secondary epilepsy the site of brain damage can be detected by current techniques including imaging, and in primary epilepsy it cannot (or at least has not) been, by definition. Genes predisposing to seizure disorders have been identified, but the mechanisms by which these genes reduce the threshold for fits have not been established. Fits during high fevers are much more common in children than in adults, but a history of febrile or other childhood seizures may provide an explanation (or at least a justification) for an adult seizure disorder.

During seizures, the energy demands of the overactive brain cells typically outrun the supply of glucose and oxygen from the blood. Demand increases more than supply can. If the seizures last long enough or recur frequently enough, brain damage can occur. It resembles the ischemic brain damage that occurs when the supply of glucose and oxygen is inadequate because of reduced blood flow. (See Chap. 9, Cerebrovascular Disorders.) Thus, seizures can themselves lead to a susceptibility to seizures. The mesial portion of the hippocampus, within the temporal lobe, is particularly sensitive to ischemia. Repeated seizures result in *mesial temporal sclerosis*. Repeated seizures involving this part of the temporal lobe can also lead to the formation of a similar seizure focus in the opposite part of the brain, that is, a *mirror focus*. Status epilepticus can lead to more diffuse damage to the brain, by the same underlying mechanisms of *relative ischemia*. The prevention of brain damage is one of the reasons to treat seizures. That is particularly true for status epilepticus.

Seizures can be manifestations of other brain diseases that lead to dysregulation of electrical activity, often by scarring the brain. A first seizure in a person over 60 years old raises a strong suspicion of cancer in the brain. Other causes include strokes. MRI or other imaging study can reveal the diagnosis. Trauma can also cause seizures. Sometimes it is hard to find out whether trauma to the head preceded a seizure or occurred in a fall due to the seizure. Careful history of what substances were ingested prior to a seizure is also important, particularly in younger people with no seizure history. Fits often occur during alcohol withdrawal (delirium tremens). Some drugs of abuse can precipitate seizures. That is a particularly important consideration in some settings, including care of young people who attend "raves." (See Chap. 14, Disorders of Conduct.) Seizures can be the signal clinical manifestations of a number of other abnormalities of the nervous system as well, including abscesses and other infections.

Treatment

The treatment of seizure disorders is a highly specialized field with a highly specialized body of knowledge that continues to develop and change rapidly. These disorders should be treated primarily by neurologists. If a seizure disorder proves hard to treat, the patient needs to be referred to a neurologist with a special interest and expertise in epilepsy. Epilepsy centers in academic medical centers provide a major resource.

However, general clinicians do have important responsibilities in the care of these patients. One is making sure that patients stay on their anti-seizure medications as prescribed. Another is being sensitive to the side effects of anti-epileptic medications. Many standard anti-epileptic drugs can have important and sometimes dangerous side effects.

Table 10-4 lists anti-seizure medications in wide use at the present time. The association of specific anti-epileptic drugs with specific types of seizures is only rough. Typical doses are listed only to provide information about the relative size of the dose in patients who appear to be developing side effects. Table 10-4 is *not* a reliable guide to therapy. The treating neurologist should decide on the drug or where necessary drugs and on the dosage(s). If possible, the neurologist should have a special interest in seizures. The important thing for each specific patient is obviously what works in that patient. That is decided by trial and error informed by knowledge of the field, i.e. by empiricism informed by theory. The list of anti-seizure medications in Table 10-4 is not exhaustive. Older anti-epileptic medications such as *primidone* (Mysoline) are still in use by some neurologists, and newer anticonvulsants are being approved regularly. Antiepileptic drugs that are used primarily in children are not listed—for instance *ethosuximide* (Zarontin), used largely for absence seizures (Petit Mal). Experts keep up with the newer drugs and their toxicities.

The side effects of the anti-epileptic drugs differ among the specific medications and medication classes, as is expected. The following paragraphs summarize the side effects specific to the more commonly used anti-seizure drugs. In addition, all anti-seizure medications are to some extent central nervous system depressants, and drowsiness and other manifestations of reduced activation of the brain are therefore expected

TABLE 10-4
Common antiseizure medications

Common name	Trade name	Types of seizures often treated	Dosage*
Carbamazepine	Tegretol	tonic-clonic (grand mal); complex partial	600-1200
Valproate	Depakote (Depakene)	tonic-clonic (grand mal); complex partial; myoclonic	1000-3000
Phenytoin	Dilantin	tonic-clonic; complex partial	300-400
Lamotrigine	Lamictal	generalized	3-500
Topiramate	Topamax	partial	400
Gabapentin	Neurontin	partial	00-1800
Benzodiazepines	Librium, Valium	tonic-clonic (grand mal); complex partial	varies with drug
Phenobarbital	Luminal	tonic-clonic; simple and complex	90-200

*typical dosage in mg/day, for adults

side effects of this group of medications. That effect is much more marked for some of these drugs—like phenobarbital—than for newer medications such as carbamazepine. That is one of the reasons that many specialists now pick carbamazepine or valproate as their first drug of choice in treating patients with new onset seizures.

Carbamazepine (Tegretol): Absorption of this drug after an oral dose can take hours and sometimes up to a day. Metabolism is by the CYP3A4 system, and so it interacts with other drugs using this system.

Chronic use can lead to drowsiness, as well as incoordination (*ataxia*), double vision and blurred vision. Other side effects can include nausea and vomiting. Clinically unimportant alterations in liver enzymes can occur, particularly early in treatment. Occasional abnormalities occur in the function of the pancreas. Some people retain water after prolonged treatment with this drug. That can be a problem particularly in people with heart disease.

Tegretol causes severe bone marrow suppression (*aplastic anemia*) in about 1out of 200,000 patients. This much-feared side effect can of course be fatal. It is too rare to discourage most clinicians from prescribing this drug. Carbamazepine can cause a transient fall in white cell count that persists in some users and leads to withdrawal of the drug.

Overdose of carbamazepine can lead to irritability and convulsions, stupor and coma, and respiratory depression. Overdose is an important consideration, since this is as effective a medication against mania as lithium. Patients with bipolar disease are of course at high risk for overdoses. (See Chap. 3, Mood Disorders.)

Valproate (Depakote, Depakene): This medication is rapidly and efficiently absorbed after oral doses. It is metabolized primarily in the liver, but not in the P-450 system.

Drowsiness, incoordination, and tremor probably indicate over dosage and typically respond to reducing the amount taken. Transient gastrointestinal side effects occur in about 15% of patients. They include loss of appetite (*anorexia*), nausea, and vomiting. Transient elevations of liver enzymes occur in almost half the patients, but serious liver disease (*fulminant hepatitis*) has been reported only in children under 10 years old.

Valproate, like carbamazepine, is as effective as lithium in treating bipolar (manic-depressive) disorder in controlled studies. Its use in mental illness of course also incurs a risk of overdose.

Phenytoin (Dilantin): This widely used medication is the most common of several chemically related hydantoins that have been used to treat seizures. A water-soluble prodrug, *fosphenytoin*, is available for IV use. Discovery of the anti-epileptic activity of phenytoin by Merritt and Putnam in 1938 was a creative use of an animal model for drug testing, and it ushered in a new era in the treatment of seizures. Dilantin has been in widespread use for nearly 70 years, and its properties including its side effects are well documented.

This drug is tightly bound to plasma proteins so a distinction exists between its total and free levels in plasma. Absorption into cells is largely from the free plasma pool.

Metabolism is largely by the cytochrome P-450 system, in particular by CYP2C9/10 and also by CYP2C19. As a result, the metabolism of other drugs metabolized by these systems can be slowed by the administration of phenytoin, and the administration of such drugs can slow the metabolism of Dilantin until toxic blood and tissue levels are reached. For instance, doses of warfarin (coumadin) and Dilantin have to be adjusted to stay at therapeutic levels when both medications are administered to the same patient. Administration of Dilantin can also induce the parts of the P-450 system that degrade it, thereby leading to accelerated metabolism of other drugs used by the same system. A practically important instance is oral contraceptives. Women on Dilantin can become inadvertently pregnant if doses of their oral contraceptive are not adjusted properly. Clinical pharmacology has demonstrated the existence of people with an intrinsically reduced ability to metabolize Dilantin, presumably based on genetic variation. Recognition that a patient is a "slow metabolizer" can both explain and help to avoid side effects.

Chronic use of phenytoin can lead to a number of unpleasant side effects. These are in general dose-related and usually respond to reductions in the amount taken. Acute overdose causes primarily cerebellar incoordination (ataxia; see Chap. 11, Disorders of Motility). Chronically excessive doses of Dilantin can cause the cerebellum to atrophy. Table 10-5 lists other side effects of chronic use of Dilantin. As with other drugs, allergic reactions can occur and can be serious and even life-threatening.

This medication acts on the heart as well as the brain. Therapeutically, it is used to treat certain cardiac arrhythmias. In excessive doses, particularly IV doses of the water soluble prodrug fosphenytoin, this potential anti-arrhythmic can also cause cardiac arrhythmias.

Lamotrigine (Lamictal): This relatively new drug is used both alone and as add-on therapy with other anti-epileptic medications. It is efficiently absorbed when taken by mouth, and is metabolized largely by being made more soluble in water by being coupled with an acidic sugar (*glucuronidation*). Drug interactions include a reduction in the plasma concentration of valproate and a tendency to promote the toxicity of carbamazepine.

TABLE 10–5
Chronic side effects of phenytoin (Dilantin)

Behavioral abnormalities
Increase in the frequency of seizures
Overgrowth of the gums (gingival hyperplasia)
Excess growth of hair (hirsutism, a problem primarily for women)
Gastrointestinal problems
Loss of bone (osteomalacia; usually responding to high doses of vitamin D)
Anemia (megaloblastic anemia usually responding to treatment with folate)

Side effects are more common when lamotrigine is added to another drug. They include dizziness, incoordination, blurred or double vision, nausea, vomiting, and rash. Rare reports of disseminated intravascular coagulation or *Stevens-Johnson syndrome* may reflect individual sensitivity, perhaps due to unrecognized genetic variations.

Gabapentin (Neurontin): This versatile medicine is used not only to treat seizures—often in combination with another medication—but also to treat pain and bipolar disorder (manic-depressive disease). It is particularly effective in treating certain types of neuropathic pain including pain from migraines. (See Chap. 7, Pain).

Gabapentin is well-absorbed after being taken orally and is excreted unchanged. It has minimal interaction with other medications.

As for other depressants of the central nervous system, the side effects of gabapentin include drowsiness, fatigue, dizziness, and incoordination (ataxia). They usually resolve within 2 weeks of starting the medication.

Topiramate (Topamax) is approved for use with other anti-epileptics but is not usually used alone. It is well absorbed after oral doses and tends to have fewer drug interactions than carbamazepine (Tegretol), or hydantoin. Reported side effects have usually been mild, and include drowsiness, weight loss, fatigue, and nervousness.

Phenobarbital: This and other barbiturates were among the first drugs used to treat epilepsy and are still in use. They are discussed in Chap. 6 (Anxiety) and Chap. 8 (Sleep). Barbiturates used primarily to treat seizures include *mephobarbital* (Mebaral) and *Primidone* (Mysoline). The barbiturates are generally well absorbed orally. They are metabolized by the P-450 system and have extensive interactions with other drugs. Drowsiness is a prominent side effect of phenobarbital when it is used against seizures. (This is of course a desirable effect when it is used to induce sleep.) The barbiturates have the other side effects associated with central nervous system depressants, as noted earlier. These drugs can also cause folate-responsive *megaloblastic anemia* and vitamin D-responsive *osteomalacia.* Allergic reactions occur in perhaps 1% of people taking these medicines.

Benzodiazepines: These widely used group of medications have potent but relatively transient anti-seizure effects. They are drugs of choice, however, for treating status epilepticus, as discussed below. Chap. 6 (Anxiety) discusses the pharmacology of this group of medications. These drugs are habituating, so that a clinical decision has to be made about whether their use in a particular patient has advantages that outweigh their risks.

Status Epilepticus: This medical emergency often has to be treated by general clinicians. The generalist may have to initiate treatment before the arrival of a neurologist or other specialist. A number of regimens are in use to treat status epilepticus. The following approach is that recommended by Victor and Roper.[5]

Treatment starts by maintaining an airway, establishing an adequate IV line, and obtaining blood samples for a metabolic profile that specifically includes glucose, BUN (blood urea nitrogen), and electrolytes as well as a screen for drugs. As promptly as possible, diazepam (Valium) is administered IV at 2 mg/minute until seizures stop or a total dose of 20 mg has been administered. (An alternative is lorazepam [Ativan] at 0.1 mg/kg at a maximal rate of 2 mg/minute. Lorazepam is a longer acting benzodiazepine, and overdoses can be problematic.) A loading dose of fosphenytoin or phenytoin (15–18 mg/kg) is then administered IV. Phenytoin is less soluble than fosphenytoin and must be given in normal saline in a freely running IV line. Phenytoin cannot be given by IM injection, but fosphenytoin can. If the patient is already taking an anticonvulsant, the dose of fosphenytoin or phenytoin is reduced accordingly, so as not to reach toxic blood levels. These maneuvers are usually adequate to stop the fits. If they do not, further efforts can include infusion of *midazolam* (0.2 mg/kg loading dose followed by infusing 0.1–0.4 mg/kg/hour as needed clinically). Midazolam is a powerful benzodiazepine that can have powerful side effects, including in too large doses a heart attack. An alternative is IV phenobarbital (100 mg/min until the seizures stop or a total dose of 20 mg/kg has been reached). If neither of these treatments stop the status, then anesthesia is needed. Usually that is given IV rather than by inhalation (mask). Pentobarbital is often used, in an initial dose of 5 mg/kg IV followed by 0.5–2 mg/kg/hour. Hopefully, by the time anesthesia is being used a neurologist, anesthetist, or other specialist will be present to direct the treatment. Therapy is the same for patients who are having continuous seizure activity but without muscular involvement.

Behavioral Manifestations: "Psychiatric" manifestations of epilepsy and particularly those of temporal lobe epilepsy can be very difficult to treat. This is not an activity suitable for easily discouraged clinicians. These patients can behave weirdly and unpredicatably, particularly if their seizures are poorly controlled. They can be difficult to help. The use of psychotropic agents to treat specific behavioral manifestations is best done by or in collaboration with a specialist, since many psychotropic medications can alter seizure thresholds.

Surgery: Brain surgery is sometimes the best way to help a patient with epilepsy. If the epileptogenic focus can be removed without undue damage to brain function, and if other significant foci are not present, the results of surgery can be enormously gratifying to the patient, the family, and the medical staff. Obviously, this drastic and irreversible approach is best considered in centers with special experience and expertise in epilepsy and in its medical and surgical management. Arguments about the degree of localization of neurological function and the validity of concepts of "total brain mass" now largely favors the localizers, supporting the idea that cutting out diseased parts of the brain can have relatively few general effects on behavior. Observationally, however, people who have had large pieces of their brain cut out tend to lose abilities compared to people who still have their whole brains intact. Specialized centers treating seizures also have available other less invasive techniques for treating epilepsy including stimulation of the vagus nerve or of the cerebellum. Success with these methods is variable. Sometimes they provide profound relief to patients with previously intractable seizures.

Pathological Inattentiveness

Patients can lose awareness of their surroundings, including of the physicians who are trying to examine them, without losing consciousness. Sometimes inattentiveness indicates nothing more than a person concentrating on something of interest to him or her but not to the other people around.[6] "Absent minded professors" are often accused, justly, of being so occupied with their own thoughts that they do not pay attention to the people or events around them. Thomas Edison famously said that being deaf was what allowed him to invent, since it helped him to avoid distractions. However, inattentiveness can reach a point where it is so debilitating for a person and his or her contacts that it is clearly pathological.[7] Such severe inability to pay attention is characteristic of delirium ("confusion;" see Chap. 5, Cognitive Disorders) and of certain psychoses (notably thought disorders with hallucinations; see Chap. 4, Thought Disorders). Sometimes a psychotic patient is so involved in his or her hallucinations that it is hard to keep their attention for any length of time.

Akinetic mutism is a descriptive term that has been used historically in Neurology for two types of patients. One group are patients who appear aware but are unresponsive and in fact do not perceive what is going on around them. (The French use a more accurate term for this state, *coma vigile*). Patients with this type of akinetic mutism may be highly treatable—for instance, by removing fluid from a cyst at the level of the third ventricle. A second group with "akinetic mutism" are pathologically apathetic. Typically this is due to lesions of the anterior parts of the frontal lobes. Physicians who remember patients who underwent frontal lobectomies for intractable psychiatric disease will have seen this syndrome. Hollywood showed a version of it at the end of the movie, "One Flew Over the Cuckoo's Nest." A Latin term for such total lack of motivation is *abulia*.

A number of other conditions where a patient may appear to be or may actually be unaware are discussed later.

STUPOR

In stupor, consciousness is by definition impaired to the point where patients respond only to intense stimuli such as significant pain (e.g., pin prick, pinching, pressing on a bone). Stupor is a state intermediate between delirium and coma. In this monograph, the discussion of delirium is in Chap. 5 (Cognitive Disorders), rather than in this chapter on Disorders of Awareness. That organization is somewhat arbitrary; arguments are available to defend discussing stupor and delirium together. The causes, mechanisms, and treatments of stupor are in general similar to those in delirium, except more severe, and to those in coma, but less severe. Those are discussed in more detail in the section below as well as in Chap. 5 (Cognitive Disorders).

COMA

In coma, patients are by definition so deeply unconscious that they do not respond even to painful stimuli. Clearly, the borderline between coma and stupor can be blurry. How painful does a stimulus have to be for lack of a response to it to define the state as coma? How purposive and organized does a patient's response have to be to call the condition stupor? As usual, definitions are much less important than finding out what is wrong with the patient and how one can usefully try to help.

General clinicians will see patients in coma. About 3% of patients who arrive in a typical American emergency room are in coma. Perhaps 20% of patients who die in a hospital in the United States go into coma before they expire.

Classification and Diagnosis

The two major causes of coma are severe metabolic insults to the brain (in about two-thirds of comatose patients) and mass lesions affecting the brain (in about one-third). Metabolic insults include overdoses of drugs, therapeutic or recreational—alcohol (ethanol) being an important offender. They also include diseases that impair brain metabolism. Mass lesions include swelling after strokes and hemorrhages into the brain as well as other conditions such as tumors or infections. As discussed below, expanding space-occupying lesions in the brain can be deadly by squeezing the brains stem down leading to its compression in a narrow bony space at the base of the skull (*brain stem herniation* or, in medical slang, *coning*). The brain stem contains structures that regulate breathing and heart rate, and interfering with these basic vegetative functions can obviously be deadly.

Other causes of coma can occur with significant incidence, depending on the sources of referral to a particular institution (e.g., a hospital's catchment area.). Head trauma including closed head trauma may be important in a center which receives many traumatic injuries–for instance, a trauma center near a major highway. The immobility of catatonia and other manifestations of psychiatric disease can be mistaken for coma. Even migraine headache can be associated with apparent coma.

Determining the cause of coma can be easy or can be very hard indeed. As with other dysfunction of the nervous system, history is critical. Since a comatose patient is by definition not talking, history must be obtained from family or other informants. It is important to talk to the person or people who bring the patient in to the emergency room, if they volunteer or can be induced to stay.[8] For instance, in a patient who became comatose suddenly during or after an auto accident, the cause of the coma is likely to be head trauma. In a diabetic, hypoglycemia has to be strongly considered. And so on. Table 10-6 lists some common causes of coma.

TABLE 10–6
Common causes of coma

Disorder	Distinguishing manifestations
Stroke and other vascular diseases	See Chap. 9 (Cerebrovascular Disorders) Hemorrhage, massive stroke, certain focal strokes (e.g., basilar artery), subdural hematomas, hypertensive encephalopathy, and eclampsia can all present clinically as coma Timely brain scanning can be a major aid to diagnosis and treatment
CO	Cherry-red skin; history
Thiamin (B_1) deficiency	History of malnutrition, eye signs, tremor; response to intravenous thiamin
Other hypoxias	History; exposure to mitochondrial toxins such as metformin; often lactic acidosis
Drug overdoses	
Alcohol (ethanol)	Alcohol on breath; signs of liver disease
Methanol	Metabolic acidosis, with rapid respiration
Ethylene glycol	Metabolic acidosis, with rapid respiration
Opiates	Pinpoint pupils; slow and shallow breathing; multiple injection tracks; response to naloxone
Sedative overdose	Low body temperature, shallow breathing, history of medication use (e.g., barbiturates, antipsychotics, antihistaminics [including over-the-counter], other central nervous system depressants)
Recreational drugs	History and social setting of drug abuse
Uremia	Urine smell to breath; often high blood pressure; dry skin; often twitching
Liver failure (hepatic coma)	Other signs of liver disease (enlarged liver, jaundice, ascites; blood tests); elevated blood ammonia; asterixis (liver flap) if testing is possible
Diabetic coma	Fruity breath; acidosis with rapid breathing; glucose and ketone bodies in urine (and elevated in blood); dehydrated
Low blood sugar	Response to intravenous glucose; often rigidity, seizures, (hypoglycemia) myoclonus; often history of diabetes;
Trauma to the brain	Other evidence of injury, on history and physical examination

(*Continued*)

TABLE 10–6
Common causes of coma (*Continued*)

Disorder	Distinguishing manifestations
Lung failure with CO_2 (hypercapnia)	History, other signs of lung disease; papilledema; asterixis; myoclonus
Shock	
Hypovolemic	Other signs of shock (e.g., sweating, rapid heartbeat, feeble pulse, low blood pressure, evidence of bleeding)
Septic	
Meningitis	Fever; stiff neck; leukocytosis; abnormal spinal fluid
Brain abscess	Fever; abnormal brain imaging
Brain tumor	History; localizing neurological signs; evidence of brain stem compression
Heat stroke	History, elevated body temperature, dehydration
Other conditions	History, physical exam, and clinical laboratory tests (e.g., electrolyte imbalance, hypercalcemia, etc.)

The patient who arrives at a medical facility in coma taxes the full abilities of the clinician, the way a patient with a fever of unknown origin or chest pain does. A full discussion of the differential diagnosis of stupor and coma has, in fact, required a whole book. Plum and Posner's *The Diagnosis of Stupor and Coma*[9] provides a complete discussion, much more complete than can be included here. Despite advances in neurobiology since its publication, the discussion of clinical issues in that book is up-to-date, including "clinical pearls" that aid in differential diagnosis and in treatment. These issues are also discussed in textbooks of Neurology.

Neurobiology

Coma and stupor are manifestations of impairment of the systems that maintain consciousness. These systems are widely distributed anatomically. Consciousness as usually thought of depends on the function of the cerebral cortex, and diffuse impairments of cerebral cortical function impair at least the manifestations of consciousness. The *reticular activating system* plays a critical role in maintaining awareness—"consciousness." Anatomically, this system consists of a set of neural structures extending from the brain stem through the midbrain to the thalamus.

These relatively poorly specified structures receive sensory input from lower centers and pass information on to higher centers in the cortex.

The drugs or other toxins that induce coma typically cause widespread reduction in brain activity including that of the cerebral cortex and of the reticular activating formation. This effect is useful medically for the induction of anesthesia. When it happens on its own it is inherently dangerous, since it interferes with a person's ability to care for himself or herself. Swelling—for instance, secondary to a hemorrhage into the brain—can also impair brain function widely, both by the effect of the swelling itself and by the pressure put on intact structures pressed against the bony box of the skull. Swelling of the higher levels of the brain can lead to squeezing the parts of the brain containing the reticular activating formation down into bony cavities that do not have room for them. This can lead to fatal compression of the brain stem and of the vegetative centers it contains that are necessary for maintaining life.

Treatment

The treatment of stupor and coma includes three broad goals: treatment of the underlying disease causing the clouding of consciousness; maintenance of physiological functions while the patient is unconscious; and rapid and effective treatment of brain stem compression (coning) if it occurs.

Underlying Disease: Treatment of the disease underlying a coma is part of general medicine, surgery, and neurology. Discussion of treatment of all of the major diseases that can cause coma is beyond the scope of this monograph.

Sometimes the treatment of the underlying disease requires simply maintaining life support until a potentially fatal overdose of a medication or other toxin has been metabolized or otherwise removed by the body. Sometimes an acceptably safe antidote to a drug that has put a patient into coma is available—for instance, naloxone for opiate overdose. Even then, however, it is important not to over titrate the dose of antidote—for instance, putting a patient into an opium withdrawal syndrome. (See Chap. 5, Cognitive Disorders; Chap. 7, Pain; and Chap. 14, Disorders of Conduct).

Sometimes treatment of the underlying disease causing the coma needs to be more active. Infections including specifically meningitis and other infections of the brain should be treated promptly and as effectively as possible. In addition to antibiotics against bacteria and drugs against fungi, agents are now available that act against certain viral diseases of the nervous system including herpes. These agents and their use are well known to general clinicians. If a patient in coma has a low blood sugar, the treatment is of course injection of glucose (usually 50 ml of 50% glucose by IV injection, after prior injection of 100 mg of thiamin (vitamin B_1). The treatment for thiamin deficiency is injection of thiamin (usually 100 mg of the HCl salt IV). Treatment of diabetic coma requires reducing blood sugar and thereby blood glucose and correcting acidosis and other electrolyte abnormalities, including hyperosmolarity. Treatment of hepatic coma includes reducing sources of nitrogen and maintaining nutrition. Branched chain keto acids can be strikingly useful in the subgroup of patients in hepatic coma in whom that treatment works. Sometimes the only hope for patients with liver failure is liver transplantation. Treatment of vascular accidents is discussed in Chap. 9 (Cerebrovascular Diseases). Just as diagnosis of coma can tax the full diagnostic abilities of a physician, the treatment of the underlying disease can tax his or her full therapeutic knowledge and abilities. Textbooks of Medicine and Neurology provide detailed discussions of how to manage patients with the relevant diseases.

Maintenance of Physiological Functions: Patients in coma need nursing and medical care to maintain their vital functions. Deep coma may include depression of respiration severe enough to require *intubation* and assisted breathing. Patients in deep coma are at risk of not moving their chests and therefore lungs adequately, and they are at high risk of pneumonia or other lung infection. Appropriate pulmonary physical therapy reduces that risk. Comatose patients are also unlikely to move the rest of their bodies adequately, and are therefore at risk for break down of skin from pressure sores and subsequent infections (*bed sores*). These patients cannot eat and drink. That creates a risk of nutritional deficiencies, including dehydration and other abnormalities in water and salt metabolism. Feeding tubes can be useful, but the patients must also be protected against getting food or drink into their lungs (*aspiration*). (Intubation normally does that.) A "PEG" tube inserted surgically through the skin directly into the stomach can reduce the risk of aspiration. Regular passive motion of the limbs is necessary to prevent contractures in patients who do not move spontaneously. The body temperatures of patients in coma can rise or fall to dangerous levels. If so, measures to heat or cool them are appropriate. Their bladders are likely to become distended, and catheterization is often indicated. Attentive medical and nursing care of these patients is necessary to avoid secondary but potentially serious and even fatal problems, while the basic condition causing the coma is being treated, where that is possible. As emphasized below, brain stem compression (herniation, coning) is a life-threatening emergency that requires immediate medical and often surgical treatment.

BRAIN STEM COMPRESSION (HERNIATION, "CONING")

Compression of the base of the brain, the *brain stem,* is a life-threatening complication and a medical-surgical emergency. It often requires immediate medical intervention by the general physician as well as immediate (stat) neurosurgical consultation.

Diagnosis

The early clinical manifestations of significant brain stem compression include headache before the onset of the coma, vomiting, blood pressures consistently higher than the patient's normal level, and retinal hemorrhages. These are particularly reliable in cases of bleeding into the brain.

Observation of the Eyes and of Eye Movements: Recognizing changes in the eyes (*eye signs)* is critical in recognizing brain stem compression. The nerve cells that give rise to the cranial nerves that control eye movements are located in the structures that are compressed during "*coning*." On occasion *metabolic coma* may be so severe that even the motor cells of the eyes in the midbrain become inactive, so that eye signs characteristic of coning may also be present in severe metabolic coma.

Loss of the normal regulation of the size and motion of the eyes is a prominent sign of brain stem compression. Large dilated pupils are characteristic of coning. In patients close to dying, the dilated pupils may decrease a little in size from about 9 mm to perhaps 7 mm. Unilateral enlargement of a pupil also indicates damage to a cranial nerve, often due to compression.

Loss of the "dolls eyes" reflex is usually an indication of midbrain and brain stem compression. This *oculocephalic reflex* occurs in comatose but not intact people. It is elicited by the examiner rapidly turning the head to one side; in a comatose person without brain stem compression, the eyes roll to the opposite side. This reflex presumably reflects loss of input from the cerebral cortex to intact oculomotor nuclei in the midbrain. As compression of the brain stem progresses, the doll's head reflex is lost. In normal people, irrigating an ear with cold or room temperature water causes the eyes to deviate to the irrigated side rapidly followed with subsequent *nystagmus* ("bouncing" eye movements as seen in *cerebellar ataxia*). Irrigation of the ear with warm water leads to the eyes moving away from the irrigated side. With brain stem compression, the adjustment phase (nystagmus) is lost and the eyes stay tonically deflected to the side that was irrigated, often for 2–3 minutes. Loss of the adjustment phase of this *caloric response* is a sign of dysfunction of the relevant structures at the base of the brain, from compression or from metabolic or other impairment.

Loss of the margin of the optic disc as viewed through an ophthalmoscope (i.e., *papilledema*) is an important sign of increased intracranial pressure. It can develop relatively rapidly—that is, within less than a day—but is often a sign of chronic disease such as a tumor or brain abscess.

A reliable indicator of loss of brain stem function from compression is reduced blinking—loss of blink in response to touching an eyelid, and finally loss of blink from touching the cornea with a soft object such as a tiny wisp of cotton. Loss of this *corneal reflex* is a reliable sign of deep coma.

Abnormal Posture and Movements: Deepening coma, including that due to brain stem compression, can often lead to abnormal postures and movements. A comatose patient who moves on one side but not the other is likely to have a lesion in the part of the brain that normally controls the immobile side. That is often a bleed or a clot, but can be another lesion such as a tumor or abscess. *Decerebrate rigidity* is a characteristic posture in brain damage that includes the brain stem. The jaws and all limbs are held stiffly, with the arms rotated inwards and the feet pointing down (plantar flexion). In this state, inhibitory input from higher centers to the motor neurons in the spinal cord is lost, and all muscles contract. The peculiar position of the arms and the feet reflects the greater strength of certain muscle groups compared to others. For instance, the muscles that lift us on our toes when we walk (*plantar flex* our feet) are strong compared to other muscles moving our feet.

Heart Rate: Heart beat can rise as well as fall in comatose patients, but a progressive fall in heart beat (*bradycardia*) often indicates progressive pressure or other damage to the structures (*nuclei*) in the brain stem that normally control heart rate. It is a bad prognostic sign.

Breathing Impairment: Loss of the ability to breathe is a typical cause of death in comatose patients who cone. The mechanism is impairment of the respiratory centers in the base of the brain (in the pontine and medullary tegmentum). In *Cheyne-Stokes respiration*, periods of over breathing (*hyperventilation*) alternate with periods of under breathing (*hypoventilation*) and even with brief periods of no breathing at all (*apnea*). This respiratory pattern is common in comatose patients who are "coning" but is not itself a reliable indicator of this complication. A bad prognostic sign is conversion of the usual type of Cheyne-Stokes respiration to *apneustic breathing*, in which a few breaths alternate with periods of apnea. (Another name for apneustic respiration is "short cycle" Cheyne Stokes respiration.) When apnea takes over, the patient dies—unless maintained on a breathing machine.

Newer Techniques: Techniques that allow relatively precise diagnosis of brain stem compression are imaging and direct measurement of intracranial pressure (ICP) by monitoring. Repeat imaging of the brain can show directly whether or not the brain is swelling and whether or not the midbrain and medulla are being compressed. ICP monitoring gives a direct measure of whether the pressure within the skull is rising or falling. These techniques have moved the diagnosis of brain stem compression from purely clinical to clinical buttressed by objective measurements.

Neurobiology

The skull is a bony box that protects the brain substance but provides limited space for the brain to expand if bleeding, swelling, or a space-occupying lesion occur. In these situations, intracranial pressure (ICP) can rise to the point where it eventually pushes the brain stem down and compresses it against bone. The brain stem contains vital neural centers that support critical, basic physiological functions including breathing. Compression of these centers can interfere with their function to the point that the patient dies.

Treatment

Acute Medical Treatment: Acute medical treatment of brain stem compression consists of drawing water out of the swollen brain by making the blood hyperosmolar to the brain fluid. The sugar derivative mannitol, which does not cross into the brain, is injected IV; a common dose is 25–50 g of a 20% solution injected over 10–20 minutes. Other osmotic diuretics—urea, glycerin, and isosorbide—are now rarely used to treat brain stem compression. In patients with brain swelling, the osmolarity of the blood should be maintained at a high physiological level, with serum sodium values not under 138 mEq/L. Sometimes diuretics such as furosemide are necessary to achieve that goal.

Corticosteroids: Corticosteroids are another treatment for more prolonged brain swelling, for instance, after head injury. Corticosteroids shrink brain, decrease transport of fluid across the endothelial cells of blood vessels, and reduce edema associated with vascular dysregulation. A typical dose is dexamethasone 4 mg every 6 hours by mouth, if the patient can swallow. Much larger doses are sometimes beneficial—as much as 100 mg a day or even more. Other corticosteroids can be used instead in therapeutically equivalent doses. Prolonged use of these high doses of course risks the complications of steroid therapy, which are well known to general clinicians.

Hyperventilation: Reducing the CO_2 by increasing the rate of breathing (hyperventilation) also reduces ICP. This is relatively easy in a patient already on a respirator. Often this effect is relatively transient, lasting less than hour (because equilibration of CO_2 across fluid compartments is relatively rapid). Obviously, if more definitive treatment becomes available during the hour, this intervention can be life-saving.

Cooling: Reducing body temperature below normal (*hypothermia*) may also slow the effects of increased ICP. It is a standard method for reducing the rate of brain damage. Certainly, fevers should be treated effectively in these patients.

Surgery: Surgery to open the skull and dura and relieve the pressure on the brain seems an obvious treatment, but results have been mixed[10,11] That may in part be due to the seriousness of the underlying illnesses. Anecdotal reports of dramatic benefits are widespread. At least one widely publicized neurosurgeon removes a large portion of the bony cranium; his patients who recovered well have appeared on television to describe how grateful they are for his vigorous interventions. The results of controlled trials are awaited.

OTHER CONDITIONS

General physicians need to be aware of several other conditions that can mimic coma or result from coma, because of the therapeutic implications of these diagnoses.[12,13] These include locked-in syndrome, minimally conscious state, chronic vegetative state, and brain death. As discussed below, these diagnoses are best made by a qualified neurologist, for legal as well as medical reasons.

Locked-In Syndrome

This tragic condition occurs in patients who are conscious but cannot voluntarily move anything but their eyelids. It is also called the *deefferented state*. The most common cause of this syndrome is a basilar artery stroke that effectively cuts the descending motor (corticobulbar and corticospinal) pathways without disrupting the ascending pathways that mediate arousal. Other causes are severe wide-spread damage to peripheral nerves (neuropathy, including Guillain-Barré syndrome [see Chap. 11, Disorders of Motility]) and rarer syndromes that are discussed in textbooks of Neurology and Medicine (such as pontine myelinosis and periodic paralysis). The treatment of locked-in state is the treatment, to the extent possible, of the underlying disease. Locked-in syndrome due to a basilar artery stroke may be treatable only by the general measures used to support life in patients who cannot move by themselves. The term *akinetic mutism* is not conventionally used in Neurology to refer to the locked-in syndrome, although in fact it does describe the state of these patients.

Active people including physicians may assume that locked-in syndrome is so horrible that the people with it would rather be allowed to die. Empirical studies, however, do not bear out that lugubrious assumption. Many of them want to live despite their physical limitations.[12] That attitude justifies active nursing and medical care for them. Even with devoted care, however, their prospects of living for many years are limited.

Minimally Conscious State

This is a condition in which consciousness is by definition severely altered in people whose behavior nevertheless provides definite if often minimal evidence that they are aware of their own selves and of their environment.[13] These patients open their eyes spontaneously and have sleep-wake cycles. They are typically obtunded ("out of it"), but most of them will have at least short periods of normal arousal.

Persistent Vegetative State (PVS)

Patients with this condition retain vegetative functions such as breathing but show no evidence of awareness and lack purposeful behavior of any kind. Other, older terms for this dreadful outcome of brain damage are *neocortical death* and *apallic syndrome*. A pitfall in recognizing this syndrome is mistaking automatic, more or less reflex behavior for purposive behavior. For instance, after Bobby Kennedy was shot, he grasped a rosary put in his hand because of a forced grasp reflex; the media widely misinterpreted this primitive reflex as a sign that he was regaining consciousness.[14] Apparent arousal or wakefulness and cycles of greater and lesser arousal do not rule out this diagnosis. Nor does the patient grinding his or her teeth (*bruxism*). The cause of this unfortunate state is usually widespread damage to the cerebral cortex and/or thalamus.

The prognosis is bad. Of patients who wake after 1 week, perhaps 10% will have good outcomes and another 20% will survive. Perhaps another 1–5% will wake up between 1 and 2 weeks. After 2 weeks, recovery is at best a statistical rarity. Of critical importance is being confident that the condition is not due to the lingering effects of a medication or other substance that has depressed the function of the cerebral cortex and is being slowly removed or otherwise detoxified by the patient's body.

Diagnosis and management of this condition is best left to neurologists or other qualified specialists, because of the controversial issues this condition raises. Nursing and medical care like that for patients in deep coma is appropriate until the diagnosis has been confidently established. After that, deciding how much care to give is polluted by political calculations and religious beliefs masquerading as political convictions.[15]

Brain Death

This vexatious problem results from the successes of modern medicine, particularly in developing techniques to support life while patients recover from deep coma or other neurological conditions.[16] Before effective life-support techniques became widely available, when the brain died the person died. Now, the heart and lungs can be kept going when a patient has no brain left. The term *brain death* is used for this state. (The earlier French term was "past coma," i.e., *coma dépassé*.) Controversy about whether or not a patient is brain dead can come down technically to a dispute over whether the patient is in a minimally conscious state or a persistent vegetative state.

The determination of brain death should be done by a neurologist. In some states, a neurologist is by law required to be in attendance and agree when a patient is declared brain dead. Formal criteria are discussed elsewhere. They include: (1) lack of evidence of cortical function, (2) lack of evidence of brain stem function as documented by an apnea test (inability of the patient to breathe spontaneously even with elevated CO_2 levels), and (3) irreversibility of the state. As with chronic vegetative state, it is critical to be sure that the evidence of brain death is not due to an overdose of a drug or of other substance suppressing brain function. Normally, the diagnosis also involves a flat EEG, but a flat EEG is *not* by itself adequate evidence of brain death. Often the evidence of overwhelming brain damage from a known cause—such as a massive hemorrhage—clarifies the diagnosis.

Controversial Public Issues

How much care should be given to people in a chronic vegetative state or who are brain dead is a societal and political concern rather than a medical problem in the limited sense. American society, however, in its bitter divisiveness has largely dumped this problem on doctors.[16] A consensus has formed in the United States on how much to do medically for people who are conscious and not psychiatrically unable to make decisions—namely, do what the patient wants. No consensus has yet formed about how much to do for people who can not express what they want—which of course includes people in coma or in a chronic vegetative state. Even when patients have written down their wishes previously in a legally binding form, interpretation of their "living will" can become fraught. In practice, it comes down to the family and the doctor coming to agreement. Fortunately, that is usually possible. In these discussions, the physician needs to listen with a sympathetic ear to what the family and its individual members are saying, both verbally and non-verbally.

When family members are fighting among themselves, resolution can become very difficult. Disagreements can be insoluble if the people involved believe that God has told them what to do, and said so in simple, declarative English sentences. These social and religious issues are even harder than the technical issues in caring for these patients.[17] Perhaps the best general guideline is that the welfare of the patient should trump ideology.

REFERENCES

1. Perry SW, Kenny RA. Drop attacks in older adults: systemic assessment has a high diagnostic yield. *J Am Geriat Soc.* 2005;53:74–78. See also commentary: Rich MW. Drop attacks revisited: yet another manifestation of cardiovascular disease? *J Am Geriat Soc.* 2005;53:161–162.
2. Stone J, Smyth R, Carson A, et al. The systematic review of misdiagnosis of conversion symptoms and "hysteria" *BMJ.* 2005;331(7523):989. The women in Charcot's classic studies of hysteria apparently included Parisian streetwalkers, who mimicked hysterical manifestations in order to have a warm bed and three meals a day. These women were professionals at giving a man what he wanted—in this instance, by feigning hysteria for the Professor. Some of their "hysterical" poses were suggestive if not frankly erotic, that being something they were good at. At the time Charcot worked there, the Salpétrière was a poorhouse as well as a chronic disease hospital.
3. Functional imaging studies have suggested that the temporal lobe is the part of the brain most involved in religious experiences. These include religious visions (for instance, the perception of the presence of Jesus). That observation does not deny the reality of these religious experiences any more than the association of activity in the visual cortex with sight negates that one is looking at real things when the visual cortex is activated. Aberrant electric activity in the visual systems in the brain can, of course, lead to aberrant visual experiences associated with *visual epilepsy*. Aberrant temporal lobe activity may have an analogous relationship to some religious experiences.
4. The diagnosis was confirmed by EEG, including nasopharyngeal leads to detect aberrant temporal lobe activity. More important, this previously "untreatable" patient responded to anti-seizure medication—finishing college, marrying, and holding a responsible job while raising children.
5. Victor M, Ropper AH. *Principles of Neurology.* 7th ed. McGraw Hill, NY, 2001, pp. 361–362.
6. People from primitive societies can be particularly skilled at retreating into fantasies because they find their present situation uncomfortable. That situation sometimes includes ignoring a physician who asks them questions they do not want to answer. Whether this is cultural conditioning, willfulness, or psychiatric disease is still a matter of debate. Perhaps all three.

7. My working definition of pathological inattentiveness is lack of awareness worse than what I inflict on my family and coworkers. By my definition, I am neuropsychologically healthy. By my definition, to be sick you have to be worse off than I am.
8. Of course, this is not always helpful. One of my first patients was delivered to a city hospital in New York by a very cooperative policeman. The history was, almost exactly, "This fellow collapsed while he was in line to get into the Muni (Municipal Lodging House). By the time he hit the ground, the other drunken bums had lifted everything from his pockets." The patient turned out to have had a massive and untreatable cerebral hemorrhage, apparently hypertensive in origin without any head trauma. He died.
9. Plum F, Posner JB. *The Diagnosis of Stupor and Coma*. 3d ed. Saunders, Philadelphia, PA; 1982.
10. Ziai WC, Port JD, Cowan JA, et al. Decompressive craniectomy for intractable cerebral edema: experience of a single center. *J Neurosurg Anesthesiol*. 2003;15:25–32.
11. Hutchinson PJ, Kirkpatrick PJ. Decompressive craniectomy in head injury. *Curr Opin Crit Care*. 2004;10:101–104.
12. von Wild KR. Functional neurorehabilitation in locked-in syndrome following C0-C1 decompression. *Acta Neurochir Suppl*. 2005;93:169–75.
13. Giacino JT. Disorders of consciousness: differential diagnosis and neuropathologic features. *Semin Neurol*. 1997;17:105–111.
14. At the time, a distinguished neurosurgeon had the courage to say on national TV, "The man is dead. Stop misleading the American people."
15. The comments of largely retired cardiac surgeons who have not themselves seen the patient have no legal or medical standing, even in politicized cases like the late Terri Schiavo, and even if the MDs have earned high political rank.
16. Consensus can be easier to achieve in more homogeneous societies—for instance, in Denmark before the current spate of immigration. When 98+% of the people were Lutherans of the same ethnic stock, there was wide agreement on how to deliver end-of-life care.
17. Religious convictions can of course differ even among people of the same faith, and specifically among people who describe themselves as Christians. A Catholic priest from Ireland whom I met at a bioethical conference condemned the maintenance of biological life for people who were brain dead or in a chronic vegetative state. He said, "You're keeping their souls in Limbo." This priest was a devout Catholic with a strong faith in the immortality of the soul. A number of avowed and vocal Christians in the United States, both Catholic and Protestant, now appear to feel strongly that society has a duty to maintain biological human life even when awareness and purposefulness have become impossible due to brain damage. The role of medical knowledge in this debate is uncertain.

CHAPTER ELEVEN

Disorders of Motility: Including Parkinson Disease and Other Movement Disorders

A number of disorders of the nervous system affect motility so much more than they do other aspects of nervous system function that they can be considered, to a first approximation, to be disorders of motility. In fact, however, meticulous neurological history and examination often uncovers other neurological problems as well. For instance, severe weakness of a limb can often lead to pain from contractures. Stiff muscles tend to ache. Sometimes brain damage is so localized to systems subsuming movement that the result appears to be a disorder of motility. That can, for instance, occur with some relatively small strokes. A patient with one of these disorders is likely to present to his or her physician complaining of weakness or poor coordination rather than a more generalized neurological problem. In this clinically oriented book, it is therefore convenient to discuss these disorders together. This chapter deals with the more common disorders that affect movement but have little effect on sensation or mentation.

Patients with disorders of mobility of acute onset, such as those due to stroke or trauma, may require immediate care by general clinicians even before a neurologist or neurosurgeon becomes available. That may involve treatment to prevent excess damage due to edema or bleeding. Such care is discussed at the end of Chapter 10 (Disorders of Awareness), in the discussion of coma and brain stem compression. More chronic disorders of mobility typically require evaluation and treatment by a neurologist. Optimal care for these disorders requires the participation of a specialist who will provide the general physician with detailed information on the condition being cared for. The discussion in this monograph is therefore relatively brief. More thorough, deeper discussions of these conditions are available in textbooks of Neurology.

The term *disorder of mobility* is used here in preference to *movement disorder*. The latter phrase is often understood in a more limited sense, to refer to a subgroup of disorders of motility resulting in adventitious movements, often associated with disease of the basal ganglia.

CLASSIFICATION AND DIAGNOSIS

The classification and diagnosis of disorders of motility has two major aspects: description of the abnormal movements or lack of movements in neurological terminology; and, deciphering the cause of the abnormality. The latter sometimes involves biological mechanisms, but sometimes is simply citing the syndrome in the literature that the patient most resembles. Often such a syndrome includes a description of the neuropathology. Often it is named for the person who first described it (i.e., is eponymic). Examples include Parkinson disease and Friedreich ataxia. (The latter is now also defined at a molecular genetic level).

There are many different ways to classify movement abnormalities. The following discussion first classifies them by the type of abnormal movement, since specific types of abnormal movements are likely to be what brings a patient afflicted with one of these conditions to the attention of a general physician. It then goes on to discuss classifications based on the biological abnormality or the syndrome. Yet other classifications are by the part(s) of the nervous system primarily involved, e.g., basal ganglia disorders or cerebellar disorders. Still another is by etiology, including specific abnormalities in specific genes where these are known. Although discussed briefly here, detailed classification in terms of specific syndrome or part of the nervous system involved or of the cause of the damage is best left to a neurologist, as is the choice of treatment.

Chronic disorders of motility fall roughly into two groups: those where patients move too little and those where they move too much. In some diseases both abnormalities occur. For instance, Parkinson disease is associated with reduced movements and rigidity but also with a resting tremor.

Reduced Movements can vary from total paralysis to relatively mild reductions in movement due to chronic increases in muscle tone.

Paralysis

In medical usage, the term *paralysis* refers to complete loss of motor (or sensory) function. *Plegia* is a synonym for paralysis that is used particularly in compound terms. *Monoplegia* refers to complete paralysis of a single limb, with or without atrophy of the muscles of that limb. *Hemiplegia* is paralysis of both an arm and a leg on one side of the body. *Paraplegia* is paralysis of both legs, and *quadriplegia* is complete loss of motor function of all four limbs. *Palsy* is an older synonym for paralysis, now little used.

Paralyses can be *flaccid* or *spastic*. In *flaccid paralysis*, tone is markedly reduced and deep tendon reflexes are lost. In *spastic paralysis*, tone is markedly increased, with increased deep tendon reflexes and upgoing toes ("extensor plantar responses"). When all the muscles of a limb are contracting (spastic) at the same time, the stronger muscles exert more force than the weaker ones. In the arms the stronger muscles are those of flexion (which bend the elbow), and in the legs those of extension (which straighten the leg and allow us to stand). Spastic paralysis can therefore lead to limbs that are contracted, with the arms in flexion and the legs and feet in extension. The contractures can themselves be both disabling and painful. (See below.) *Decerebrate rigidity* is a type of spastic paralysis that occurs when the brain stem is intact but higher centers are severely damaged. These unfortunate patients typically end up with severe contractures unless they receive excellent and continuing nursing care.

<u>Sensory paralysis</u> refers to complete loss of sensation. Derivative terms describing the location of the sensory loss are analogous to those for motor loss. *Sensory hemiplegia* refers to loss of all sensation on one

side of the body, and *sensory paraplegia* to loss of sensation in both legs. Disorders that primarily affect sensation are the subject of Chapter 12 (Disorders of Sensation).

Paresis

In medical usage, this term refers to incomplete loss of motor (or sensory) function as distinct from the total loss of function in paralysis. Subclassifications of paresis are analogous to those for paralysis. Thus, *hemiparesis* means weakness of an arm and a limb on one side. *Paraparesis* is weakness of both legs, and *quadriparesis* weakness of all four limbs. Paresis, like paralysis, can be flaccid or spastic.

Weakness

Weakness, or sometimes *fatigue,* is the usual term used by patients to refer to decreased mobility due to primary disease of muscle. Both weakness and fatigue can be documented during physical examination by formal muscle testing, which needs to take no more than a few minutes. If the examination reveals no abnormalities, other causes for the patient's complaint should be sought. As a generalization, muscle diseases tend to manifest themselves clinically first as problems with the larger (proximal) muscles in the upper arm or leg, while diseases of peripheral nerves tend to affect first the smaller (distal) muscles in the lower arm or leg. However, that generalization is no more true in detail than most other generalizations. In fact, a specific type of muscle disease (*Welander dystrophy*) characteristically begins in the small muscles of the hands and then spreads to the distal muscles of the legs as well. Differential diagnosis of myopathies and their treatment is usually done by neurologists, unless the problem is due to a systemic disease such as thyroid imbalance or a collagen vascular disease (e.g., *polymyositis, dermatomyositis*). Even then a consultation with an expert in muscle disease can be well advised. The distinction between primary disease of muscle and that of peripheral nerves innervating the muscles is often difficult. Neurologists specializing in muscle diseases have available special techniques to aid in the differential diagnosis, including electrophysiological techniques (*electromyography*) and analysis of muscle biopsies including special immunochemical stains and electron microscopy.

Certain muscle diseases of adults have clinical patterns that allow their recognition even before special tests are done. *Myotonic dystrophy* typically involves first the small muscles of the hands and muscles of the eyes and face, giving the patients a characteristic appearance. A weak and monotonous voice results from weakness of the throat and larynx. A characteristic finding is slow contraction of muscle; this can be elicited by tapping a muscle with a reflex hammer. *Periodic paralyses* are, as the name indicates, attacks of weakness that typically last hours to days and usually occur every few weeks. Several forms are known, most of which involve alterations in potassium regulation. Responsible genes have been described. A general discussion of the types of muscle disease and their diagnosis is beyond the scope of this monograph. The appropriate differential diagnoses are best made by neurologists with special interest in these diseases.

Hypokinesia

Hypokinesia refers to poverty of movement without weakness. Akinesia is more or less a synonym, despite the distinction in meaning between the Greek roots. Hypokinesia reveals itself prominently in loss of normal movements accompanying an action. Such "accessory movements" include, for instance, swinging the arms while walking or moving one's legs before arising from a chair. *Hypomimia* is hypokinesia of the facial muscles that are involved in the physical expression of emotion. Hypokinesia is often the first sign of Parkinson disease, as discussed below.

Bradykinesia

Bradykinesia is slowness of movements, typically affecting the same activities as hypokinesia. Bradykinesia affects initiation of movements. Thinking about the action is typically not slow, but initiating it and doing it are. However, slowness of thinking—*bradyphrenia*—does tend to accompany bradykinesia in the later stages of Parkinson disease. (See below).

Impairments of Posture

Impairments of Posture include disordered postural fixation, equilibrium, and righting reflexes. These often occur in syndromes that also include bradykinesia/hypokinesia and rigidity, including Parkinson disease.

Rigidity

Rigidity occurs when muscles are continuously tensed, even in people who otherwise appear relaxed. Test of passive movement can distinguish rigidity from spasticity. Spastic muscles provide a "free interval" before tension is felt; rigid muscles are tense from the get-go. *Cogwheel rigidity* is a ratchet-like resistance to movement. It may represent a tremor concealed at rest by the rigidity of the musculature. Cogwheel rigidity is common in Parkinson disease. *Gegenhalten* (paratonia; oppositional resistance) is resistance to passive movement that cannot be accounted for by rigidity or spasticity. Characteristically, the patient can eliminate gegenhalten at least briefly by concentrating on not resisting the passive movement. Muscle strength is typically normal in patients with gegenhalten.

Hypotonia

Hypotonia is the opposite of rigidity. Hypotonic muscles have decreased tone. Like rigidity, hypotonia does not imply decreased strength although the two may occur together (e.g., in a flaccid paralysis).

Apraxia

Apraxia refers to the inability to carry out a skilled action not due to weakness or other motor disability. Examples are loss of ability to button clothes or to use a computer keyboard. Apraxias are subclassified as ideational, ideomotor, or kinetic. Patients with *ideational apraxia* are unable to conceive of the affected action, either spontaneously or on command. Those with *ideomotor apraxia* can conceive of it but can not do it. In kinetic apraxia, the patient can do it but only clumsily.

Increased movements can vary in severity from socially embarrassing (e.g., mild *essential tremor*) to severely disabling (e.g., *hemiballismus*). The specific types of increased movements listed below are essentially involuntary, although sometimes concentrated conscious effort can diminish their intensity for a time. Sometimes patients with abnormal involuntary movements may try to act as if the movements were voluntary, to reduce social embarrassment. This can occur in patients with *chorea* or *athetosis*, as described below.

Tremors

Tremors are regular, rhythmic, bidirectional movements. *Rest tremors* occur at rest; voluntary movements diminish or abolish them. The *"pill-rolling" tremor* of Parkinson disease is a typical rest tremor. (See below.) Action tremors occur with voluntary action but not at rest. *Postural tremor* is an alternative term for action tremors involving the limbs or trunk. In general medical usage, action tremor refers to a tremor of lesser magnitude than the *intention tremors* characteristic of disease of the cerebellum and discussed below.

Essential tremor is a form of action tremor, usually affecting the arms and specifically the hands more than the legs. Essential tremor usually does not lead to clinically important problems. With progression, however, it can come to interfere with life—eventually even with such critical skilled motor activities as feeding oneself. *Familial tremor* refers to essential tremor that runs in families. *Senile tremor* is essential tremor that starts in late life. The unusual essential tremor that affects the legs more than the arms is called *orthostatic tremor*.

Emotional tremor of the hands is so common that its mild form is a statistically normal form of human behavior. Tremor as a major manifestation of an emotional state has been referred to as *hysterical tremor*.[1]

Action tremors can also result from a number of neurological conditions that are discussed below later and elsewhere in this monograph. (See especially Chap. 7, Anxiety; Chap. 12, Disorders of Sensation; Chap. 13, Disorders of Both Motility and Sensation; and discussions of the effects of medications and recreational drugs in Chap. 4, Thought Disorders, and in Chap. 14, Disorders of Conduct.) These include neuropathies, intoxications, demyelinating disease, and infections.

Asterixis

Asterixis is a loss of postural control during extended static movement, most often due to a metabolic disease of the brain. The typical test to elicit asterixis is to hold the arms in front of one with the wrists flexed. Asterixis manifests itself by loss of the sustained dorsiflexion, i.e., the hands "flap." *Liver flap* is asterixis associated with brain disease due to liver disease (*hepatic encephalopathy;* see Chap. 5, Disorders of Cognition.).

Chorea

Chorea refers to abrupt, rapid, jerky movements, typically involving the limbs and/or face. Muscle tone is typically reduced (hypotonia), but muscle strength is not.

Athetosis

Athetosis refers to slow, writhing, purposeless movements. They typically involve the fingers and hands; often the toes, tongue, and throat; and to a lesser extent muscle groups in other areas.

Choreoathetosis

Choreoathetosis is a combination of choreic and athetotic movements. In patients with choreoathetosis, the two types of movements are so mixed that trying to make a distinction between them is not clinically useful.

Clonus

Clonus is a rhythmic contraction of a muscle or group of muscles in only one direction. It contrasts with tremor, which is in both directions. A wide variety of diseases of the nervous system can cause this movement abnormality. Clonus in response to elicitation of reflexes is commonly a sign of severe spasticity—for instance, after a severe stroke.

Myoclonus

Myoclonus refers to asynchronous, asymmetrical, sudden, irregular contractions of a muscle or group of muscles. Segmental myoclonus (*myoclonus simplex*) is myoclonus affecting only a restricted group of muscles, such as those in a single limb. Polymyoclonus (*myoclonus multiplex*) is widespread myoclonus.

Ataxia

Ataxia refers to a group of abnormalities in the rate, range, and force of movements. The abnormal movements that characterize ataxia typically result from disease of the cerebellum and its extensions.

- "Dysmetria" is trouble hitting a mark—for instance, touching one's nose with an outstretched finger.
- "Intention tremor," mentioned above, may be related functionally to dysmetria. It is thought to arise from "overshooting" a mark and then correcting the overshoot with movements of decreasing amplitude, until the target is reached.
- "Titubation" is a rhythmic (~3/second) tremor of the head and/or upper body. It is related to "wing-beating tremor," a coarse, irregular tremor that develops when the afflicted patient activates certain limb muscles, even for posture.
- "Cerebellar speech" (*scanning speech*) is typically jerky and poorly modulated.
- "Cerebellar gait" is typically wide-based and unsteady. The patient may have trouble turning around or walking heel-to-toe along a straight line. A somewhat similar disorder, "sensory ataxia," is due to impairment of position sense.
- "Disdiadokokinesia" refers to loss of rhythm in carrying out repetitive movements.
- "Nystagmus" is excessive *"saccadic"* movements of the eye when trying to fix on an object. Nystagmus probably represents the ocular analogue of intention tremor. In other words, it reflects dysmetria of eye movements. The patient with nystagmus overshoots the position of fixation and then readjusts with eye motions of less amplitude until fixation is achieved. The extraneous movements are often called *"beats" of nystagmus.* The number of beats is often used as one of the measures of the severity of the abnormality.

Ballism

Ballism refers to flinging movements. (The term is derived from the same sources as the words for throwing a ball.) These movements are typically on one side of the body only (unilateral). While unintentional—not "willed"—these are typically so strong as to be "violent." Severe ballismus can be so disabling that surgery to paralyze an affected limb has been a rational therapy. Once seen, severe ballismus is unmistakable.

Dystonia

Dystonia is a persistent imbalance of muscle contractions such that the afflicted patient assumes bizarre postures or carries out strange, undesired movements. Early manifestations of dystonia can be mistaken for an annoying or hysterical mannerism, particularly if the dystonia decreases when the patient focuses attention on some other stimulus.[1] Severe and persistent dystonia, particularly of large muscle groups, can lead to bizarre, unattractive deformities and severe disability. *Dyskinesias* are localized forms of dystonia. These can involve the muscles of the eye lid (blepharospasm), of the hand (e.g., writer's cramp), of the neck (spasmodic torticollis), or of other muscle groups.

Paroxysmal Choreoathetosis and Dystonia

Paroxysmal choreoathetosis and dystonia are episodes of these abnormal movements. They can be a consequence of many types of brain damage. Two rare but well-characterized inherited forms are known. One is precipitated by startle or rapid movement (*paroxysmal kinesigenic choreoathetosis*), and the other by coffee, tea, or fatigue (*dystonic spasms*).

Fasciculations

Fasciculations are localized muscle twitches. They represent contractions of single motor units. Fasciculations typically look like muscle quivering or ripples under the skin. They are often accompanied by other signs of abnormalities of the affected muscle units, as discussed below.

Tics and Habit Spasms

Tics and habit spasms are more or less normal movements that become unusually habitual. They sometimes annoy individuals with tics. Perhaps more often, they annoy others, who find tics to be irritating "bad habits."

Mild to moderate tics are hardly a source of medical concern. They may interfere with life for those in positions in society that require relatively rigid adherence to prescribed codes of behavior. For instance, tics may be or relatively great concern to people in professions that involve public appearances, such as acting or politics.[2] Gilles de la Tourette described an unusual form of tic-like disorder that is often treated with medication or even neurosurgery but can be accepted in highly tolerant societies; it is discussed below.

In some cases of severe brain disease, repetitive tic-like motions can become potentially harmful. For instance, autistic individuals who bang their heads incessantly may have to wear helmets. People with severe, widespread damage to the cerebral cortex and other centers controlling volition can develop habits that deeply bother their caregivers or family—for instance, frequent public masturbation by a severely brain damaged woman who was "a perfect lady" when healthy. Whether this is a medical problem or a problem of educating caregivers is a matter of judgment. If it interferes with care, it becomes a medical problem.

Gait Disorders

Difficulty with walking is often the presenting complaint in a patient with a chronic disorder of motility. A fluid, coordinated gait requires the participation of most or all of the motor systems in the nervous system. Gait disorders can be characteristic of particular types of brain damage, although overlapping and intermediate forms are also common. Close observation of a patient's gait can provide valuable information on which motor system or combination of motor systems is impaired.[3,4]

Paretic (paralytic) Gait: Paretic *(paralytic)* gait is slow, stiff, and scraping. The leg tends to be swung out and then in (*circumduction*). The toe and outer sole of the shoe are often worn away. Weakness can affect one or both legs. If weakness affects the arm as well, arm swing is reduced.

Foot-Drop: Dropping the foot is a characteristic result of damage to lower motor neurons or to the peripheral nerves that carry their axons. A *steppage* or *equine gait* can result, in which the leg is lifted abnormally high and the foot makes a slapping sound when it hits the ground.

Waddling Gait: A number of muscle diseases, including progressive muscular dystrophy, make the affected patients waddle when they walk.

Cerebellar Gait: Cerebellar gait is often described as "drunken" or 'reeling." It is wide-based, irregular, and unsteady, often with a tendency to veer to one side. It is typically accompanied by other evidence of cerebellar dysfunction. The superficially similar gait abnormality of alcohol intoxication tends to be more haphazardly abnormal than does cerebellar gait. A wide-based gait due to loss of position sense (*sensory ataxia*) reveals itself in a positive Romberg test: the patient can not maintain a stable position if standing with the feet together and eyes closed.

Parkinsonian Gait: The typical gait in patients with Parkinson disease is typically slow and hesitant, but accelerates as the patient moves. It is described as a *festinating gait*, from the Latin word for accelerate. Other characteristics are reduced arm swing, turning the whole body in a block, shuffling, and freezing.

Choreoathetotic Gaits: These are due to the distortions of movements that characterized the choreoathetosis. They include jerks, grimacing, squirming, and abnormal positions of the legs, feet, or other parts of the body. The gait abnormality can be the first clinically evident manifestation of a choreoathetotic disorder. Observing the patient when walking can provide the clue to the diagnosis.

Magnetic Gait: In a magnetic gait the feet seem glued to the floor. It can be a manifestation of hydrocephalus, including low-pressure hydrocephalus, where it is typically associated with incontinence and impairment of cognition. It may be a manifestation of hyperactive plantar reflexes.

Frontal Gait: The gait impairment associated with damage to the brain's frontal lobes typically appears first as hesitancy in walking. Patients stoop forward and seem unsure of their footing and other actions. As more is lost of what we learned as babies about how to walk and to carry out other actions, impairments become more profound. In the last stages of movement apraxias, the ability to sit, stand, or even turn over in bed can be lost.

Aged Gait: Elderly people frequently lose the fluid ease with which younger people walk. Sometimes *senile gait* appears to be a mild form of Parkinsonian gait, sometimes a mild form of frontal gait apraxia, sometimes an adaptation to poorer position sense, sometimes an adaptation to loss of muscle (notably of the quadriceps femoris and other leg muscles), and often enough a combination of a number of these and other problems.

Fortunately, most old people who are mentally intact learn to walk carefully. More systematic and detailed classifications of gait disorders including gait disorders of aging are available in the medical literature.[3,4]

DIAGNOSTIC CONSIDERATIONS FOR DISORDERS OF MOTILITY INVOLVE BOTH QUESTIONS OF MECHANISM AND RECOGNITION OF CERTAIN COMMON SYNDROMES (CLINICAL ENTITIES)

The same two major questions apply to a chronic disorder of motility as to other neurological or psychiatric disorders seen by a general clinician. Is there an acute process that requires treatment even before a neurologist or neurosurgeon becomes available? Should the condition be referred to a neurologist or other specialist? Sometimes a relatively chronic disorder of motility results from a lesion that deserves prompt medical attention. A tumor in the spinal cord is a classic example. Even there, however, if the signs and symptoms have had an insidious onset and slow progression, there is usually time for consultation with a specialist.

Certain diagnostic generalizations are straightforward even if they may prove misleading in individual cases. A family history of a movement disorder raises the suspicion of a genetic condition, particularly if the patient admits having something like what his or her relatives had. Spastic weakness is typically associated with damage to the upper motor neuron unit and flaccid paresis with damage to the lower motor unit. In spastic paralysis, slow pressure to move a paralyzed limb can typically lead to a sudden release of tension—a "clasp-knife response" that helps to distinguish spasticity from the "cog-wheeling" resistance to passive motion characteristic of Parkinson disease and other diseases of the basal ganglia. (See below). As noted above, atrophy predominantly in the proximal muscles tends to reflect muscle disease, perhaps because the proximal muscles are bulkier and therefore provide more space for things to go wrong. Atrophy primarily of the distal muscles tends to reflect disease of peripheral nerve, perhaps because the nerves running to the distal muscles are longer than to the proximal muscles and therefore provide more space for abnormalities to make themselves evident clinically. Fasciculations are characteristic of primary disease of nerve rather than muscle, particularly when they are associated with weakness and atrophy—for instance, in Amyotrophic Lateral Sclerosis (ALS; see below). Ataxia calls attention to the cerebellum. Ataxia can also result from abnormalities of sensory systems, particularly of the long sensory tracts in the spinal cord (the *posterior columns*). These patients have trouble putting their hands or feet where they want them, because their brains do not receive adequate information about where their hands or feet are. Parkinsonian signs and symptoms call attention to the basal ganglia. Few diseases of peripheral nerve cause weakness with little or no change in sensation. The exceptions can include poisoning with certain heavy metals, notably lead or gold. Lead poisoning characteristically manifests itself in other parts of the body, with such signs as basophilic stippling of red blood cells and a lead line in the gums. Gold poisoning is typically the result of excessively vigorous use of gold salts to treat rheumatoid arthritis or related diseases. Weakness and fatigue are easily confused by patients and can refer to a number of conditions. A motor examination including tests of muscle strength and fatigability, which can be done in under five minutes, provides a relatively definitive answer to what if anything is wrong with a patient's muscles.

The generalizations in the two previous paragraphs do not make diagnosing the cause of the damage to the nervous system or muscle easy. Doing so confidently requires special expertise. For instance, although fasciculations in the muscles of the arms or legs are characteristic of primary disease of the lower motor neuron (e.g., ALS), fasciculations also occur with other diseases that affect the motor unit (Table 11-1). Optimal work-up requires the skills and knowledge of a specialist. It is not good medical practice to present a frightening diagnosis like ALS to a patient

TABLE 11–1
Common causes of fasciculations

Motor neuron disease (ALS, other variants)
Spinal cord tumors
Syringomyelia (affecting spinal gray matter)
Damage to motor roots (for instance, due to disc disease)
Peripheral nerve damage
Electrolyte imbalance (including severe dehydration)
Toxins (e.g., organophosphates)
Medicines (e.g., neostigmine)
Syndrome of generalized muscular hyperactivity

simply on the basis of weakness and fasciculations. Before the bad news is presented to the patient and family, a specialist should have confirmed the diagnosis after appropriate testing.

A number of laboratory tests aid in the diagnosis of a disorder of motility, beyond what can be gained from history and examination by a trained neurologist. These tests are normally part of the specialist's work-up. Imaging studies (CT or MRI) are useful for disorders of the spine as well as of higher parts of the nervous system. They can, of course, detect strokes as well as space occupying lesions and other lesions of various types including less common conditions such as *syringomyelia*. *Electromyography* and related electrophysiological studies are useful particularly in the differential diagnosis of disorders of the lower motor unit—spinal motor neurons, peripheral nerves, and muscle. Muscle biopsy with appropriate special tissue staining, including immunohistochemistry, can provide a relatively definitive diagnosis, particularly in primary disorders of muscle.

Focused molecular genetic testing can provide firm confirmation of a diagnosis that is clearly associated with a particular site of mutation in DNA—for instance, in Huntington disease. However, two clinical caveats need to be emphasized about genetic testing. In diseases that presdispose to mental instability, like Huntington disease, a positive genetic diagnosis has to be communicated to the patient with great care so as not to raise the risk of suicide. Also, some "well-defined" genetic abnormalities have been associated with so many different clinical syndromes that there is an element of conjecture in linking the abnormality in DNA to the clinical disabilities. These include *mitochondrial myopathies* that are attributed to mutations in mitochondrial DNA (mtDNA).

As discussed above, a variety of medical conditions can predispose to the development of disorders of motility. Table 11-2 is a partial list of some of them that fall within the province of the internist or other general clinician. Information from an appropriate medical evaluation including indicated laboratory tests helps the consultant neurologist make a diagnosis.

Common syndromes of disordered motility can easily be recognized by generalists, even though consultation with a neurologist is wise to confirm the diagnosis and rule out odd diagnoses that can appear to mimic common disorders ("zebras" masquerading as horses.) Four conditions that involve primarily motility are so common that they deserve separate if brief description here: Parkinson disease and related syndromes; myasthenia gravis; acute inflammatory polyneuropathy, also called Guillaine-Barré syndrome; and motor neuron disease (amyotrophic lateral sclerosis,

TABLE 11–2
Medical causes of disorders of motility

- Physician-induced (iatrogenic)
  - Neuroleptic drugs (haldoperidol, risperidone, phenothiazines, and so on)
  - Some seizure medications (e.g., Dilantin)
  - Lithium toxicity
  - Oral contraceptives
  - Other drugs
- Endocrine diseases
  - Thyroid disease (thyrotoxicosis)
  - Diabetes
    - Hypoglycemia
    - Nonketotic hyperosmolar hyperglycemia
- Cancers
  - Direct effects (metastases)
  - Metabolic derangements (e.g., electrolyte disorders)
  - Paraneoplastic syndromes
- Nutritional Disorders
  - Vitamin B_1 (thiamin) deficiency
  - Vitamin B_3 (niacin) deficiency
  - Magnesium deficiency
- Collagen-vascular disease (e.g., systemic lupus)
- Blood diseases
  - Acanthocytosis (neuro form)
  - Polycythemia vera
- Other Conditions
  - Wilson disease
  - Hypoxia
  - Uremia
  - Toxins

ALS; Lou Gehrig disease). Several other conditions are rarer and mentioned only briefly.

Parkinsonian Syndromes

These are among the most common neurological disorders seen by clinicians. The clinical picture is characteristic and is described above. It includes muscle rigidity often with cog-wheeling, poverty of motion, a "festinating," unsteady gait with small steps, a typical 3 per second, "pill-rolling" tremor of the hands and eventually other parts of the body, and slowness of response first in motor activities including speaking and eventually often in thinking as well.

Parkinson disease in its most common form is typically a disease of older age. The neuropathology involves loss of neurons in the substantia nigra with the accumulation of characteristic *Lewy bodies*. The latter contain the protein synuclein among other constituents. The course of this disease varies, but typically involves years or even decades until total disability. Many elderly patients die before they reach that point. Modern treatments discussed below are effective at reducing disability—or, more accurately, at postponing disability.

Other Parkinsonian syndromes typically have clinical manifestations superficially similar to "Parkinson's disease" but different clinical courses and less satisfactory responses to medication. Even in expert settings, perhaps a quarter of the patients who receive the diagnosis of "classic" Parkinson disease turn out at autopsy to have neuropathological abnormalities other than those predicted by the clinical diagnosis.[5]

Striatonigral Degeneration

This exists in a variety of forms. The clinical syndrome is easily taken for drug-unresponsive Parkinson disease with relatively little tremor. The pathology involves marked atrophy of specific parts of the brain, notably the basal ganglia including the putamen as well as of the substantia nigra in the base of the brain. In *Shy-Drager* syndrome, striatonigral degeneration is combined with damage to neurons of the brain stem and therefore with dysfunction of the autonomic system. In addition to the motor symptoms, patients suffer from various combinations of low blood pressure with fainting particularly when standing up (*orthostatic hypotension*), impotence, dry mouth, and difficulty urinating or urinary incontinence. *Multiple system disease* is, as its name suggests, a yet more wide spread disorder of the nervous system. In addition to the brain damage and resultant symptoms seen in Shy-Drager syndrome, there is damage to the other parts of the brain, notably the cerebellum and pons. The clinical picture varies. Usually Parkinsonian signs other than tremor are prominent. So are cerebellar signs, i.e., ataxia. Often Parkinsonian and cerebellar signs occur together, but sometimes one or the other predominates. Patients with multiple system disease are likely to be severely disabled within five years of the onset of clinical abnormalities. Many are in wheel chairs. MRI can help to make the diagnosis by revealing atrophy of the pons and cerebellum. Intermediate forms of striatonigral degenerations are not rare. As the disease progresses and new symptoms and signs appear, changes in diagnostic label can become appropriate. Some neurologists group the striatonigral degenerations together as one disorder, while others prefer to distinguish among them. These arguments about classification are best left to interested specialists.

Cortical-Basal-Ganglionic Syndrome

This syndrome is another Parkinsonian variant with a poor prognosis. These patients are typically elderly. They develop a combination of degeneration of the basal ganglia in the brain and of degeneration of the long motor tracts in the spinal cord. The former lead to Parkinsonian manifestations and the latter to a spastic, upper-motor neuron type paralysis. Sometimes, as the disease progresses, some involvement of lower motor (spinal) neurons also occurs with resulting muscle atrophy. Some patients develop mental problems late in the course. Total disability usually occurs within five years. Fortunately, this condition is relatively rare.

Progressive Supranuclear Palsy

Progressive Supranuclear Palsy (PSP) is yet another variant of Parkinsonism. (Its older, eponymic name is Richardson-Steele-Olszewski Syndrome). These patients also tend to be elderly. Their earliest clinical abnormality is often a tendency to fall. That frequently precedes clear Parkinsonian manifestations. The characteristic neurological sign is difficulty with moving the eyes, particularly vertically (i.e., vertical gaze palsy). Many but not all patients with PSP go on to develop evidence of dysfunction of the cerebral cortex, including difficulties with thinking that can progress to clear-cut dementia. (See Chapter 5, Cognitive Disorders.) Failure to move the eyes up and down (*vertical gaze paralysis*) in a demented patient should alert clinicians to the possibility of this diagnosis. MRI helps with diagnosis particularly in the later stages of the disease, where the form of atrophy of the midbrain is reasonably characteristic.

Chronic liver disease

Chronic liver disease can lead to chronic dysfunction of the basal ganglia. This condition is attributed to chronic elevation of blood ammonia. The manifestations of *chronic hepatocerebral degeneration* are chronic versions of those of acute hepatic encephalopathy, including "liver flap." (See

Chapter 5, Cognitive Disorders.) Wilson's disease, which is well known to general clinicians, is an important form of hepatocerebral degeneration to recognize. This disease is an inherited error of copper metabolism that can be well treated in its earlier stages by appropriate therapy to remove the excess copper, with chelators. A diagnostic clue is provided by the characteristic dark Kayiser-Fleischer ring" in the eye.

Myasthenia Gravis

Myasthenia gravis is the most common disorder of the connections (synapses) between nerves and muscles (neuromuscular junctions). Even so, it is still, fortunately, an uncommon condition. As discussed above, myasthenia gravis is an autoimmune disease in which antibodies are directed against the neuromuscular junction. It is often associated with other disorders of the immune system, and particularly with tumors of the thymus.

The onset can be insidious or sudden, and all ages and both sexes are susceptible. Myasthenia gravis typically begins with weakness of muscles that control eye movements. These small muscles are rich in neuromuscular junctions. The combination of double vision and drooping eyelids (*ptosis*) with normal reactions of the pupil to light and accommodation is almost diagnostic of myasthenia gravis. The disease typically goes on to involve other muscles, although in some patients, clinically significant manifestations stay limited to the eyes. As myasthenia gravis progresses, the autonomic nervous system often also becomes impaired. The disorder is typically chronic and potentially fatal but can be effectively treated, as discussed below. Patients with myasthenia typically die from either respiratory or cardiac complications. *Myasthenic crisis* is a rapid deterioration of the afflicted patient that can lead to respiratory crisis within hours. Intercurrent infection or inappropriate medication or other toxins can be the precipitating event, but crisis can occur for no obvious reason. Aspiration pneumonia is sometimes the presenting event.

Clinical and laboratory tests are useful to confirm the diagnosis. The standard bedside test is transient but definite improvement following injection of a short-acting peripheral cholinesterase inhibitor, usually edrophonium (Tensilon) and sometimes neostigmine (Prostigmin). A rare complication of this test is potentially fatal ventricular fibrillation, so testing should be done in hospitals where equipment and staff for resuscitation are available. The increase in strength needs to be documented objectively, by the examiner and/or electrophysiologically. A statement by a patient that he or she "feels stronger" does not by itself constitute a positive result. Electrophysiological testing can be diagnostic, either a decrementing response on electromyography or characteristic "jitter" on recordings from single muscle fibers. Normalization of these abnormalities by edrophonium secures the diagnosis. Most patients with generalized myasthenia have detectable antibodies to the acetylcholine receptor in their blood. Such antibodies are identifiable in half or more of patients with myasthenia limited to the eye muscles.

Lambert-Eaton syndrome

Lambert-Eaton syndrome is a form of myasthenia that affects the muscles of the trunk and legs more prominently and earlier than the small muscles of the eyes. It, too, is often associated with other immunological abnormalities. Normally these involve calcium channels in the nerve endings rather than the acetylcholine receptor in the muscles. Lambert-Eaton syndrome is associated with oat cell cancer of the lungs so frequently that the diagnosis requires a search for such a cancer. Since the cancer is often small, repeated examinations can be needed. Formal studies have not yet determined whether the newer spiral MRIs of the lungs will help in finding very small cancers in people with this syndrome.

More than 30 known drugs can precipitate myasthenia. Table 11-3 lists some of them.

Acute Inflammatory Polyneuropathy

Acute inflammatory polyneuropathy (Guillain-Barré syndrome; Landry-Guillain-Barré-Strohl syndrome) is an immune-modulated paralysis of relatively acute onset. The disorder typically begins in the legs and ascends to involve the arms, respiratory muscles, and often muscles innervated by cranial nerves, such as the muscles of the face. Often but not invariably, a history is available of viral or other illness a few weeks before the onset of the paralysis. Typically, protein is elevated in the spinal fluid without significant elevation of cells. Electromyography reveals characteristic findings. The clinically prominent abnormalities are primarily motor, although involvement of the autonomic nervous system and complaints of pain are not rare. The disease is normally self-limited, although there is a form in which nerve processes (axons) are so damaged that recovery is incomplete. Death can result acutely from respiratory insufficiency; perhaps a third or more of these patients require mechanical ventilation to survive the severe phase of their disease. As many as 5% of these patients die even with excellent care, some of them from cardiac instability. A number of other conditions that can cause similar paralyses are important in the differential diagnosis. They include acute spinal cord disease, basilar artery stroke,

TABLE 11–3
Drugs and toxins inducing or exacerbating myasthenia

Antibiotics
Neomycin
Kanamycin
Colistin
Streptomycin
Polymyxin B
Tetracyclines
Cholinesterase inhibitors
Botulinum toxin
Tubocurarine
Suxamethonium
Decamethonium
Other Medications
D penicillamine
Toxins
Black widow spider venom and certain other spider venoms
Tick bites (some)
Snake bites (some)
Malathion
Parathion
Organophosphate insecticides
Some military nerve gasses

botulism, poliomyelitis and other infections of motor neurons, acute onset of myasthenia gravis, tick paralysis, and motor neuropathies associated with various forms of severe medical illness. Examination of the spinal fluid and electromyography help in the differential diagnosis. For instance, they help in differentiating immune modulated acute paralysis from the clinically almost identical syndrome resulting from tick bites. (Of course, finding the tick can also help in recognizing tick paralysis.)

Motor Neuron Disease

There are a group of essentially untreatable diseases that lead to the death of motor neurons. There are minimal or no clinically notable alterations in sensation, except perhaps some secondary to weakness and resulting strains on muscle and joints. The causes are unknown except for rare genetic forms. Specific syndromes have been delineated, based on which group of motor neurons are affected most prominently.

Amyotrophic lateral sclerosis (ALS) is the most common of these syndromes. In America this is still sometimes called Lou Gehrig disease, after the prominent baseball player who suffered from it. The disease often begins with problems with the fine muscles of the hands. The diagnosis then becomes relatively obvious, with the development of the triad of atrophic weakness of the hands and forearms, slight spastic weakness of the arms and legs, and increased reflexes, without impairments of sensation. Typically, fasciculations occur. However, as mentioned above, it is a diagnostic error to make the diagnosis primarily on the basis of these abnormal muscle movements. Many things can cause fasciculations (Table 11-1). In the so-called Mills variant of ALS, the pattern of weakness involves an arm and a leg on the same side. Patients with ALS tend to live no more than 3 to 6 years from the onset of clinically apparent illness.

Many of these patients develop problems with thinking as their disease progresses, probably because of loss or damage spreading to include nerve cells that are involved in functions other than movement. Problems have been reported in attention, concentration, and working memory; dementia when it occurs has been reported to often resemble the *frontotemporal* type.[6] (See Chapter 5, Cognitive Disorders.)

Progressive muscular atrophy is more slowly progressive than ALS, with some patients living 15 years or more. *Progressive bulbar palsy* first involves muscles of the jaw, face, tongue, and larynx, which are enervated by motor neurons in the lower brainstem. The course is more rapid, with the patient usually dying within 2 to 3 years of disease onset.

Primary lateral sclerosis is a form of motor neuron disease in which loss of upper motor neurons in the brain precedes prominent loss of lower motor neurons of the spinal cord by up to a year. If signs of lower motor neuron disease such as muscle atrophy and fasciculations do not appear within a year, the disorder may actually be multiple sclerosis or a primary disease of the spinal cord. Patients with this form of motor neuron disease can survive for years.

Clinical history and physical examination can provide the diagnosis of motor neuron disease. Electrodiagnostic techniques available through neurological consultation can confirm it.

Mixed Disorders

Mixed disorders involving motility and sensation are not rare, as mentioned above. Sensory and motor systems and particularly their axonal connections are close to each other in many parts of the nervous system. It is therefore not surprising that many lesions of the nervous system present clinically with a mixture of motor and sensory disabilities. Chap.13 (Disorders of Both Sensation and Motility) discusses several such conditions not discussed elsewhere in this monograph. They include multiple sclerosis and other disorders that primarily affect the material that sheathes nerves (*myelin*) as well as primary afflictions of the peripheral nerves. Some of the conditions discussed in Chapter 13 are of particular concern to general physicians because they are associated with diseases normally treated by generalists. A screen for toxins is a standard part of the evaluation of weakness that can be attributed to damage to peripheral nerves.

NEUROBIOLOGY

For chronic disorders of motility, as for other disorders of the nervous system, the term "cause" (*etiology*) is used in at least two ways. One is what part of the nervous system is affected (the localization of the damage). The other is what it is affected by (the disease causing the damage). Both meanings are useful when considering the etiology of disorders of motility.

Localization of function within the parts of the nervous system controlling movement has been gratifyingly successful. As a result, detailed neurological examination often allows relatively precise mapping of the part of the nervous system involved in an abnormality of mobility. Motor systems are conveniently divided into *primary* and *secondary*. Disorders of the first most often lead to reduced movement, and to either spastic or flaccid paresis or paralysis. Disorders of the second most often lead to extraneous movements, and can be associated with either increased muscle tone (rigidity and hypokinesia), or with decreased muscle tone (hypotonia).

The primary motor system initiates and carries out movements. It includes: the *upper motor neurons* of the "*motor strip*," that lies just posterior to the fissure of Roland in the cerebral cortex; their long processes (*axons*), that form the cerebrospinal tracts in the spinal cord; their connections (*synapses*) onto the primary motor neurons in the spinal cord; the primary motor neurons in the spinal cord; their long axons, that extend through the anterior roots of the spinal cord to form *peripheral nerves*; the synapses of those nerves onto *muscle receptors*; and the muscle fibers. Disease of the upper motor neurons or their axonal projections and synapses typically leads to *spastic paresis* or *paralysis* (see above) of the affected limbs or other muscle groups. The reason is that the inhibitory effects of the upper motor neurons normally predominate over the excitatory. The result is that loss of upper motor neuron innervation increases the resting activity of the lower motor neurons that directly innervate the muscles, with resultant increases in the tonic contraction of muscles.[7] Upper motor neuron lesions lead to release of inhibition of *deep tendon reflexes*, such as the knee jerk and the infantile form of the *Babinski reflex*. Deep tendon reflexes therefore typically increase in magnitude, and the Babinski sign becomes positive (i.e., toes become upgoing). In contrast, *flaccid* weakness is the typical consequence of damage to the lower motor neurons, of the peripheral nerves that contain their extended axons, and of their synapses on muscle fibers or of the muscle fibers themselves. Reflexes tend to be diminished or lost in lower motor neuron disease.

The secondary or "accessory" motor systems are involved in the modulation of movements. They are required for smooth and coordinated movements. They include *the basal ganglia* and the *cerebellum*, among other structures in the brain. Different kinds of movement disorders tend to be associated with different structures. In the basal ganglia, under-activity of the caudate tends to lead to a Parkinson-like picture, with rigidity and rest tremor. (See below.) Hypokinesia and bradykinesia are prominent and usually more disabling than the tremor. Under-activity of the caudate can be due to loss of innervation from structures that project to caudate neurons. Parkinson disease, for instance, is associated with loss of cells located in the pars compacta of the substantia nigra in the midbrain. Overactivity of the basal ganglia tends to cause chorea or choreoathetosis. Ballismus is typically the consequence of a lesion of the subthalamic nucleus, although lesions of other parts of the nervous system are known to lead to more transient forms of this condition.

Disorders of the cerebellum typically present clinically with a mixture of the signs and symptoms of ataxia, the motor signs of which are described above. Specific manifestations have been related to dysfunction of specific parts of the cerebellum, and that knowledge is useful for specialists managing these diseases.

Apraxias typically result from dysfunction of parts of the cerebral cortex that feed information about learned activities into the primary and secondary motor systems. The parietal cortex, which lies behind (*caudal to*) the motor strip, is typically involved in apraxias.

Gait abnormalities reflect the part or parts of the nervous system that are impaired. Total paralysis of one or both legs due to stroke or other damage to the central nervous system is incompatible with unassisted walking. Paresis (partial paralysis) of a leg is a frequent result of less extensive central nervous system damage of the same type. Damage to upper motor neurons in the motor cortex or to their axons normally causes the leg to be weak but stiff (spastic); damage to lower motor neurons or their axons or synapses leads to a leg that is both weak and flaccid. It can lead to a *steppage gait*, described above. Muscle disease typically leads to a *waddling gait*, due in part to diminished ability to contract the gluteal muscles of the buttocks. *Cerebellar gait* is a typical manifestation of disease of the cerebellum, particularly disease involving the cerebellar vermis. *Sensory ataxia* is due to loss of position sense and therefore to damage anywhere in the relevant ascending sensory pathways or, rarely, to bilateral lesions of the parietal cortex involved in organizing that sensory information. The *tabetic gait* characteristic of late stage (tertiary) syphilis is a form of sensory ataxia. (See Chapter 12, Disorders of Sensation.) Cerebellar gait and sensory ataxia occur together in a number of diseases, notably Friedreich's ataxia, that are now defined by molecular genetics.[8] (See Chapter 13, Combined Disorders of Sensation and Motility.) Damage to the cerebellum and/or brain stem can also lead to tottering and falling (*toppling gait*), as can dizziness and vertigo and certain other neurological diseases such as *Progressive Supranuclear Palsy*. (See above.) *Parkinsonian gait* is typically due to damage to the basal ganglia; in Parkinson disease the *pars compacta* of the *substantia nigra* is also damaged. A *wide-based gait* in which the feet appear to be "stuck" to the floor is thought to be characteristic of *hydrocephalus*, including low-pressure hydrocephalus. It is associated with white matter dysfunction due to pressure from the spinal fluid in the cerebral ventricles. The abnormality in lifting the feet (*magnetic gait*) has been attributed to an overactive but otherwise normal adult plantar (Babinski) reflex. Magnetic gait can also be part of *gait apraxias* (loss of knowing how to walk); gait apraxias are a frequent and sometimes severe effect of damage to the frontal lobes. This gait is sometimes seen accompanying widespread vascular damage to white matter (*leukoaraiosis; Binswanger disease*). The gait abnormality of hydrocephalus may be due in part to damage to white matter connections to the frontal lobe. Alzheimer disease and a variety of other conditions that can damage the frontal lobes can also lead to this gait abnormality. Aged gait is a poorly defined condition, both clinically and in terms of etiology. Its appearance resembles that of a mild Parkinsonian gait.

Causes of chronic disorders of motility vary widely. As usual, they include both genetic and environmental factors, alone and in different combinations. As mentioned earlier, sometimes "cause" in Neurology still consists of grouping the patient with other patients in an eponymic syndrome.

Hereditary Disorders

Hereditary disorders of motility are well known, and in some the responsible gene has been identified.

In a number of these, the genetic defect is an expansion of a triplet repeat in the DNA encoding the abnormal gene product. Often these are repeats of the "CAG" triplet, which encodes the amino acid glutamine. The results are abnormally long stretches of glutamine residues in the protein encoded in the affected gene. The best known of these conditions is Huntington disease, in which the affected protein is *huntingtin*. Pathological CAG expansions are also responsible for a variety of rare hereditary *spinocerebellar ataxias*. The clinical manifestations of the different hereditary ataxic syndromes overlap widely.[8] Another, relatively common form of spinocerebellar ataxia still has the eponymic name of *"Friedreich's ataxia."* It typically results from any of a variety of mutations in the *FRAX* gene that encodes a mitochondrial protein, frataxin. Some episodic ataxias are associated with mutations in potassium channel or calcium channel genes.

Rare hereditary forms of Parkinsonism have been associated with several abnormal genes. The extent to which these movement disorders mimic the common form of late-onset Parkinson disease is a matter of debate. Most Parkinson disease appears to be more the result of environmental than genetic factors, although genetic predispositions may still play a part.[9]

Muscular dystrophies are caused by mutations in a number of genes, most of which have been well characterized. The most common form of muscular dystrophy is caused by mutations in the dystrophin (*DMD*) gene, the largest human gene yet characterized. Genes causing other forms of muscle disease such as myotonic dystrophy are also well characterized. Defects in the DNA of mitochondria (mtDNA) cause a number of relatively rare but extensively studied syndromes. Hereditary disorders including hereditary disorders of muscle are likely to become clinically important in childhood or adolescence rather than first causing trouble during adult life.

In many hereditary disorders of motility, a single abnormal gene can lead to clinical manifestations ("dominant inheritance"), although sometimes both copies of the gene must be abnormal ("recessive inheritance"). In Huntington disease, two copies of an abnormal gene do not lead to a worse clinical syndrome than does a single mutated gene.

Injuries

Injuries can, of course, impair motility by damaging neurological or musculoskeletal systems or both. Minor back injuries are so common in our society as to be statistically normal, even though they often need some kind of treatment. (See Chapter 7, Pain.) Major injuries that impair motility, for instance from auto accidents, are unfortunately not rare. Repeated blows to the head are not good for the brain, whether they come from boxing, heading the ball in soccer, or other sports. The risk of mental impairment appears to be greater in people who carry the ε-4 allele of the *APOE* gene. Most sports injuries are, however, more likely to be orthopedic than neurological.

Intercurrent Diseases

Intercurrent diseases can lead to chronic impairments of motility. Some of these diseases tend to be associated with damage to particular parts of the nervous system and therefore with typical behavioral read-outs.

Vascular diseases are frequently involved with stroke or other damage to upper motor neurons in the cerebral cortex, although they certainly can affect the accessory motor areas and lower motor neurons in the spinal cord as well.

Infections can cause chronic problems with motility. Viral infections are often associated with damage to lower motor neurons, for instance in *poliomyelitis*. However, they can certainly affect other parts of the nervous system as well in various forms of *encephalitis*. Von Economo described encephalitis which led to a severe form of Parkinson's disease. This condition is now happily rare. Bacterial and fungal infections can affect any part of the nervous system, including the meninges. The sequelae of poorly treated meningitis can involve severe motor disabilities. Syphilis and its neurological sequelae are happily less common than they were a century and more ago, but *borreliosis* from Lyme disease is a major problem particularly in areas such as the Northeastern United States where it is endemic. As emphasized in Chap. 5, patients with neurological or psychiatric disease deserve a blood test for syphilis, which used to be known as "the great imitator" of other diseases. Syphilis, now rarer than a century ago, can still remain unsuspected, particularly in patients whose disorder is "typical" for another condition.[4,10] Among infections of muscle are parasitic infections such as *trichinosis* and *toxoplasmosis*.

The AIDS virus infects muscle and can lead to significant muscle weakness. Unfortunately, so do some of the antiviral agents used to treat AIDS.

Toxins including medications can damage neurological systems involved in movement. Antipsychotic drugs are a common cause of movement disorders, particularly extrapyramidal ("Parkinson-like") syndromes. (See Chapter 4, Thought Disorders.) Both older and newer neuroleptics can have this unfortunate side effect. Environmental poisoning, notably with magnesium, can also lead to an extrapyramidal syndrome. The suggestion has been made that the common form of Parkinson disease results from some form(s) of environmental pollution that became common with the industrial revolution. Parkinson described this disorder in 1817, in the early days of the industrial revolution in England. Surprisingly, earlier medical writings provide no clear description of this hard-to-miss syndrome. That contrasts with conditions like stroke and epilepsy, which were well described thousands of years ago. Specific industrial toxin(s) have not been identified. Toxins are also classic causes of peripheral neuropathy and can sometimes be identified in individual cases.

Certain toxins usually cause predominantly motor weakness without much sensory loss. For instance, lead neuropathy tends to lead to wrist drop and finger drop, due to relatively selective damage to the motor fibers of the radial nerve. Foot drop can also occur.

Table 11-4 lists drugs and other toxins that are important causes of muscle disease. It is, of course, only a partial list. Perhaps 100 substances have been identified as causing muscle disease. Outbreaks have been traced to odd materials, such as rapeseed oil and a contaminant in a commercial batch of tryptophan. Sometimes the same drugs that are used to treat a disease that can cause muscle weakness can themselves cause muscle weakness. Examples include steroids for dermatomyositis and other inflammatory myopathies and *zidovudine* to treat AIDS myopathy. These situations are difficult to decipher unless reducing or withdrawing the drug ameliorates the muscle weakness. Withdrawing the drug may, of course, exacerbate the muscle weakness by reducing the effectiveness of treatment.

Cancers can cause disorders of motility both by their direct (mass) effects on the appropriate parts of the nervous system and also by immunological mechanisms (*paraneoplastic syndromes*).[11,12] (See below.)

Nutritional disorders can lead to weakness, such as the peripheral nerve disease associated with deficiency of thiamin (vitamin B_1).

Endocrine disorders frequently lead to motor manifestations, such as the tremor of hyperthyroidism or the neuropathy that accompanies diabetes. Both too much thyroid hormone (hyperthyroidism) and too

TABLE 11–4
Drugs and toxins causing muscle disease

Statins (lovastatin, pravastatin, simvastatin)
Corticosteroids (often associated with critical illness)
Diuretics (hypokalemic weakness)
Laxatives (with loss of potassium from diarrhea)
Licorice
Clofibrate
Malnutrition
Ipecac, other materials that cause vomiting
Excess vitamin E (hypervitaminosis E)
Organophosphates
Some snake venoms
Some mushroom poisoning (including *A. Phalloides*)
Alcohol abuse (acute or chronic)
Cocaine abuse
Chloroquine and other antimalarial drugs
Penicillamine
Zidovudine
Rifampin
Amiodarone

little (*hypothyroidism*) can cause muscle weakness, as can too little parthyroid hormone (*hypoparathyroidism).*

Autoimmune disorders can affect both nerve and muscle. One of the best known of these, *myasthenia gravis*, results from autoantibodies to the receptors in the synapses of peripheral nerves onto muscles (i.e., antibodies to the *neuromuscular junction*). A variety of paraneoplastic syndromes are associated with antibodies that arise in patients with cancer and cross- react with constituents of the nervous system.[11,12] Typical manifestations can include ataxias of various forms, peripheral neuropathy that is often sensory but sometimes primarily motor or autonomic, spinal cord disease including damage to white matter and sometimes to motor neurons, and occasionally damage to the retina. Because cancer is not rare, these syndromes are also not rare.

Autoimmune disorders that characteristically affect muscle include *polymyositis* and *dermatomyositis*. Both are well known to general clinicians. Dermatomyositis in adults is often associated with cancer, sometimes occult cancer; reported incidences vary from 10% of adult patients with this disease to 50% or more.

Primary degenerative diseases can be associated with more or less specific constellations of signs and symptoms. Parkinson disease and other "Parkinsonian syndromes" are a classic example. (See below.) Spastic weakness so often develops in progressive multiple sclerosis that it is one of the characteristic findings in this disorder, as in other conditions that damage myelin. (See Chapter 12, Combined Disorders of Sensation and Motility.)

Hysterical disorders of motility have been extensively discussed, by Freud among others. The conventional explanation for these disorders is that the patients gain in some way from their difficulty with movement. Sometimes the gain is monetary, as in *compensation neurosis* after an injury for which an employer or someone else is financially liable. Sometimes it involves other motivations, including rage or sexual desires that make the patient uncomfortable. As discussed below, the diagnosis of hysterical movement disorder should be made by a specialist. Hysteria has proven to be an easily made but risky diagnosis.[1]

Identifying the disease or other condition that damages the nervous system and leads to a disorder of motility is often challenging—sometimes even more challenging than identifying the part of the brain involved. Therefore, as discussed below, a thorough medical examination including appropriate laboratory tests is part of the evaluation of a patient with a chronic disorder of motility.

TREATMENT

The treatment of chronic disorders of motility is best done by or in consultation with a neurologist. The state of the art is changing rapidly for a number of common conditions, and specialists are obligated to stay up to date with those advances. However, these disorders are so common that general clinicians will almost certainly have patients receiving medications originally prescribed by neurologists or rehabilitation physicians. General physicians need to know about these agents and to be familiar with their side effects, since generalists are likely to care for patients taking these medications (e.g., older people with spastic paralysis from strokes or with Parkinson disease).

Interventions other than drugs are very important in caring for patients with disorders of motility. Severely afflicted patients need to be turned and moved so as to prevent bed sores and resultant infections and to mobilize secretions from their lungs. Special diets and eventually surgery can help patients who can no longer control swallowing and are in danger of food or other inappropriate material passing into their lungs instead of their stomachs (*aspirating*). Rehabilitation techniques that can help to maximize residual function include not only braces and other prostheses but also a variety of other specialized devices and procedures, including such newer developments as robotics. Occupational therapists can teach patients and their families techniques and introduce tools that allow the afflicted person more or less to "get around" the disability. These non-pharmacological interventions are critical to the care of these patients, and general clinicians should become reasonably familiar with them. However, they fall outside the scope of this monograph.

Paralysis and Paresis

Motor weaknesses are treated with drugs to reduce their complications. As yet, transplantation of stem cells and pharmacological treatments to restore damaged motor neurons remain "exciting, innovative research frontiers," far removed from actual medical practice.

Spastic paralysis or paresis can raise problems related to the spasticity itself. Medications are available to relieve spasticity (Table 11-5). Except for botulinum toxin, all of these agents reduce activity not only of the motor system but of other parts of the nervous system as well. Their

TABLE 11–5
Medications for spasticity and their major side effects

Agent	Side effects
Baclofen	Sedation, dizziness, tiredness, confusion, seizures, hallucinations, paresthesias, nausea, low blood pressure
Tizanidine	Sedation, dizziness, fatigue, hallucinations, dry skin, low blood pressure, liver damage
Benzodiazepines	Sedation, confusion, drooling, depression (diazepam [Valium]) (see Chap. 6, Anxiety)
Dantrolene	Weakness, drowsiness, headaches, nausea, diarrhea, paresthesias, liver damage
Botulinum toxin A	Uncommon. Occ. transient flu-like syndrome, occ. transient headache
Others (e.g., phenol)	Not recommended

side effects include drowsiness and other signs of central nervous system depression. When a patient taking one of these medicines becomes confused, it is important to lower the dose or stop the medicine and see if the patient improves before attributing the confusion to "a new stroke" or to other progression of the primary brain disease.

Baclofen (Lioresal) acts on receptors for the neurotransmitter γ-aminobutyric acid (GABA), which classically inhibits the activity of nerve cells. Side effects of this medication include drowsiness, confusion, and seizures, among others. The typical starting dose of baclofen is 5 mg –10 mg a day, but the medication can be titrated up to doses 20 times that high (100–200 mg a day) unless side effects supervene. Baclofen can be given directly into the spinal fluid, typically via an indwelling pump, but too much of the medicine can easily reach the brain stem, depress vital functions, and kill the patient. Such intrathecal administration of baclofen should be done ***only by experts***.

Tizanidine (Zanaflex) acts in the central nervous system to decrease the activity of motor neurons. It does so by activating the appropriate α-adrenergic receptors. Side effects again include liver damage as well as drowsiness and other side effects associated with baclofen. The starting dose is typically 2 to 4 mg a day, with carefully titrated increases until side effects appear. These patients should have periodic tests of liver function.

Benzodiazepines (e.g., clonazepam, Klonipin) also relieve spasticity. Their use and side effects are discussed in Chapter 6 (Anxiety). Too much benzodiazepine is a classic cause of confusion, particularly in brain-damaged people. (See Chapter 5, Cognitive Disorders.)

Dantrolene (Dantrium) acts primarily on muscle rather than on the nervous system itself. It interferes with calcium fluxes necessary for muscle contraction. It can therefore exacerbate muscle weakness. Despite its peripheral action, it, too, can cause drowsiness and related problems. This drug can be toxic to the liver, and patients put on it should have liver function tests before starting the medicine and periodically thereafter.

Botulinum toxin (Botox) acts primarily on receptors at the neuromuscular junction. It is given by injection directly into the affected spastic muscles. The properties and the relatively mild side effects of this medication are now widely known to general clinicians, since this substance is now so widely used in cosmetic surgery.

Flaccid paralysis is treated primarily by non-pharmacologic means, such as providing optimal prosthetics and moving the patients to prevent break down of the skin and infection. When bed sores occur, their treatment with antibiotics and other approaches are well known to general clinicians.

Specific treatments are available for some forms of flaccid paralysis due to intercurrent disease. For instance, steroids can be very beneficial in patients with weakness due to peripheral nerve damage from a vasculitis or autoimmune disorder (other than Guillain-Barré syndrome). Removing toxins can benefit patients with toxic neuropathic weakness. Lead toxicity is well treated with *penicillamine*, an agent that removes lead; *British snti-Lewisite* (BAL) is an alternative if penicillamine is not tolerated. The general clinician is likely to be able to develop a suspicion of the existence of such exogenous disorders on the basis of their other manifestations. An example is the gastrointestinal symptoms of arsenic poisoning. Another is the anemia, stomach cramps, and "lead line" on the gums that frequently result from lead poisoning.

Hypotonia

Hypotonia not due to paresis is treated by management of the cause—for instance, letting a medication or toxin that blocks neuromuscular transmission wear off. Sometimes an effective antitoxin is available—for instance, a cholinergic blocking agent in patients with muscle weakness due to organic phosphate poisoning. Over-titration of an antidote is always a risk, however. Optimally, the possibility of going to supportive measures such as mechanical ventilation should also be readily available.

Hypokinesia, bradykinesia, and rigidity are discussed below with the treatment of Parkinson disease.

Postural Disturbances

Postural disturbances are treated as part of the neurological syndromes in which they occur. Sometimes postural disturbances are associated with disorders of consciousness, as discussed in Chapter 10 (Disorders of Awareness). Falls in the elderly are common, can be dangerous, and typically arise from a combination of causes. Only about a third of falls in the elderly are due to neurological disease.[13] These include Parkinsonism or sequelae of strokes. The primary causes of old people falling often relate to problems with the heart or the muscles, joints, and skeleton. For instance, poor regulation of blood pressure after meals can lead to repetitive but preventable falls by patients in nursing homes. Prevention can be achieved by having these patients sit or lie down for the appropriate time after meals, particularly after lunch. There is now an extensive literature on prevention of falls in the elderly and the clinical management of falls when they occur.[13]

Apraxias

Apraxias are normally treated not by drugs but by occupational therapy or other techniques to try to train the patient to find a way around his or her disability. For apraxias that are triggered by toxins, drug side effects, or metabolic disease, treatment of the underlying disease is obviously in order.

Muscle Disorders

Muscle disorders are sometimes highly treatable and sometimes unfortunately still effectively untreatable. Unfortunately, muscular dystrophies usually fall into the untreatable group.

Secondary disorders of muscle are treated by ameliorating the primary disease as well as possible. Myopathies due to toxins or side effects of drugs are treated primarily by stopping exposure to the offending material. The treatment of muscle weakness due to thyroid imbalance is treatment of the thyroid problem. The treatment of parasitic infections of muscle (E.G., *trichinosis*, *toxoplasmosis*, etc) is treatment of the infection, by methods well known to general internists. In treating these unusual infections, consultations with specialists in infectious disease can be useful. "Recommended" treatments for these conditions change as new medications come on the market and consensus conferences announce their opinions.

Inflammatory muscle disease is typically treated with anti-inflammatory drugs, usually steroids. A typical dose for patients with polymyositis or dermatomyositis is high dose prednisone (1 mg/kg body weight daily) until strength increases adequately, followed by maintenance doses (often about 20 mg/day of prednisone or equivalent doses of another corticosteroid). Measurements of the activity of creatine kinase (CK), an enzyme that leaks from injured muscle into blood, are helpful in regulating dosage. CK activity tends to come down even before muscle strength increases and to rise even before weakness increases during a relapse. Relapses of course suggest increases in steroid dosage. General clinicians are familiar with the uses and complications of chronic steroid therapy, including specifically the use of steroids to treat collagen-vascular diseases that lead to muscle weakness.

The treatment of periodic paralysis depends on the specific form of this condition. For the hypokalemic form, the frequency of attacks can usually be dramatically reduced by treatment with *acetazolamide* (Diamox), 250 mg 3 times a day. An alternative is dietary alterations that raise serum potassium, such as taking 5–10 gm of KCl in an (unsweetened) solution every day, or switching to a low Nacl, high KCl diet with addition of diuretics when necessary. For acute attacks, the treatment is supplemental potassium by mouth (PO) if possible (0.25 meq KCl/kg body weight) or, where necessary, intravenously IV (0.05 to 0.1 meq/kg initially, followed by maintenance KCl until the disorder has cleared). It is critically important to remember that too much KCl intravenously too fast kills people by stopping their hearts; it is a favored means of execution of criminals in the United States today. By contrast, attacks of periodic paralysis are rarely life threatening by themselves. The muscle weakness that follows repeated attacks of hypokalemic periodic paralysis has been reported to respond to treatment with a carbonic anhydrase inhibitor, specifically *dichlorphenamide* (Daranide). The treatment of the hyperkalemic form associated with too much potassium is, reasonably enough, more or less the opposite of the treatment of the more common hypokalemic form associated with too little potassium. Keeping the serum potassium below 5 meq/kg generally prevents attacks. *Diuretics* (e.g., hydrochlorothiazide, [500 mg/day p.o.], or other thiazides) can achieve this. Appropriate diet is sometimes all that is needed. Fortunately, in many patients attacks of this form of periodic paralysis are so brief that treatment is often unnecessary.

Other specific muscle diseases respond to specific treatments. The rare disorders associated with hereditary defects in the ability of muscle to oxidize fatty acids often respond to a low fat, high carbohydrate diet and to the avoidance of too strenuous exercise. ("Too strenuous" is strenuous enough to bring on an attack.) A rare form of familial myotonia responds to acetazolamide. As noted above, the diagnosis and at least initiation of treatment for these unusual conditions is best left to specialists.

Tremors

Tremors frequently respond to medication. The treatment of the tremor of Parkinson disease is discussed below, with therapy for that entity.

Familial and essential tremors usually respond to medication. With treatment, they typically diminish and become less disabling even if they do not disappear entirely. Most people with these problems have noticed that their tremor gets better after they drink alcohol but sometimes gets even worse when the effect of the alcohol wears off. A longer lasting treatment although one with more side effects is *β-adrenergic blockade*. *Propranolol* is useful in a majority but not all patients, in divided doses of 120–300 mg/day or as a sustained release preparation. Other β-adrenergic blocking drugs have also been found useful (e.g., metoprolol, nadolol). General physicians are familiar with the properties and side effects of this group of medications. An alternative for the minority of patients who do not respond to or cannot tolerate β-adrenergic blockade are anticonvulsants. *Primidone* (Mysoline) tends to be useful for tremor in the arms or hands and *valproate* and *clonazepam* in the rare patients with *orthostatic tremor* of the legs. These medications are discussed in this monograph in Chap. 10, Disorders of Awareness. Sometimes giving *amantadine* along with other medication helps.

Withdrawal syndromes including alcoholic withdrawal (delirium tremens) typically cause tremulousness. Mild alcohol withdrawal symptoms are unpleasant but not serious. Full-blown delirium tremens is life-threatening. Its treatment is discussed in Chap. 14 (Disorders of Conduct) and Chap. 5 (Cognitive Disorders, in the section of treatment of delirium).

Asterixis

Asterixis typically responds to treatment of the underlying disease. "Liver flap" is treated by methods to reduce ammonia toxicity—protein restriction, reducing urease-producing bacteria in the colon by treatment with neomycin or kanamycin or with non-absorbable antibiotics, and with enemas. The use of *branched-chain keto acids* is controversial, since effects are variable among patients and higher mortality has been reported. On the other hand, the response of patients who do regularly respond to ingesting branched chain keto acids can be very satisfying to both the patient and the physician. (See discussion of treatments for delirium, in Chap. 5 [Cognitive Disorders].)

Chorea

Chorea including the movement disorder of Huntington disease sometimes responds symptomatically to dopamine depleting agents such as reserpine.

Tetrabenazine has been reported to be effective but is not approved in the United States for other than investigational use. (It is available in Canada and the United Kingdom.) These medications do not slow the degeneration of brain tissue. They can have serious side effects including precipitating depression in Huntington patients who are already at risk of suicide. Treatment of chorea should be left whenever possible to neurologists or other specialists. That includes the treatment of the psychiatric complications that often accompany Huntington disease and often other forms of chorea.

Athetosis and Choreoathetosis

Athetosis and choreoathetosis can respond to treatment of a disease which underlies them—for instance, a metabolic disease. Symptomatic treatments for chorea, discussed immediately above, can be tried.

Myoclonus

Myoclonus is treated in different ways depending on the underlying cause. Relatively mild hereditary myoclonus often requires no intervention beyond teaching the patient how to live with the disability. Myoclonus secondary to a metabolic disease is managed by treating the underlying metabolic disease, when possible. In *Hashimoto encephalopathy*, myoclonus is associated with antithyroid antibodies although usually not with abnormalities of thyroid function; it typically responds well to steroids or other treatments of the autoimmune disorder. For myoclonic epilepsy, the anticonvulsant of choice is valproate. An alternate where necessary is lamotrigine, particularly in the juvenile form of this condition. These agents are discussed in Chap. 10, Disorders of Awareness.

Ataxia

Ataxia due to an underlying toxic or other disorder is treated by managing the underlying disorder. A staggering drunk needs to be put into a safe situation while the effect of the alcohol wears off. In many cases, nutritional supplementation particularly with B vitamins is needed. Ataxia in acute Wernicke-Korsakoff syndrome typically responds rapidly to treatment with intravenous thiamin (vitamin B_1). A conventional dose is 100 mg of thiamine hydrochloride IV followed by oral supplementation. (See Chap. 5, Cognitive Disorders.) Vitamin B_{12} deficiency causing *combined systems disease* can lead to a sensory ataxia, where staggering is due to loss of position sense. Unfortunately, the neurological abnormalities of vitamin B_{12} deficiency, unlike the blood disease, do not characteristically respond well to replenishment of the vitamin. Ataxia due to a genetic abnormality is treated with rehabilitation techniques to lessen the effect of the disability. Ataxia due to a tumor or bleeding or other mechanical lesion of the cerebellum is typically treated surgically. The cerebellum is located in the posterior fossa, and mass lesions in the posterior fossa are potentially life threatening. If they expand and compress the brain stem, they damage structures needed to maintain vital functions such as breathing.

Ballismus

Ballismus usually responds to treatment with standard doses of a *butyrophenone* (e.g., haloperidol [Haldol]) or a phenothiazine (e.g., chlorpromazine [Thorazine] or fluphenazine [Prolixin]). These antipsychotic agents are discussed in Chap. 3, Thought Disorders. Severe ballismus that persists despite drug therapy may require surgery to ablate the relevant motor centers. Uncontrolled ballismus can kill the victim from exhaustion.

Dystonia

Dystonia is hard to treat, unless the cause of the dystonia is an intercurrent condition that can be treated effectively. Dystonia that is a side effect of excessive treatment with antipsychotics (*dyskinesia tardive*) often responds well to reducing or discontinuing the offending medication. (See Chap. 4, Thought Disorders). The response can take months. Clozapine can be substituted for other antipsychotics, since it has little tendency to cause dystonic movements. So can quetiapine. For unclear reasons, the response to reducing the antipsychotic medication can be a paradoxical worsening of the movement disorder, which then responds to increasing doses of the "offending" antipsychotic drug. Sometimes the syndrome is helped by medications that deplete dopamine, such as reserpine (Serpasil). Tetrabenazine (Nitoman) has also been reported to be useful, but is not available in the United States except as part study protocols approved by the FDA (U.S. Food & Drug Administration). Dystonia that occurs soon after starting an antipsychotic medication often responds well to treatment with intravenous *diphenhydramine* (Benadryl), in ordinary doses (e.g., 25–50 mg IV, repeated once after 2 hours). Dystonia can be due to irreversible brain damage from *Wilson Disease* or *kernicterus* or episodes of hypoxia; in these cases, the underlying condition should of course be treated as well as possible even if the movement disorder does not improve. Some authors have reported successes in treating primary dystonias with massive doses of cholinergic agents (*trihexyphenidyl* [Artane], *ethopropazine* [Parsidol]) or with very low doses of DOPA/Sinemet (see treatment of Parkinsonism, below).

Fasciculations

Fasciculations can be benign although they can also be associated with severe diseases of the nervous system, such as motor neuron disease (ALS) and occasionally with *stiff man syndrome*. (See above.) When fasciculations are severe enough to deserve treatment by themselves, anticonvulsants can be effective, notably carbamazepine (Tegretol) or phenytoin (Dilantin), in conventional doses. (See Chap. 10, Disorders of Awareness, for information on these agents.)

Tics

Tics are often exacerbated by anxiety, but they usually have so little clinical significance that treatment with anxiolytic medications hardly seems appropriate. In social situations, a glass of wine or other mild alcoholic beverage can sometimes make tics milder and therefore less offensive to people who are offended by them.

The tic-like behavior of Gilles de la Tourette syndrome needs pharmacological treatment only if it is severe enough to cause disability in the social situation in which such a patient finds himself or herself. These tics typically respond to *haloperidol* (Haldol). Treatment should begin with no more than 0.25 mg daily, titrating up as needed to as much as 5–10 mg a day. Alternatives for non-responders include the neuroleptic *pimozide* (starting at 0.5 mg a day and titrating up as needed to 8 or 9 mg a day), with *naltrexone* (50 mg/day), and according to a few case reports with some anti-seizure medications. This complex, rare, but striking neurological syndrome should whenever possible be treated by or in consultation with a neurologist. Patients refractory to medical therapies may benefit from neurosurgical approaches. Resort to neurosurgery is, of course, justified only for disabilities severe enough to warrant making a hole in the skull.

Parkinson Disease

Parkinson disease should also be treated by or in collaboration with a neurologist or other specialist. Parkinsonism is normally a chronic condition of gradual onset, and there is time for a referral before initiating therapy. As noted above, accurate differential diagnosis among the Parkinsonian syndromes is not trivial. New medications are being introduced continually, and the state of the art in treatment keeps changing. Simply prescribing DOPA/carbidopa to people who appear Parkinsonian is not good medical practice in this new millennium. In the discussion below, dosages are not discussed, although they are presented in Table 11-6. The assumption in this discussion is that treatment will be initiated and supervised by a specialist familiar with the appropriate doses and their adjustment for individual patients.

Table 11-6 lists medications now used to treat Parkinson disease. The main deficiency in Parkinson disease is in the neurotransmitter dopamine, and the most common treatments of this disorder attempt to modify that deficit or its effects.

L-DOPA/carbidopa is the most effective single treatment for Parkinson disease. It is based on replacement of the deficient dopamine neurotransmitter by feeding its precursor, L-DOPA (L-dihydroxy phenylacetic acid). Nowadays, L-DOPA is normally prescribed along with carbidopa in a combined formulation. The original formulation carried the name *Sinemet.* Carbidopa inhibits the conversion of L-DOPA to dopamine in the periphery and therefore reduces peripheral side effects. It does not enter the brain with any efficiency and therefore does not inhibit the therapeutically desirable conversion of L-DOPA to dopamine in the damaged parts of the brain. Its typical combinations with carbidopa are in ratios of 4:1 (e.g., Sinemet 100:25) or 10:1 (e.g., Sinemet 250:25). Long-acting preparations are also available. The introduction of L-DOPA/carbidopa treatment revolutionized the therapy of Parkinson disease. When first used it benefits a large majority of patients, often dramatically. The combination of L-DOPA and carbidopa induces fewer side effects than feeding L-DOPA alone, and allows the use of lower doses.

Side effects can still be troubling, however, although taking the medication with food tends to reduce them. Nausea and other gastrointestinal side effects are usually mild and self limited, but may require treatment with

TABLE 11–6
Medications for Parkinson disease

Medication	Dosage
Neurotransmitter replacement	
Levodopa/Carbidopa (Sinemet)	tabs 1 (25/100), 2-3 day, titrating up to 2-12 tabs/day sustained release form (50/200), 2id going to 1-6/day
Direct dopamine agonists	
Bromocriptine (Parlodel)	1.25 mg, 2id, titrating slowly up to 3.75-40 mg/day
Pergolide (Permax)	0.05 mg/day, titrating slowly up to 0.75-5.0 mg/day
Ropinirole (Requip)	0.25 mg, 3id, titrating up to 1.5-2.4 mg/day
Pramipexole (Mirapex)	0.125 mg, 3id, titrating up to 1.5-4.5 mg/day
Cabergoline (Dostinex)	titrate up to 2.5-3.0 mg/day
COMT inhibitors	
Entacapone (Comtan)	200 mg with each dose of Sinemet, titrating to 600-2000 mg/day
Tolcapone (Tasmar)	100 mg, 2id, titrating up to 200-600 mg/day (potential liver toxicity)
MAO inhibitors	
Selegiline (Deprenyl)	2.5 mg once a day or 2id
Direct cholinergic muscarinic antagonists	
Trihexyphenidyl (Artane)	1 mg, 2id, titrating up to 15 mg/day
Benztropine (Cogentin)	1-4 mg, 3-4/day
Diphenhydramine (Benadryl)	25-50 mg, 3-4/day
Other mechanism of action	
Amantidine (Symmetrel)	100 mg, once a day or 2id

domperidone to antagonize the responsible dopaminergic receptors or with supplemental carbidopa to diminish conversion of L-DOPA to dopamine in the periphery. Hypotension, particularly postural hypotension, can be troublesome. It is treated when necessary by the usual medical modalities.

Hallucinations, depression, or other psychiatric manifestations are not rare. The extent to which they are due to the medication can be hard to determine, since they are also typical complications of the disease itself. Sometimes they respond to lowering the dosage, without undue worsening of the manifestations of Parkinson disease. Sometimes the dose cannot be lowered without the development of unacceptably severe motor disabilities.

Hallucinations and other psychotic manifestations appear to be mediated by stimulation of dopaminergic receptors other than those primarily involved in movement. The psychiatric symptoms of Parkinson disease reportedly respond to newer antipsychotics, notably *quietapine*.[14] *Clozapine* is also effective and reportedly reduces the L-DOPA–induced dyskinesias discussed below.[15] However, clozapine can suppress the bone marrow raising a risk of agranulocytosis. Regular blood tests are necessary to use clozapine safely. Haloperidol and risperidone typically make parkinsonism worse. Sharp reductions in dopaminergic tone can precipitate a potentially fatal complication, *neuroleptic malignant syndrome*, which is well known to general clinicians. Such reductions can arise from sharp reductions in or failure to take L-DOPA as prescribed as well as from treatment with dopamine-blocking neuroleptic medications. (For details, see Chap. 4, Thought Disorders.)

Unfortunately, the majority of patients with Parkinson disease tend to "break through" DOPA/carbidopa treatment within 5 years after starting it. They develop some mixture of over action of the drug shortly after a dose is taken and wearing off of the beneficial effects before the next dose is taken. The former effect leads to troublesome dyskinetic movements, and the latter to periods of return of disabling rigidity and tremor. This "on-off phenomenon" can be extremely troubling. Various ways have been used to treat it. They include more frequent but smaller doses, use of slow-release preparations, and combinations with other medications. Although useful, no single one of these treatments is fully satisfactory for the majority of patients.

A theoretical concern with treatment with L-DOPA is that it may accelerate the damage to the vulnerable neurons, specifically those that take up and use dopamine. A major pathway for the removal of dopamine is oxidation. One of the products of this reaction, catalyzed by the enzyme monoamine oxidase, is a free radical that may itself be harmful to cells. Although controlled studies have not documented that early treatment with L-DOPA (Sinemet) accelerates the progression of Parkinson disease in groups of human patients, the concern about this treatment in individual patients persists and strongly influences some neurologists' choices of treatment in the earlier stages of the disease.

Direct dopaminergic agonists can ameliorate the functional deficiency of dopamine in Parkinson disease, providing an alternate to treatments designed to increase the supply of dopamine itself. Both the older and the newer drugs have some side effects in common. Those include nausea, fatigue, hallucinations, perhaps increased sexuality, and with longer use episodes of hypotension or exacerbation of orthostatic hypotension. The side effects with the first direct dopaminergic agonists were so troublesome as to limit their use. These drugs, *bromocriptine* (Parlodel), *pergolide* (Permax), and *lisuride* (lysuride; Dopergin, Revanil), are ergotamine derivatives that can induce serious elevations of blood pressure, as well as troublesome nausea and fatigue. These medications have to be started at low doses and titrated up slowly. Pergolide use is associated with subclinical damage to heart valves detectable by cardiac imaging but rarely reaching clinical significance. These medications were typically used when treatment with Sinemet was no longer adequate, and then used with caution.

The newer direct dopaminergic agonists have proven more useful. They are *ropinirole* (Requip), *pramipexole* (Mirapex), and *cabergoline* (Dostinex). These medications can be titrated to full doses rapidly without causing severe hypertension. They often cause transient and relatively mild nausea and fatigue. In some patients, they can cause episodes of intense sleepiness similar to narcolepsy. (See Chap. 8, Sleep.) The side effects of these newer direct dopamine agonists are mild enough that they are being increasingly used as first line therapy in Parkinson disease, in preference to L-DOPA (Sinemet). For instance, the Parkinson Disease Study Group concluded, from a 4-year controlled comparison, that initial treatment with L-DOPA and with dopaminergic agonist pramipexole led to similar qualities of life for the patients.

> Initial treatment with pramipexole resulted in lower incidences of dyskinesias and wearing off compared with initial treatment with levodopa. Initial treatment with levodopa resulted in lower incidences of freezing, somnolence, and edema and provided for better symptomatic control, as measured by the Unified Parkinson's Disease Rating Scale, compared with initial treatment with pramipexole. Both options resulted in similar quality of life. Levodopa and pramipexole both appear to be reasonable options as initial dopaminergic therapy for Parkinson disease, but they are associated with different efficacy and adverse-effect profiles.[16]

A 5-year study comparing the dopaminergic agonist cabergoline to L-DOPA came to much the same conclusion.

> . . . compared with levodopa, initial therapy with cabergoline in patients with Parkinson's disease is associated with a lower risk of response Fluctuations at the cost of a marginally reduced symptomatic improvement and some tolerability disadvantages that are mostly limited to a significantly higher frequency of peripheral edema.[17]

COMT Inhibitors One of the pathways for inactivation of dopamine involves the enzyme catechol O-methyl transferase (COMT), and inhibitors of this pathway have been used to treat dopamine deficiency. Some patients respond well to adding a COMT inhibitor to DOPA/carbidopa. Presumably, they are people whose genes lead to the COMT-containing pathway being a major route for inactivation of the already deficient neurotransmitter. On the whole, however, results with COMT inhibitors have not been impressive. A recent, double-blind, multicenter study concluded that adding entacapone to Sinemet in Parkinson patients did not improve motor function, although it may have helped "quality of life."[18]

MAO Inhibitors Dopamine is chemically a monoamine, and monoamine oxidases (MAOs) inactivate it. They simultaneously produce a toxic free radical, hydrogen peroxide (H_2O_2). Treatment with an MAO inhibitor becomes a rational approach to increasing the amount of the deficient neurotransmitter and decreasing the amount of the harmful free radical. The MAO inhibitor of choice has been Selegiline, an MAO-B inhibitor that is less dangerous to use without strict dietary control than are compounds that also inhibit MAO-A. (The MAO inhibitors are discussed in Chap. 3, Mood. Disorders.) Early trials indicated that this treatment could slow the progression of Parkinson disease relatively briefly, but longer term follow-up showed that MAO inhibition had little or no effect on the disease in the longer term.[19] MAO inhibition now tends not to be widely used by experts in the treatment of this disease.

Acetylcholine Antagonists The use of these agents in Parkinson disease depends on the finding that healthy brain function normally requires a balance between systems using acetylcholine as a neurotransmitter and systems using dopamine or other catecholamine as neurotransmitter. If dopaminergic tone falls and cholinergic tone remains the same, then cholinergic transmission can become functionally excessive. This appears to happen in Parkinson disease. Medications that are antagonists at muscarinic cholinergic receptors were used to treat Parkinson disease before the introduction of L-DOPA and direct dopaminergic agonists. They include *trihexyphenidyl* (Artane), *benztropine* (Cogentin), and the antihistaminic *diphenhydramine* (Benadryl). In some patients, the effects of these agents are gratifying. These medications can still be useful, particularly when they are added to the regimen for patients in whom DOPA/carbidopa or direct dopaminergic agonists no longer provide satisfactory control by themselves.

As with all anticholinergic medications, side effects can be troublesome. Systemic effects include dry mouth, constipation, blurred vision (from *mydriasis*), and sometimes urinary retention. A troublesome side effect referable to the nervous system is impairment of cognition. This can be particularly troublesome in patients in whom Parkinson disease is associated with some degree of dementia. (See the discussion of Lewy Body Dementia in Chap. 5, Cognitive Disorders.)

Amantadine is an older treatment for Parkinson disease that can still be useful, particularly as an addition to newer treatments such as Sinemet or dopaminergic agonists. It is believed to act by at least two mechanisms. It favors the release of dopamine and also has anticholinergic effects. The effects of amantadine by itself tend to be mild, but as mentioned it can be a useful adjunct.

Initial treatment of Parkinson disease is a topic on which there is no clear consensus. Some clinicians believe L-DOPA/carbidopa should be started early,[20] while others are concerned that doing so will lead to greater cell damage in part due to dopamine metabolism with generation of H_2O_2. Some clinicians now start with direct dopaminergic agonists. Some start with a cholinergic agonist or even amantadine and only move on to direct dopaminergic therapy when necessary. Some experienced clinicians hold off all treatment until disability becomes relatively troublesome. This uncertainty is another reason for the treatment of this chronic disorder to be undertaken by or in consultation with a specialist who can have a fully informed opinion on how to treat (and has the qualifications for his or her choice to be defended in a malpractice suit).

A situation where prompt treatment of Parkinson disease is, however, necessary, is in the rare form of severe Parkinsonism of sudden onset due to a toxin to dopaminergic cells. These patients are so stiff ("rigid") that they need prompt treatment to maintain important functions such as nutrition. The classic case of this kind was in a young man exposed to a contaminant of a "designer recreational drug" he was trying to synthesize chemically. He was in the San Francisco area, and could be seen promptly by specialists who not only treated him effectively but also worked out the basis of his unusual syndrome.

Innovative techniques to treat Parkinson disease are under development. Repetitive transcranial magnetic stimulation is under study but appears not to have effects long lasting enough to make this technique clinically useful. Deep brain stimulation of the subthalamic nucleus has been reported to improve function even 4 years after surgery.[21] Despite encouraging initial reports, benefits from cell transplantations have been inconsistent.[22]

Other Parkinsonian Syndromes

Other Parkinsonian syndromes typically do not respond to L-DOPA as well as Parkinson disease itself does. The difference is so marked that lack of response to this medication has been used as support for the diagnosis of one of these syndromes. Progressive Supranuclear Palsy has no established treatment, although anecdotal reports have suggested possible benefits from the use of serotonergic, noradrenergic, or GABA agonists (benzodiazepines). Response to cholinergic agonists—notably physostigmine—has not been impressive. Cortical Basal Ganglionic syndrome sometimes responds relatively transiently to L-DOPA. In contrast, treatment with L-DOPA tends to worsen striatonigral degenerations, particularly in the early stages of these disorders. The disabilities due to autonomic failure as in Shy-Drager syndrome can be treated symptomatically—for instance, support stockings and other appropriate measures in patients with postural hypotension. The difficulties in treating these syndromes have encouraged speculation that newer techniques like stem cell therapy might help people suffering from them.

Myasthenia Gravis

Myasthenia gravis is another disorder of motility that should, whenever possible, be treated by or in collaboration with a neurologist or other specialist experienced in the complex clinical management of this disorder. Myasthenic patients can get weaker from either too much or too little of their cholinergic medication. That clinical judgment is not easy. If the physician is wrong, the patient can get dangerously worse very fast.

Treatment of myasthenia involves three approaches:

- enhancing neuromuscular transmission, normally by inhibiting the breakdown of the neurotransmitter involved, acetylcholine, with acetylcholinesterases;
- reducing the inappropriate, autoimmune process; and,
- supportive measures such as assisted ventilation to prevent death from acute exacerbations.

Acetylcholinesterases used to treat myasthenia are designed to be active in the periphery without entering the central nervous system. The most commonly used drug is *pyridostigmine* (Mestinon), although *neostigmine* (Prostigmin) is also widely used. Optimal doses vary widely from patient to patient and can vary widely for a single patient. Some patients require as little as 30 mg of Mestinon 4 times a day; others need as much as 120 mg every 3 hours. Too little of the medication permits excessive weakness to persist. Too much leads to cholinergic crisis, where excessive and often life-threatening weakness is due to continuous activation of the neuromuscular receptors by over stimulation without the possibility of muscle recovering (*repolarizing*) so that it can contract again.

Cholinergic crisis is typically associated with other evidence of excessive activity of cholinergic systems. This can include gastrointestinal troubles (nausea, vomiting, diarrhea, cramps), sweating, salivating, pale skin, and slow heart rate. Constriction of the pupils is a relatively reliable sign, particularly constriction to less than 2 mm. Failure to respond with increased strength to the short-acting cholinesterase inhibitor *edrophonium* is often used as a way to show that too much rather than too little anticholinesterase medication is in the patient, that is, to validate the presence of cholinergic crisis. However, some clinicians familiar with this disease do not trust edrophonium testing to distinguish cholinergic crisis from other causes of decreasing strength in these patients, such as progression of the autoimmune process or the presence of intercurrent infections or other diseases that can cause myasthenic crises. Cholinergic crisis can be treated with anticholinergics—for instance with *atropine* in small doses (e.g., up to 0.6 mg atropine IV, given slowly). The therapeutic trap is, of course, over-titration of antagonist with the temptation to then give more agonist which, if over-titrated, then raises the temptation to give more antagonist, and so on. Patients of course do not usually do well when subjected to this type of meddlesome medicine.

Modern treatment of Lambert-Eaton syndrome utilizes a combination of Mestinon and *3,4-diaminopyridine* (3, 4-DAP). The latter enhances neurotransmitter action by binding to appropriate potassium channels. The conventional dose of 3, 4-DAP is 20 mg 5 times a day, PO.

Treatment of the autoimmune process involves procedures well known to general clinicians. Because of the interaction between myasthenia and the thymus gland, the thymus is removed in most myasthenics over the age of puberty whose disease is not limited to the eye muscles. Complete remission occurs in about a third of the patients, and a total of 80% or more tend to improve at least somewhat. Corticosteroids typically help myasthenic patients. Doses have been as high as 50–60 mg of prednisone a day. Such treatment incurs the usual complications of steroid therapy so well known to general clinicians. Steroid-induced myopathy can be particularly dangerous in these patients who already suffer from muscle weakness that can be life-threatening. Therefore, as usual, doses of steroids are reduced to the lowest levels compatible with adequate therapeutic effects. Every other day dosage or daily alternations between higher and lower doses can be used to try to limit side effects. Immunosuppressants such as *azathioprine* (Imuran) and *cyclosporine* can be effective in myasthenia. Some patients have done well treated with azathioprine alone, in doses titrated up to 3 mg/kg per day, that is, 150–250 mg daily. Intravenous immune globulin can provide useful short term benefits, particularly in patients who have had not had thymectomies and are undergoing rapid exacerbations.[23] Dosage is about 2 g/kg in divided doses over the course of 3–5 days. Plasma exchange can be life-saving. It has proven useful even in patients with steroid-induced myopathies.

Supportive therapies include mechanical support of breathing when respirations become dangerously weak. This is an area well known to general clinicians, including the indications for assisted ventilation. Some patients with myasthenia prove difficult to wean off the respirator. These include elderly patients with steroid-induced muscle weakness. Many clinicians stop cholinesterase inhibitors in patients on respirators. The dosages needed when the patients come off the respirators may be much less than those needed before they go on.

In summary, myasthenia gravis is a chronic disease that is not easy to treat. Mistakes can easily cause "preventable deaths." The management of this disease is best left to those skilled in the art.

Acute Inflammatory Polyneuropathies

Acute inflammatory polyneuropathies in their milder forms can be treated directly with intravenous immune globulin (0.4 g/kg a day consecutively for 5 days) or with plasma exchange.[23] Sometimes these procedures need to be repeated. Controlled studies suggest that corticosteroid treatment is of relatively little use, despite positive anecdotal results observed by many clinicians who have treated patients with this disorder.

The more severe forms require supportive care, often intensive supportive care. The procedures are familiar to general physicians, particularly those who specialize in intensive care. Many of these patients need assisted ventilation. Sometimes intubation is necessary to prevent aspiration, even before respiratory failure. If blood pressure drops, it needs to be maintained by volume repletion and where necessary by drugs. Significant elevations of blood pressure also need to be treated medically. Short acting drugs to increase or decrease blood pressure are advisable, since shifts from pressures that are too high to those that are too low and vice versa can happen quickly. Other aspects of intensive care also require attention. As usual, these include among other issues electrolyte balance, venous thromboses with the risk of pulmonary emboli, maintaining nutrition while avoiding complications of feeding tubes, and treatment of infections including infections of the lungs or urinary tract. Cardiac arrhythmias are a risk in this population. Even with optimal care, as many as 5% of these patients are likely to die during the acute illness. The techniques for weaning patients off respirators and the problems with the minority of patients who are hard to wean are well known to those with expertise in intensive care.

Recovery for those who survive the acute illness is usually complete or nearly complete. Recurrences occur in perhaps 5–10% of patients. Some degree of damage to nerve cell processes (*axons*) is common in severe forms of this disorder, but a small percentage of patients have such marked and persistent damage to axons that recovery is limited.

Motor Neuron Diseases

Treatment of these disorders is supportive. When spasticity is a major problem, treatment with *baclofen* can be helpful. For motor neuron disease, this is typically done *intrathecally* and needs to be supervised by a neurologist with experience in the use of this medication. Too sudden cessation of baclofen treatment—including pump failure—can induce major neurological complications. Antioxidant treatment with vitamin E has been a failure in the established disease. Data on prevention by vitamin E is controversial. Whether taking 400 mg or more vitamin E daily, PO, protects against developing motor neuron disease or tends to shorten life depends on which study one reads.

Sensitive support and counseling patients with these relatively rapidly fatal chronic diseases is important. The subject of end-of-life care goes beyond the scope of this monograph, however.

Other Disorders of Motility

Other disorders of motility can be secondary to a variety of illnesses. Relatively nonspecific acute motor neuropathy can occur secondary to a variety of severe medical illnesses. They can include cancers and paraneoplastic syndrome. Treatment is primarily treatment— if possible—of the underlying disorder. As discussed above, neuropathy can signal the presence of an occult cancer that is so small that it is still curable but not yet visible on routine X-ray. The malignancy responsible is so often cancer of the lung that using newer diagnostic techniques such as spiral MRI to search for it is probably justified. However, clinical studies to test this suggestion are not yet available. Treatments for poisoning with lead or other heavy metals are well known to general clinicians, and are touched on earlier.

Impaired mobility is, of course, a prominent manifestation of many other neurological disorders, including those discussed elsewhere in this monograph. They include stroke, tumor, demyelinating diseases, and others discussed in other chapters.

REFERENCES

1. The word *hysterical* can easily become a pejorative label, applied to patients who irritate physicians.
2. Tics do not interfere much with people who have captive audiences, such as medical school professors or other teachers.
3. Victor M, Roper AH. *Textbook of Neurology*. 7th ed. New York, NY: McGraw-Hill, 2001; p. 107.
4. See, for instance, Liston R, Mickelborough J, Bene J, et al. A new classification of higher-level gait disorders in patients with cerebral multi-infarct states. *Age Ageing*. 2003;32:252–258. A widely recognized classification of gait disorders has divided them into higher level (cortical), middle level (hemiplegic, paraplegic, cerebellar, Parkinsonian, choreic, and dystonic), and lower level (peripheral musculoskeletal and sensory disorders that can be compensated for by an intact central nervous system). Nutt JG. Classification of gait and balance disorders. *Adv Neurol*. 2001;87:135–141.
5. Hughes AJ, Daniel SE, Kilford L, et al. Accuracy of clinical diagnosis of idiopathic Parkinson's disease: A clinicopathological study of 100 cases. *J Neurol Neurosurg Psychiatry*. 1992;58:181–193.
6. Ringholz GM, Appel SH, Bradshaw M, et al. Prevalence and patterns of cognitive impairment in sporadic ALS. *Neurology*. 2005;65:586–590.
7. For a number of years, I tried to convince medical students in Southern California that inhibition was a higher function than excitation. They described me as "that prig from New England."
8. Previous attempts to define those disorders on clinical grounds into eponymic syndromes gave rise to a forest of erudition that is now primarily of historical interest.

9. Wirdefeldt K, Gatz M, Pawitan Y, et al. Risk and protective factors for Parkinson's disease: a study in Swedish twins. *Ann Neurol.* 2005;57:27–33.
10. Carr J. Neurosyphilis. *Practical Neurology.* 2003;3:328–341.
11. Dalmau JO, Posner JB Paraneoplastic syndromes. Arch Neurol. 1999;56: 405-8.
12. Darnell RB, Posner JB. Paraneoplastic syndromes affecting the nervous system. Semin Oncol. 2006;33:270-98.
13. Parry SW, Kenny RA. Drop attacks in older adults: systematic assessment has a high diagnostic yield. *J Am Geriatr Soc.* 2005;53:74–78.
14. Juncose JL, Roberts VJ, Evatt ML, et al. Quetiapine improves psychotic symptoms and cognition in Parkinson's disease. *Mov Disord.* 2004;19:29–35.
15. Durif F, Debilly B, Galitzky M, et al. Clozapine improves dyskinesias in Parkinson disease: A double-blind, placebo-controlled study. *Neurology.* 2004;62:381–388.
16. Holloway RG, Shoulson I, Fahn S, et al. and the Parkinson Study Group. Pramipexole vs. levodopa as initial treatment for Parkinson disease: a 4-year randomized controlled trial. *Arch Neurol.* 2004;61:1044–1053.
17. Bracco F, Battaglia A, Chouza C, et al. PKDS009 Study Group. The long-acting dopamine receptor agonist cabergoline in early Parkinson's disease: final results of a 5-year, double-blind, levodopa-controlled study. *CNS Drugs.* 2004;18:733–746.
18. Olanow CW, Kieburtz K, Stern M, et al. US01 Study Team. Double-blind, placebo-controlled study of entacapone in levodopa-treated patients with stable Parkinson disease. *Arch Neurol.* 2004;61:1563–1568.
19. Marras C, McDermott MP, Rochon PA, et al. Parkinson Study Group. Survival in Parkinson disease: thirteen-year follow-up of the DATATOP cohort. *Neurology.* 2005;64:87–93.
20. Cederbaum JM, Gandy SE, McDowell FH. "Early" initiation of levodopa treatment does not promote the development of motor response fluctuations, dyskinesias, or dementia in Parkinson's disease. *Neurology.* 1991;41:622–628.
21. Rodriguez-Oroz MC, Zamarbide I, Guridi J, et al. Efficacy of deep brain stimulation of the subthalamic nucleus in Parkinson's disease 4 years after surgery: double blind and open label evaluation. *J Neurol Neurosurg Psychiatry.* 2004;75:1382–1385.
22. Langston JW. The promise of stem cells in Parkinson disease. *J Clin Invest.* 2005;115:23–25.
23. Dalakas MC. Intravenous immunoglobulin in autoimmune neuromuscular diseases. *JAMA.* 2004;291:2367–2375.

CHAPTER TWELVE

Disorders of Sensation

Probably the most common sensory abnormality of which patients complain to general clinicians is pain. Patients also complain frequently of other problems with sensation. A separate chapter (Chap. 7) discusses pain. Sensory problems other than pain are the subject of this chapter.

Sensory dysfunction can be a sign of disease of sensory organs as well as of disease of the central nervous system. It can signal the presence of serious brain diseases such as tumors. People can complain of decreased sensation (*hypesthesia*), of loss of sensation (*anesthesia*), or of abnormal and/or uncomfortable sensations (*paresthesias*, *dysesthesias*). These problems are usually referable to specific areas of their bodies.

Problems related to organs of sensation become very common with increasing age. Elderly people typically do not have the sight or hearing that they had as youngsters, nor for that matter as acute senses of smell and taste. Some loss of sensory sensitivity in advanced age is statistically normal, although often unpleasant and sometimes disabling.

CLASSIFICATION AND DIAGNOSIS

Clinical history and other symptoms and signs are major aids in deciding how rapidly a disorder of sensation needs to be treated. A key piece of data is whether a sensory disturbance has come on slowly or gradually. Sudden changes in sensation are more likely to signal a process that requires immediate attention—such as a vascular event, exposure to a toxin, or other acute injury. Transient abnormal sensations can accompany seizures or other transient events in the nervous system. Sensory difficulties of gradual onset are less likely to require acute intervention by the general physician. In these situations, detailed diagnosis and choice of treatment can more safely be left to specialists.

The classification of disorders of sensation presented in this chapter provides a crude framework for localizing disorders of sensation. The general clinician is probably wise to try only the more obvious, "bite-you-in-the-nose" localization of sensory abnormalities. More subtle and specific diagnoses of these problems are better left to specialists, who are quite likely to have enough trouble themselves in precisely specifying the nature of the disability. Diagnosis can be particularly difficult in anxious patients in whom the results of sensory tests are obscured by a hysterical overlay. The sensory examination is perhaps the most difficult and almost certainly the most subjective part of a neurological examination. Doing it well requires expertise. The anatomy of the sensory systems is complex. Although most of us learned it in the first year of medical school, general clinicians do not usually have to keep it in the front of their minds. Neurologists do. Electrophysiological testing can aid greatly in the differential diagnosis of sensory problems, and both the equipment for such testing and the skills needed for its interpretation are available in specialty clinics.

In the following discussion, disorders of sensation are discussed in three groups: problems with organs of special sensation, for example, eyes and ears; loss of sensation; and abnormal, unpleasant sensations.

DISORDERS OF SPECIAL SENSATIONS

The anatomy and physiology of the organs of special sensation have been well worked out and are described in specialized texts.[1] Specialties are devoted to the diagnosis and treatment of disorders of these organs. Ophthalmologists treat the eyes. Optometrists, who are not MDs, specialize in refraction and provide prescriptions for spectacles. Physicians who specialize in ears, nose and throat (ENT) deal with deafness and with disorders of the nasal mucosa that impair smell and therefore taste. Specially trained technicians assist them by providing tests of hearing and by constructing hearing aids. In disorders of special sensations, as in so many other conditions that affect the nervous system, the duty of the general physician is to recognize problems, distinguish between problems that need emergency care and those that do not, and make appropriate referrals.

Vision

Problems with vision tend to be rapidly recognized and often relatively easily localized within the nervous system. Humans tend to rely on vision in the way that bats tend to depend on hearing and dogs on smell. The primary pathways of vision are highly localized in humans, and the localization of functions has been well worked out. Referrals to experts in Ophthalmology or Neuro-ophthalmology are appropriate when a visual disturbance is chronic enough or the availability of a consultation fast enough to permit waiting for the consultant. Techniques to evaluate the eye in detail, such as slit lamp examinations, require special equipment and training. Many people need glasses to see well, but refraction and prescriptions for corrective lenses are not part of general clinical practice in the United States. Disorders of the eyes often rouse great anxiety in people, even though modern humans can live without vision.[2]

Prompt treatment is appropriate to prevent imminent and permanent damage to vision in several conditions. They include temporal arteritis, acute glaucoma, and retinal artery occlusion.

Temporal arteritis (giant cell arteritis) is associated with headache and characteristic changes in the temporal artery; it is discussed, including the need for prompt treatment with steroids, with headaches in Chap. 7 (Pain) and also in Chap. 9 (Cerebrovascular Disorders).

Glaucoma refers to increased pressure within the eye, potentially great enough to permanently damage the retina and thereby potentially lead to blindness. It is a disease of the sense organ rather than of the nervous system (retina) itself. However, it does risk loss of a critically important sense, namely vision. Acute angle-closure glaucoma can cause irreversible blindness in the affected eye within a couple of days if untreated. It typically presents clinically with a painful red eyeball and blurring of vision. Halos around lights are a common complaint. *Acute glaucoma* is a syndrome that can have a number of causes, among them inflammation of the uvea or iris. *Chronic glaucoma* can cause chronic headache and can also destroy vision, although more slowly. Glaucoma is so common in the elderly that routine measures of ocular pressure are indicated for them. As discussed below, the general physician has medications that can help to prevent damage to vision until definitive laser treatment by an ophthalmologist becomes possible.

Retinal artery occlusion should be suspected in patients with sudden painless loss of vision in an eye. *Wegener granulomatosis* or other vasculitis can be the underlying cause. Retinal artery occlusion is now treatable by dissolving the clot, if it is caught early enough.

Anatomical classification of disorders of vision into three groups is convenient: disorders of the eyes (other than disorders of the retina); disorders affecting the muscles that move the eyes or control the size of the pupils; and disorders of parts of the central nervous system that subsume vision and the processing of visual information. These include the retina, which is anatomically and physiologically part of the central nervous system.

Disorders of the eye itself are listed in Table 12-1. Texts on Ophthalmology discuss these conditions, including their diagnosis and treatment.[1] A detailed discussion is beyond the scope of this monograph. Disorders of the eye that need to be treated promptly are discussed above.

Abnormal eye motions and pupils are frequent indicators of disease of the nervous system. The typical clinical presentations are double vision (*diplopia*), drooping of an eyelid (*ptosis*), or pupils that differ markedly in size. These abnormalities can result from increase in intracranial pressure due to a tumor or other lesion. They require evaluation, optimally by a specialist.

TABLE 12–1

Common disorders of the eye itself

Lens:
Senile cataracts
Infectious
Diabetic
Other
Cornea:
Trauma
Infection (herpes zoster, trachoma)
Hereditary diseases (e.g., Wilson disease)
Anterior chamber:
Acute glaucoma
Chronic glaucoma

Double vision (*diplopia*) most often results from loss of balance among the muscles of the eye. The cause is most often disease affecting the cranial nerves that innervate these muscles, including disease of the brain stem or pons. Involuntary rhythmic movement of the eyes (*nystagmus*) is a common sign of disease of the cerebellum. Various forms of peripheral neuropathy can also affect the eyes. Double vision is a common first complaint in *multiple sclerosis* (Chap. 13, Disorders of both Sensation and Motility) or in *myasthenia gravis* (Chap. 11, Disorders of Motility). Examination by a specialist in Neurology or Neuro-Ophthalmology usually allows precise localization of the defect. For instance, palsies of lateral gaze typically implicate Cranial Nerve VI.

Drooping of the eyelids (*ptosis*) usually indicates weakness of Cranial Nerve III but can also indicate muscle weakness, as in myasthenia gravis. (See Chapter 11, Disorders of Motility.)

Abnormalities of the pupils are often very revealing. The pupils of the eyes are regularly examined in even the most cursory general physical examinations. General clinicians are familiar with the normal pupillary reactions to light and accommodation. Decreased response to light and/or inequality of the pupils (>0.5 mm) can occur in many conditions that lead to the loss of the normal functional balance of sympathetic and parasympathetic innervation to the eye. Abnormalities of a pupil can be innocuous or a sign of very serious illness. Enlargement of the pupils and loss of their reaction to light is a typical physical sign of serious compression of the brain stem and impending death. A comatose patient who arrives in an emergency ward with fixed, dilated pupils is quite likely to die in the emergency suite or during the resulting admission to the hospital.

Central nervous system disorders impairing vision can conveniently be divided into three groups. They are disorders of: (1) the retina; (2) visual functions, which are localizable in the brain; and (3) relatively poorly localizable disorders of the processing of visual information.

The retina is a part of the central nervous system, that is, it is an "outcropping of the brain." It is the only part of the brain that can be looked at directly, through an ophthalmoscope, without opening the skull. Many disease processes affecting the central nervous system can be visualized in the retina, including vascular processes. General clinicians are familiar with *hypertensive retinopathy* and with visualizing emboli in retinal arterioles. Table 12-2 lists a number of other common conditions that can be visualized in the retina.

Macular degeneration, which is the most common cause of visual failure in the elderly population, can happily now be treated with medications.

TABLE 12–2
Disorders visualizable in the retina

Increased intracranial pressure
Papilledema (various causes)
Pseudotumor cerebri
Vascular
Hypertension (including malignant hypertension)
Atherosclerosis
Aneurysms
Ischemia (retinal artery occlusion)
Infections (often associated with AIDS)
Toxoplasmosis
Cytomegalovirus (CMV)
Histoplasmosis
Syphilis
Tuberculosis
Degenerations
Retinitis pigmentosa
Nonpigmentary degenerations
Hereditary diseases (often rare, e.g., Refsum disease)

There are two forms of this condition. The dry form is atrophy. The wet form involves inappropriate new blood vessels (*neovascularization*) in the retina. The dry form is more frequent but causes relatively little disability. The wet form causes over 90% of the loss of vision due to macular degeneration. FDA (U.S. Food & Drug Administration) approved treatments for the wet form include Verteporfin with laser treatment and more recently *pegaptanib* (Macugen). Each injection of the latter now costs $1000. Active treatment of macular degeneration is appropriately left to ophthalmologists.

Lesions of the well localized visual pathways in the brain cause characteristic disabilities, depending on their location in the brain. If close to the eye, that is, before the *optic chiasm*, they typically cause loss of vision in one eye. If after the chiasm, they typically cause loss of vision in a visual field that affects both eyes. Textbooks of Neurology contain diagrams that relate specific losses of visual fields *(field cuts)* to lesions in specific parts of the visual system.

Sometimes patients see perfectly well but cannot process visual information adequately. They have *visual agnosias*. These problems typically result from diseases affecting the large parts of the posterior cortex that are involved in integrating visual stimuli. For instance, Alzheimer patients often have visual agnosias among their other problems. Specific names derived from Greek and/or Latin roots describe loses of specific abilities such as the ability to recognize faces, numbers, or letters. These terms are well known to specialists.

Seeing things that are not there constitutes visual hallucinations. Visual hallucinations are considered typical of delirium. (See Chap. 5, Cognitive Disorders). They can, however, also occur in other diseases, despite the old clinical saw that psychiatric hallucinations tend to be auditory rather than visual. (See Chap. 4, Thought Disorders.) Sometimes hallucinations result from discrete lesions in the brain, particularly in areas that are involved in the integration of visual information, such as the parietal lobes. Drugs can cause visual hallucinations, as can drug withdrawal. Visual hallucinations can occur in surprisingly large proportion of people with impaired vision; they have been reported in over 10% of visually impaired older people (*Charles Bonnet syndrome*). Often, but certainly not always, the intense emotions that accompany psychiatric hallucinations are less prominent or absent with hallucinations attributable to discrete lesions in the brain that can be identified by current techniques.

Hearing

Disorders of hearing fall conveniently into two categories: hearing too little and hearing too much.

Hearing Too Little: Deafness affects perhaps 10% of the American population. Hearing loss is conventionally divided into three types: (1) conductive deafness, (2) sensorineural deafness (also called nerve deafness), and (3) central deafness. Hearing loss is usually relatively harmless even if inconvenient. It can, however, be dangerous if it leads to accidents involving motor vehicles or other dangerous machinery. Shouted warnings can be life-saving—for instance, warning a swimmer about a shark. Decreased hearing can also be a manifestation of life threatening disease. A notable example is *acoustic neuroma*—a tumor that needs to be recognized early to be operated on safely.

Infections including meningitis can impair hearing. They need to be diagnosed promptly and treated appropriately when treatment is available—for instance, antibiotic therapy for bacterial meningitis. Hearing loss due to bacterial or other infection tends to be associated with a relatively rapid onset combined with other evidence of infection. However, chronic infections including chronic meningitis can be difficult to recognize. In the preantibiotic era, acute and chronic middle ear infections (*otitis media*) were an important source of disability and death, particularly in children.

A rather large number of relatively rare hereditary disorders can cause premature hearing loss. These include very unusual entities such as *Heredopathia Atactica Polyneuritiformis* (Refsum disease, which is treated by a special diet). The recognition of these syndromes requires the expertise of a specialist. Confirmation by molecular genetics is often possible, by specialists who are in a position to know personally the researchers specializing in studies of the relevant gene(s).

Inability to process the information from sounds occurs in a number of diseases of the brain, notably degenerative diseases such as Alzheimer disease. (See Chap. 5, Cognitive Disorders.)

Hearing too much can involve unformed sounds or formed sounds. Unformed sounds often take the form of ringing in the ears—*tinnitus*. Clinically significant tinnitus affects perhaps 10–15% of Americans. More subtle forms of tinnitus can be elicited in almost everyone. Tinnitus is usually innocuous but can be a sign of serious illness. It is a classic early sign of aspirin toxicity.

Tinnitus, typically in combination with hearing loss, can signal the presence of a tumor of the Cranial Nerve VIII, an acoustic neuroma. This tumor does not normally metastasize, but removing it surgically can be dangerous because of the risk of tugging on the brain stem. That can kill the patient, or perhaps even worse leave the patient unable to move although still conscious (*locked-in syndrome;* see Chap. 10, Disorders of Awareness). Acoustic neuroma should be diagnosed in its early stages, when this "benign" tumor is still small enough to be dissected out relatively easily.

Tinnitus and/or hearing loss combined with vertigo characterize Ménière syndrome. Chapter 10 (Disorders of Awareness) discusses this syndrome and its treatments, because the presenting complaint is often "dizziness."

Formed sounds that others do not hear are classified as auditory hallucinations. They can include not only voices but also music or other intelligible sounds. Auditory hallucinations are characteristic of "schizophrenia" and certain other psychiatric diseases. (See Chap. 4, Thought Disorders.) They can also accompany anatomically discrete lesions of parts of the brain that process sound and language, including tumors or other lesions of the pons.

Smell and Taste

These senses are conveniently considered together because they are so closely involved with each other. Perhaps 70% of the taste of food comes from volatile molecules reaching the smell receptors in the nose rather than from direct stimulation of the taste receptors ("taste buds") in the tongue. This physiology is illustrated in statements such as "the smells from the kitchen were so good, they got my taste buds tingling." The acuity of smell and taste also tends to diminish in the elderly. Old people complaining that "food does not taste as good as when I was younger" may be depressed, but they may also just be complaining about a real age-related change in their physiology.

When the sensation of smell is diminished (*hyposmia*) or lost (*anosmia*), the damage is usually bilateral. Smelling with one nostril is usually as satisfactory as smelling with two. Damage to the nasal mucosa can cause diminished ability to smell—for instance, because of smoking or chronic rhinitis. Head trauma can damage the fibers that pass from the nose through the cribriform plate of the skull. Degenerative diseases of the brain often lead to loss of the sensation of smell. Loss of the ability to distinguish smells is so common in Alzheimer disease that some workers have recommended that it be used in the early diagnosis of that common form of dementia. (See Chap. 5, Cognitive Disorders.)

Sensing smells that other people do not sense usually indicates disease of the central nervous system. Such "olfactory delusions or hallucinations" often indicate serious diseases. Temporal lobe epilepsy is characteristically associated with foul, often "undescribable" smells, particularly during the aura. Episodic occurrence of an abnormal smell can be the "tip-off" to this diagnosis in a patient with an unusual behavioral syndrome. (See Chap. 10, Disorders of Awareness.) Depressed patients often sense unpleasant smells of which others are unaware. Sometimes they are convinced that they themselves stink. Such patients can be at severe risk of suicide. (See Chap. 3, Mood Disorders.) Bizarre smells often form part of typical psychotic syndromes as well. (See Chap. 4, Thought Disorders.)

Complaints of loss of taste sensation often reflect damage to the mouth, and specifically to the taste receptors in the tongue. As noted earlier, loss of taste often reflects loss of smell. Diseases of the nose and mouth that can damage the sensory end organs for smell and taste fall within the scope of the general clinician or specialist in ENT. They are not part of the subject of this monograph. Food losing its taste can be a somatic complaint that is a clue to an underlying masked depression. (See Chap. 3, Mood Disorders.) As noted above, loss of taste sensation can accompany degenerative diseases including Alzheimer disease. Whether these reflect a primary inability to taste or smell or rather an inability to recognize tastes is a secondary consideration in the care of these patients. More important is changing the diet to accord to what a patient can still find pleasant to eat. (That often includes ice cream; see Chap. 5, Cognitive Disorders.)

Drugs can cause loss of taste or abnormal tastes. Anticholinergic drugs are classic offenders, in part because they lead to dry mouths.

Persistent abnormal tastes or smells can be a manifestation of other diseases of the brain including on occasion tumors. Temporal lobe epilepsy can be associated with unusual, often foul tastes as well as foul smells. MRI (magnetic resonance imaging) scan and—more importantly—referral to a specialist can lead to appropriate diagnosis and treatment. Not making the appropriate referral can be risky for the patient medically and for the physician medicolegally.

Disorders of Other Senses

The anatomy and physiology of general sensation, like that of special sensations, has been well worked out. Appropriate textbooks give detailed descriptions. Table 12-3 lists the sensations (*sensory modalities*) tested as part of the general neurological examination. As with other disorders of the nervous system, diagnosis involves at least two questions. What

TABLE 12–3 **Sensory modalities**
Light touch
Pain
Superficial (pinprick)
Deep (pressure pain, e.g., from bones or tendons)
Hot and cold (thermal sense)
Position (proprioception)
Vibration
Discrimination
Two-point discrimination
Figure perception (graphesthesia)
Texture
Size
Shape (stereognosis)

part of the system is not functioning well (pathoanatomy of the disorder)? Why is it not functioning well (etiology of the disorder)? This discussion outlines the crude neuroanatomic localization of lesions impairing sensation. Detailed localization is best left to specialists.

As with special senses, problems with general sensation divide themselves conveniently into too little (loss of sensation) and too much (excess, unpleasant sensations).

Sensory losses occur in patterns that reflect the part(s) of the sensory system involved.

Peripheral nerve damage usually leads to both motor and sensory abnormalities, since most nerves are mixed. However, disorders of sensory nerves with little effect on motor nerves do occur. Damage to peripheral nerves can involve one nerve (*mononeuropathy*), several nerves (*polyneuropathy*), or rapidly shifting disease affecting different nerves (*mononeuropathy multiplex*).

Sensory root or dorsal ganglion disease leads to pure sensory loss, since sensory and motor nerves separate before they enter the spinal cord. Damage to a sensory root or ganglion typically can involve all sensory modalities in the area served by those structures. An example of widespread damage to sensory roots is *tabes dorsalis*, which is often a later manifestation of syphilis.[3]

Spinal cord damage leads to different patterns of sensory loss depending on which part of the spinal cord is damaged. Complete cutting of the cord (*complete transection including functional transection*) leads to total loss of all sensory (and motor) modalities below the level of the lesion. Section of only one side of the cord typically leads to loss of position sense (*proprioception*) on the side of the lesion and pain and temperature on the opposite side, below the level of the lesion (hemisection; *Brown-Séquard syndrome*). Diseases of the center of the spinal cord—for instance, *syringomyelia*—tends to lead to loss of pain and temperature sensation without loss of light touch. Damage to the posterior columns causes loss of the sensations they carry, namely vibration and position. The rare complete lesions of the posterior columns interfere with the perception of other sensations as well.

Brain stem lesions characteristically cause "crossed sensory disturbances," with loss of pain and temperature sensation on one side of the face and the other side of the body.

Thalamic lesions can cause loss of sensation on the other side of the body, usually of position sense more than of other sensations and almost always more than of pin prick and light touch.

Cortical lesions that affect the primary sensory cortex lead to loss of sensation on the opposite side. Lesions involving accessory sensory cortex—typically the parietal lobe—can lead to loss of the ability to discriminate sensory modalities. They can also cause neglect of the opposite side, more commonly with lesions of the non-dominant (usually right) parietal lobe than of the left.

Abnormal (Excessive) Sensations (paresthesias and dysesthesias): Pathological sensations may be perceived by the patient as variants of a normal sensation or as previously unknown and therefore "undescribable" sensations. Naturally enough, people will often try to describe the latter in terms of the former. Sometimes a normal stimulus induces an inappropriate sensation. An example of such perverted sensation (*allodynia*) is burning pain in response to a light touch.

Disease of the peripheral nerves often leads to sensations described as "numbness" or of "pins and needles."

Disease of nerve roots often causes "shooting" (*lancinating*) or "burning" pains referred to the areas served by those roots. A typical and unfortunately common example is pain in the leg from *sciatica*. (See Chap. 7, Pain.)

Disease of sensory ganglia typically resembles disease of nerve roots. Relatively widespread disease of sensory ganglia can keep the victim from knowing where his or her limbs are. It can lead to a wide-based and unsteady gait—a *sensory ataxia*. This occurs, for instance, in tabes dorsalis due to later stage syphilis.[3]

Disease of the thalamus can cause pain and other unpleasant sensations. Often the threshold for sensing stimuli is raised, but the response to stimuli includes pain or other unpleasant feelings (*hyperpathia*). Those stimuli can involve organs of special sensation and/or more general sensations. For instance, loud sounds and pinprick can both cause hyperpathia in susceptible subjects.

Disease of the parietal lobe or other parts of the cortex or hippocampus system sometimes leads to unusual and unpleasant sensations. These can occur in some forms of delirium, including withdrawal states. Unpleasant skin sensations are a classic complaint in people with delirium tremens.

Mixtures of Abnormal and Lost Sensations: Often a disorder will lead to both loss of normal sensory modalities and gain of unpleasant sensation. For instance, "pins and needles" can accompany "numbness" (a term which patients sometimes use to describe what is really weakness). Both the feelings of decreased sensation and of abnormal sensation can be due to the same lesion(s) in the same location(s).

Causes of abnormalities of general sensations include the common causes of disease of other organ systems. Sudden losses of sensation can be caused by trauma, vascular compromise, or sometimes infection or toxins. Diagnosis of these problems typically depends on clinical history and other evidence of these conditions. Chapter 13 (Disorders of Both Sensation and Motility) discusses a number of disorders that can cause peripheral neuropathies that usually involve loss of sensation as well as motor strength. A clue that a nerve is being compressed—for instance, by a blood clot—is relatively greater loss of pressure sensation than pain and temperature sense.

More chronic sensory loss can arise from just as wide a spectrum of types of disease. The diagnosis of these conditions depends on the acumen and knowledge of the physician. General clinicians are skilled in recognizing diabetes, vascular disease, collagen-vascular disease, and other disorders including infections.

Syphilis and Lyme disease (*treponemal infections*) deserve special mention. Tabes dorsalis and other later complications of syphilis are much less common today than they were, because most strains of the responsible organism (*spirochete*) are still susceptible to commonly used antibiotics. However, syphilis still occurs, often together with other sexually transmitted diseases including AIDS.[4] Syphilis is, as mentioned previously in this monograph, a "great imitator." Any patient with a neurological disease about whose etiology there is any doubt deserves a blood test for syphilis.[5] Similar considerations apply to *Lyme disease*, a treponemal infection now common in many parts of the United States including suburban counties outside New York city. It is also a great imitator, often occurring without a history of the chronic ring lesion that is supposed to be its "give away sign." Again, a high index of suspicion and blood tests can be necessary to make the diagnosis and institute the appropriate antibiotic treatment to prevent the occurrence and progression of neurological and other complications. Empirical treatment may sometimes be warranted even without confirmatory laboratory studies. (See below.)

NEUROBIOLOGY

The causes of disorders of sensation cover the whole range of causes of disease in general. They go from inheritance to environmental toxins (*toxicants*). They include among others vascular disease, tumors, infections, autoimmune diseases, trauma, and degenerations including degenerations associated with aging.

Aging is associated with non-neural impairments of vision, including cataracts and deformations of the eye ball leading to *presbyopia.* While disabling and benefiting from specialized treatment when they cause disability, these conditions are so common as to be statistically normal in the elderly. There are also age-related diseases of the eye, notably the different forms of glaucoma. These threaten vision because the increased pressure inside the eye kills the cells of the retina, which like almost all other neurons do not regenerate effectively. Macular degeneration, which is basically a disease of the blood vessels of the retina, is an unfortunately common cause of blindness for which treatments are now available, as discussed above. Aging is also associated with the statistically normal decrease in hearing that typically accompanies advanced age. Some investigators attribute this loss of particularly high-tone hearing to damage from being exposed to too much loud noise for too long. A similar effect occurs in younger people who have habitually listened to over amplified music. Slowing of the processing of sensory information is a normal concomitant of human aging, at least statistically. The ability to sense vibration and position in the ankles and feet is so often decreased in older people as to be almost a physiological change of aging. Aging is sometimes associated with burning and other unpleasant sensations of the feet, more often in older women than in men.

Specific diseases and medications can damage primarily the sensory parts of peripheral nerves, as discussed below. In general, these diseases and drugs can also cause mixed sensory and motor (sensorimotor) neuropathies. Specific causes of damage to peripheral nerves (neuropathies) are discussed in more detail in Chap. 13 (Disorders of Both Sensation and Motility).

The classification of sensory disorders presented earlier can relate to etiology in the sense of localization. For instance, types of deafness can be organized according to the primary anatomic location of the lesion. *Conductive deafness* is by definition linked to disorders of the external or middle ear, which are not themselves parts of the nervous system. *Sensorineural deafness* results from damage to the cochlea or the cochlear division of cranial nerve VIII. *Central deafness* represents damage to the cochlear nucleus, its connections to the primary auditory connections in the temporal lobe of the brain, or to dysfunction of the processing of auditory stimuli in the brain. A variety of specific genetic syndromes of deafness are known, and the genes for some of these have been specified. Total tone deafness also appears to be inherited.

Diabetes can cause peripheral sensory disturbance without much impairment in motor function. The mechanism is damage to peripheral nerves. *Diabetic neuropathy* appears to involve damage to blood vessels serving the nerves. (Damage to blood vessels in general is of course a common complication of diabetes.) Clinically, the symptoms of diabetic neuropathy are typically symmetrical, often involving both feet, and not rarely going on to involve the ankles and calves and other parts of the body. Patients most commonly describe themselves as having "numbness" and "tingling," although other abnormal sensations are not rare particularly as the condition progresses. About 5–15% of diabetics complain of these problems, but careful neurological examination reportedly reveals some degree of peripheral nerve damage in perhaps half the people with diabetes severe enough to require insulin. Often occult signs of motor damage are present as well but do not bother the patient. Most general clinicians are familiar with this complication of diabetes.

Loss of sensation without much interference with motility can result from other disorders well known to general clinicians, at least in the earlier phases of these diseases. Sjögren (*sicca*) syndrome often leads to a loss of peripheral sensation as its first clinically significant manifestation, with the result that these patients are often seen first by neurologists. Other *collagen-vascular* diseases more often lead to a combination of motor and sensory disabilities but occasionally first present clinically as primarily sensory neuropathies. The nervous system manifestations of systemic (non-neural) cancers are sometimes primarily sensory.[6] Such *paraneoplastic* syndromes can be the earliest clinical manifestation of cancer, notably of cancers of the lung. They can provide a clue to diagnosis while the malignancy is still curable. Certain drugs can lead to primarily sensory abnormalities. Among the medications that can cause a primarily sensory neuropathy are antitumor agents (*cisplatin, carboplatin, taxols*), anti-infection agents (*isoniazid, chloramphenicol, metronidazole*), the anti-angina agent *perhexiline*, and even megadoses of the vitamin B_6 (*pyridoxine*). Leprosy—fortunately rare in the United States—typically causes sensory loss before its other manifestations. Other neuropathies can give rise to sensory symptoms before motor, but not so regularly as to be characteristic. (See Chap. 13, Disorders of Both Sensation and Motility.)

TREATMENT

Disorders of Special Senses

Vision: As noted earlier, several disorders of the eye require immediate treatment.

Acute angle glaucoma is best treated in most urban or suburban settings by immediate transfer of the patient to the care of an ophthalmologist. That specialist is trained and equipped to make a definitive diagnosis and start the appropriate treatment. *Definitive therapy* is reduction of the intraocular pressure by making a hole in the iris, either with a laser or surgically.

When immediate referral to an ophthalmologist is not available, medical treatment of even acute, closed-angle glaucoma can usually buy time. A *prostaglandin F2α* analogue, *latanoprost* (Xalatan), is now the favored medical treatment to alleviate the increased pressure in the eye while awaiting surgery. The recommended dose is 1 drop (1.5 μg; 50 μL) of the standard 50 μg/mL solution, no more than once a day. (The effect is reported to be decreased by more frequent dosage.) An alternative prostaglandin analogue is *unoprostone* (Rescula).

Adjunct treatments are available if latanoprost is not effective enough by itself. A common choice is the *β*-blocker *timolol* (Timoptic, Betimol). The usual dose 1–2 drops of a 0.25% ophthalmic solution of timolol maleate. Where necessary, intravenous injection of a carbonic anhydrase inhibitor can be dramatically effective. The usual intravenous dose of *acetazolamide* (Diamox) is 250 mg up to every 6 hours but not more than a gram a day. Carbonic anhydrase inhibitors (*acetazolamide*, *methazolamide* [Neptazane], *dichlorphenamide* [Daranide]) can incur side effects with which general clinicians are familiar: excessive urination, sexual impairments, weight loss, fatigue, stomach problems, depression, intolerance of aspirin, and rarely anemia or kidney problems. Textbooks of Ophthalmology and of Neurology describe other therapies, notably including eye drops that act on cholinergic innervation, as presented in textbooks of Ophthalmology. As noted earlier, chronic glaucoma is common particularly in older people and in those with a family history of this condition. Discussion of the treatment of chronic glaucomas is beyond the scope of this monograph. Glaucoma is not strictly speaking a disorder of the nervous system, and the reader is referred to specialized sources for discussions of its pathology, physiology, treatments, and the mechanisms of actions of the medications used to treat it.[1]

The treatment of temporal arteritis with steroids is discussed in Chap. 7 (Pain). First aid for toxins in the eye is generally extensive flushing with sterile saline or with clean water if saline is not available.

Nearsightedness, farsightedness, astigmatism, and other disorders requiring refraction and corrective lenses or laser treatment are conventionally referred to specialists rather than being diagnosed and treated by general physicians.

Disorders of the eye muscles leading to double vision are generally treated by specialists. The treatment of double vision due to myasthenia gravis is discussed in Chap. 11 (Disorders of Motility) and of other neuropathies and of Multiple Sclerosis in Chap. 13 (Disorders of Both Sensation and Motility).

Treatment of central disorders affecting vision depends on the nature of the disorder. Retinal artery occlusion is now treated with intra-arterial thrombolysis.[7] Chapter 9 (Cerebrovascular Disorders) discusses treatments of other strokes. Chapter 13 (Disorders of Both Sensation and Motility) discusses treatment of optic neuritis, which is a common manifestation of multiple sclerosis.

Hearing: Hearing aids are available to treat the common forms of more or less slowly progressive hearing loss, including those in the elderly. Testing and prescription of the appropriate hearing aid is the province of specialists. Hearing loss and/or tinnitus due to an acoustic neuroma or other tumor is treated surgically or, where indicated, by other modalities. The treatment of tinnitus due to too much aspirin is conventional treatment of aspirin toxicity, a subject with which general clinicians are familiar. Hearing loss due to infection is treatment of the infection, another subject familiar to general clinicians.

Precise diagnosis of a type of hereditary hearing loss can be surprisingly therapeutic, for two reasons. First, some of these conditions are treatable. For instance, a special, rather weird diet helps people with Refsum disease. Secondly, a precise genetic diagnosis can be surprisingly satisfying to a patient and family even if it does not lead to effective treatment. It documents that "everything has been done."

Smell and Taste: The treatment for loss of smell or taste due to sensory organ damage in the mouth or nose is treatment of the underlying disease, such as chronic rhinitis. The diagnosis and treatment of such conditions is part of the domain of general clinicians, as discussed above. Chap. 10 (Disorders of Awareness) discusses the treatment of abnormal smells or tastes due to temporal lobe epilepsy and Chap.3 (Mood Disorders) treatment of complaints of loss of taste due to depression.

Disorders of General Sensation

The treatment of disorders of general sensation is the treatment of the underlying disorder. The treatment of vascular, infectious, or mechanical disturbances is covered in other chapters. (See Chap. 9 [Vascular Disorders] and Chap. 11 [Disorders of Motility]) Treatment of Sjögren syndrome or other collagen-vascular diseases and of vasculitides is with steroids or other immunosuppressants and is well known to general clinicians.

Diabetic neuropathy, like other complications of diabetes, is now thought to respond well to precise control of blood sugar, i.e., to "tight diabetic control." Antidepressants including SSRIs (see Chapter 3, Mood Disorders) and amitriptyline are usually effective against the pain. Sometimes antiepileptic medications are more helpful. (See Chap. 7, Pain.)

The primary treatment for toxic neuropathies is to stop exposure to the drug or other toxin. Where available and of proven usefulness, agents that help removal from the body can be utilized. In acute situations, dialysis or *plasmapheresis* may be helpful.

For paraneoplastic syndromes, complete removal of the cancer that rouses the immune reaction often cures the disease of the nervous system. When that is not possible, treatments to modify the immune reaction can sometimes be helpful. The choice of such treatment is best left to the oncologist treating the patient. The general clinician who has primary care of the patient does, however, need to be sensitive to the side effects of the chemotherapeutic agents being used. Among ourselves, we physicians often refer to these agents as poisons, and for good reason.

Infections should be treated appropriately. Recommendations for the optimal treatment of syphilis and Lyme disease change. Clinicians should check with an infectious disease specialist or with the CDC (U.S. Centers for Disease Control and Prevention) on the changing recommendations for treating syphilis or Lyme disease before instituting treatment for these diseases. At the time of this writing, in 2005, the recommended treatment for secondary syphilis is penicillin and for Lyme disease antibiotics taken by mouth, such as cefuroxime axetil (Ceftin), amoxicillin, doxycycline, penicillin, and erythromycin (for people allergic to penicillin). Treatment of leprosy with dapsone is best left to specialized physicians and facilities.

REFERENCES

1. For instance, East DL, ed. *Oxford Textbook of Ophthalmology*, Oxford University Press, Oxford, 1999.
2. Loss of visual acuity could be life-threatening for our distant ancestors who had to hunt or forage to get enough food. Although the organs of reproduction are also not necessary for life in this era of overpopulation, problems with them also tend to rouse great anxiety. The incomes of ophthalmologists, urologists, and specialists in assisted reproduction tend to reflect these common anxieties.

3. O'Donnel JA, Emery CL. Neurosyphilis: A current review. *Curr Infect Dis Rep*. 2005;7:277–284.
4. Widespread sexual continence is, of course, not characteristic of American society today and probably never was (cf. the birth rate in colonial times). Non-venereal transmission of syphilis can occur but is not likely. The old medical saw about catching syphilis on a toilet seat still holds—possible but uncomfortable.
5. Testing for syphilis was part of the routine clinical laboratory battery used on the dementia service that the author directed for 25 years. Cases of untreated syphilis turned up even in people in their seventies. In our patients, a relevant history was not obtainable (or at least not obtained) until after the family had been informed of the laboratory diagnosis.
6. Darnell RB, Posner JB. Paraneoplastic syndromes involving the nervous system. *New Eng J Med*. 2003;349:1543–1554.
7. Arnold M, Koerner U, Remonda L, et al. Comparison of intra-arterial thrombolysis with conventional treatment in patients with acute central retinal artery occlusion. *J Neurol Neurosurg Psychiatry*. 2005;76:160–161.

CHAPTER THIRTEEN

Disorders of both Sensation and Motility: Multiple Sclerosis and Related Disorders; Neuropathies

This chapter discusses two sets of disorders not discussed elsewhere in this monograph, namely:

1. Multiple sclerosis and related disorders of myelin (Table 13-1)
2. Disorders of peripheral nerves impairing both sensory and motor functions

These conditions typically impair both motor function and sensation, at least in their later stages.

Many other disorders of the nervous system can lead to problems with both motility and sensation. They include many disorders that are

TABLE 13–1
Disorders of myelin other than multiple sclerosis

Acute disseminated encephalomyelitis
Postinfection
Postvaccination
Rabies (old vaccine)
Smallpox
Others (rare)
Necrotizing hemorrhagic encephalitis
Acute (hemorrhagic encephalopathy of Hurst)
Subacute necrotic myelopathy
Inherited
Usually in infants/children
Occasional adult forms (e.g., metachromatic leukodystrophy)

discussed elsewhere in this monograph (including in Chap. 9, Cerebrovascular Disorders; Chap. 10, Disorders of Awareness; and Chap. 14, Disorders of Conduct). For instance, patients with major strokes typically lose both the ability to move and the ability to feel on the affected side (*hemiparesis* and *hemianesthesia*). That is often combined with loss of the visual field on that side and often with difficulty in processing visual or auditory information. Similar problems can occur with tumors, infections, and a variety of other diseases and lesions that can affect in the brain. Other chapters in this monograph discuss a number of these conditions, and neurologists are by training familiar with the full panoply of disorders that can impair both motility and sensation.

MULTIPLE SCLEROSIS (MS)

The characteristic of this condition is episodes of damage to myelin. *Myelin* is the fatty sheath that surrounds nerves in both the central and peripheral nervous systems. Structures rich in myelin make up the white matter of the central nervous system. In multiple sclerosis (MS), damage to other structures including nerve cell processes (axons) also occurs but is much less prominent. By definition, MS causes loss of myelin that varies over time and over location in the central nervous system, that is, "over time and space." Since the translation of the word "sclerosis" is scarring, the words *multiple sclerosis* themselves only signify multiple scarring, and do not specify what part of the nervous system is being scarred. The British name, *disseminated sclerosis*, and the French name, *sclerose en plaques*, are hardly more descriptive. A more descriptive name for this condition would be *episodic demyelination.*

Etiology

Whether MS is one condition or a manifestation of several types of white matter damage remains unsettled. Nor has the etiology or etiologies been well defined, despite enormous amounts of research. Theories abound. The original description of MS was accompanied by a proposal that it was due to abnormal sweating. Over the years, the medical literature has contained confident statements that MS is a viral disease, that it is not a viral disease, that it is an autoimmune disease, and that it not usefully described as an autoimmune disease.

Currently, a favored possible etiology combines infectious and immune mechanisms. This theory proposes that the cause of MS is an infection that leads to the formation of antibodies and immune cells that react with one or several normal constituents of myelin. This phenomenon—where an antibody to an infective agent cross-reacts with a normal body constituent—has the name *molecular mimicry*. The nature of the infective agent or agents contributing to the development of MS remains uncertain. Infection with measles, chicken pox, or German measles can lead to antibodies in humans that react with a protein in myelin. The nature of the autoimmune process if any is also a subject of debate. Many immunologists believe that T cells are important mediators of the demyelination. The aberrant immune reaction appears to be determined in part genetically, but the specific gene or genes predisposing to MS remain unknown. Certain histocompatibility antigens (HLA types) are associated with a higher risk for MS. White people appear more susceptible than Blacks. Acute disorders of myelin that follow a known infection or vaccination lend indirect support to the possibility that the more chronic and episodic demyelination of MS also reflects molecular mimicry. According to this proposal, the etiology of MS is in some ways analogous to proven mechanisms in rheumatic heart disease or in paraneoplastic syndromes.

Empirical studies have defined risk factors for MS. They include being a woman, living or having lived in a cold climate (high latitude), and family history. The association with colder climates has been cited as support for an infectious element, but infections are at least as common in the tropics as nearer to the poles. Spouses of patients do not have a higher risk than the general population. Age at onset is most often 20–40 years.

Pathology

The fundamental finding in MS is rather sharply delineated patches in the white matter where myelin has been lost. They appear pinkish-gray rather than white on gross examination of the spinal cord and brain. The appearance of these "*plaques*" under the microscope varies with their age. Early lesions show predominantly loss of myelin with relative sparing of other structures as well as an inflammatory exudate. Somewhat older lesions also show a reaction of *microglia*—the "immune cells of the nervous system." As lesions age, scars rich in *astroglia* form. Nerve cell processes (axons) that had been surrounded by myelin degenerate. Eventually the scars become almost free of cells. Sometimes attempts at partial remyelination can be seen. Rarely, the lesion becomes a cavity.

Clinically, MS can bring a patient to the attention of a general clinician in a variety of ways. That is expected since the disorder is characterized by variability in location of the lesions in the nervous system as well as by variation over time. MS classically appears to start relatively suddenly. Sudden onset of symptoms within less than an hour can occur but it is not typical. Careful questioning often reveals milder symptoms that developed weeks before the presenting complaint. Not rarely, a previous episode of transient neurological disease occurred that the patient thinks was too unimportant to mention. A typical example is having had difficulty with vision in one eye that then cleared without any treatment.

In about half the patients, the first manifestation of MS is weakness and/or impaired sensation ("numbness") in one or more limbs. The weakness is typically *spastic* (stiff). Its extent varies from patient to patient and over time, but it can be severe. Tingling and "band-like" sensations are common. So is aching pain. Sharper, more localized, "lancinating" or burning pain occurs more rarely. It is presumably due to demyelination affecting the sensory roots. Incoordination and staggering gait are frequent. They result from diminished input of position sense through the spinal cord to the cerebellum and other parts of the brain that mediate balance.

In about a quarter of the patients, loss of vision is the first sign of MS. *Optic neuritis* results from damage to the optic nerve. It affects one eye more often than both. Typically, the initial visual problems clear at least partially. In some fortunate people, this brief problem is the only manifestation of a disease of myelin during their lifetime. In others, the transient problem with vision is a harbinger of future development of more lesions in other parts of the nervous system and eventually of permanent disabilities. Specialists debate whether a single episode of optic neuritis should be considered a manifestation of MS.

A smaller number of patients develop lesions at a single level of the spinal cord. This so-called *transverse myelitis* involves the long tracts of the spinal cord. It can have a relatively sudden onset. In some patients, it is followed eventually by other demyelinating lesions. In others, it is not. Specialists also debate the relation of this condition to "classic" MS. As expected from the fact that variation is characteristic of this disease, it can start in a variety of other ways, depending on which part of the nervous system is first involved and how badly. Double vision (*diplopia*) is a common clinical presentation. Other presentations include disorders of urination, staggering (*ataxia*), difficulty in speaking (*dysarthria*), and dizziness (*vertigo*). Other variants also deserve mention. "Acute MS" can lead to death during the first episode; whether these patients should receive the diagnosis of MS is debated. In *neuromyelitis optica* (Devic disease), both the optic nerves and the spinal cord are simultaneously or successively involved in a single episode. Experts debate whether this is a form of "true MS." Massive demyelination in children or adolescents characterizes Diffuse Cerebral Sclerosis (Schilder disease; *encephalitis periaxialis diffusa*).

As MS goes on, disabilities tend to increase. Problems with bladder control become common, with attendant medical complications. After 25 years, about one-third of the patients are still working and about one-third of patients are in wheel chairs.

Impairments in cognition and psychiatric disabilities also tend to appear as the disease progresses. Memory difficulties are present in many patients particularly in later stages of MS, but often show some response to treatment. (See below.) Depression is very common. While having MS may seem to justify feelings of loss, helplessness, and anger, damage to parts of the nervous system mediating mood ("affect") almost certainly contributes. Depression is more common in patients with MS than in paraplegics. Estimates are that perhaps as many as half of patients with MS suffer from depression during their lifetimes and 20% in any given year. Fortunately, the depression of MS tends to respond to adequate treatment. (See Chap 3, Mood Disorders and below.)

Neurological examinations in MS patients vary among patients and in the same patient over time, just as the disease does. Abnormalities on neurological examination usually reflect lesions visible on MRI scan in the central nervous system, but the opposite is not true. Examination by MRI or at autopsy tends to find many more lesions in the brain than were evident during clinical examination. Thus, MRI or autopsy examination tends to identify "clinically silent plaques" in addition to symptomatic plaques. Lesions in the spinal cord tend to relate more predictably with the development of clinical disabilities than do lesions in the white matter of the brain.

Certain findings on neurological examination raise a high suspicion of the diagnosis of MS. The patient with early MS typically complains of symptoms in only one leg but has neurological signs in both. In many patients, passive flexion of the neck induces "electric" sensations in the shoulder, often the back, and sometimes even the thighs (*Lhermitte sign*). A specific type of weakness of the eye muscles in a young person is almost diagnostic of MS (*bilateral internuclear ophthalmoplegia*).

Laboratory tests provide useful information. MRI imaging of the brain reveals multiple areas of demyelination in 80–98% of MS patients. The demyelinated lesions are particularly clear on T 2 weighted scans. Certain findings are recognized by neuroradiologists and neurologists as almost diagnostic of MS (e.g., *Dawson fingers*). MRI scans are also useful to follow the biological progress of the underlying disease, independent of clinical complaints.

Examination of the cerebrospinal fluid (CSF) is usually revealing in these patients. Over 90% of MS patients have abnormal γ-globulins in their CSF that are recognized in the clinical laboratory as *oligoclonal bands*. Total γ-globulins are increased in the CSF in about 65% of MS patients, total protein in about 40%, and mononuclear cells in about 30%.

Electrophysiological studies can also aid diagnosis. Evoked visual and sensory potentials tend to be abnormal in half to two-thirds or more of MS patients. That occurs because once a nerve has lost its myelin sheath (been *demyelinated*), it conducts nerve impulses more slowly even if its myelin sheath is more or less reformed (*remyelinated*). The slowing may be measured in thousands of a second differences—for instance, in comparing responses of the two eyes by visual evoked potentials. Like MRI and CT imaging, electrophysiological studies can provide evidence of neurological damage that did not come to the attention of the patient nor to that of the physician doing a routine neurological examination.

In patients with psychiatric problems or difficulties with memory, the appropriate testing instruments will document the abnormalities. Recognizing and documenting these disabilities is often useful in guiding care even when it does not add to the precision of the diagnosis.

Differential diagnosis in MS should be made by a neurologist—where convenient, a neurologist specializing in this and related demyelinating diseases. Differential diagnosis at presentation includes *disseminated lupus* or other *vasculitis/collagen vascular disease*, infections including *syphilis*, hereditary disorders including *hereditary ataxias*, and the *disseminated encephalomyelitis* discussed below.

Treatment of MS and related disorders of myelin is best left to a neurologist, when that is feasible. A neurologist specializing in these diseases is usually the optimal choice. MS and related disorders are typically chronic conditions. They are difficult to manage clinically. Research on new treatments continues, and keeping up with the vast literature in this area is a challenge.[1,2] Unfortunately, the Internet and other forms of public information tout a variety of poorly documented "therapies." Patients who happened to go into a remission after indulging in one of these nostrums may provide enthusiastic endorsements that seem convincing to other patients and their families. Specialists are in a good position to be aware of this "information" and to be able to discourage patients from experimenting with putative remedies that may harm their health as well as their finances. Much of the treatment of MS depends on "clinical experience" rather than on data from formal clinical trials. Of course, clinical trials are difficult in a disease like MS that is characterized by variability.

Steroids

Steroids are the treatment of choice for acute attacks or exacerbations of MS. Methylprednisolone, prednisone, or ACTH (*adrenocorticotropic hormone*) are all used. The regimen is typically high doses with a rapid taper. A typical dosage schedule is intravenous or if necessary oral methylprednisolone (0.5–1.0 g/day for 3 days), followed by prednisone starting at 60–80 mg/day and tapering over a period of 2 weeks. General clinicians are familiar with the potential side effects, complications, and contraindications of steroid therapy, including short-term high-dose treatment. These do not need to be belabored here.

Interferon Beta-1a

Interferon beta-1a injections are now an accepted part of the treatment of chronic relapsing MS. Controlled studies have confirmed that this agent tends to reduce the number of relapses and to slow the progression of the disease as determined by MRI scanning of the brain.[3,4] Unfortunately, there is no convincing evidence that this therapy slows progression to disability. (The progression is so variable in this disease that it is hard to study.) The use of interferon is logical according to the current theories of the mechanism of the MS, since interferon has both antiviral and immunomodulating activities. Unfortunately, the use of interferon does not come free. A characteristic, transient, unpleasant, but relatively unimportant side effect is a flu-like syndrome that typically occurs and resolves within a day or two after the injection of interferon. The intensity of this reaction usually lessens with repeated treatments. Ordinary anti-inflammatories tend to reduce the intensity of the reaction. Some people, however, find interferon treatment intolerable even with anti-inflammatories.

More serious side effects of interferon also occur (Table 13-2). The general clinician is likely to be familiar with these potential complications since interferon therapy is now used to treat a number of "medical" illnesses, including viral illnesses and malignancies. MS is a common disease, and general clinicians are likely to be providing medical care for patients with MS who are being treated chronically with interferon and therefore may develop its side effects. They are in an excellent position to pick up the early manifestations of interferon toxicity to the heart or kidney or other organs. The generalist is likely to be more familiar with and focused on dysfunction of these organs than the treating neurologist is.

Immunosuppressants

Medications other than steroids that diminish the immune response are widely used to treat MS. However, support for their use comes more from "clinical experience" than from controlled clinical trials—from clinical lore rather than from clinical science.[5] Not all neurologists are convinced of their usefulness. A Cochrane data base study did not find convincing evidence for the use of methotrexate in MS.[6] Some specialists use high dose immunotherapy for *refractory MS* that is not controlled by interferon.[7] This therapy entails many risks and is best left to specialists experienced in its use, to whom such patients can be referred. Occasional patients described in the medical literature appear to have made a remarkable recovery after *plasmapheresis* to remove antibodies from their blood stream, but occasional patients with MS have made remarkable recoveries without plasmapheresis.

TABLE 13–2
Major side effects of interferon

Major side effects of interferon
Flu-like syndrome after injection (transient)
Fever
Chills
Headache
Gastrointestinal (nausea, vomiting, diarrhea)
Bone marrow suppression
Granulotocytopenia
Thrombocytopenia
Neurotoxicity
Sleepiness
Confusion
Seizures
Fatigue (excessive)
Other behavioral abnormalities
Weight loss
Autoimmune reactions
Thyroiditis
Other autoantibodies
Cardiovascular abnormalities
Low blood pressure
Rapid heart rate
Kidney disease
Interstitial nephritis
Proteinuria
Azotemia
Fertility problems
(safety during pregnancy undetermined)
Hair loss (alopecia)
Liver damage

In laboratory models and according to some anecdotal reports, statins can be as effective as interferon against demyelinating disease.[8,9] Formal clinical trials are being started. If the initial enthusiasm proves correct, these relatively safe medications will be a valuable addition to the armamentarium of treatments for MS.

Other potential therapies are also being tested. They include monoclonal antibodies (e.g., alemtuzumab, daclizumab, natalizumab, and rituximab), mycophenolate, antibiotics, and antivirals. Centers that specialize in the treatment of MS are likely to be participating in structured clinical trials of these and other agents. An important responsibility of the staff of these centers is to keep up with the literature on these newer agents, so as to know as soon as possible which are useful and which are useless or harmful.

Cannabinoids

Cannabinoids (i.e., marijuana derivatives) have been claimed in anecdotal reports and a few animal studies to have a protective effect in MS.[10] General physicians need to know about these claims, since their patients are likely to. Currently available data do not make clear whether the patients improved biologically or were just less bothered about having MS. Of course, use of marijuana or related substances is not an approved therapy for this condition. In almost all states, its use is against the law.

Complications of MS

Complications of MS can usually be treated usefully by standard treatments for the specific problems. Memory problems in patients with multiple sclerosis (MS) reportedly responded to donepezil (10 mg/daily), in a small, double-blind, placebo-controlled trial.[11] Donepezil (Aricept) has been approved for the memory disorder of Alzheimer disease (Chap. 5, Cognitive Disorders) and also appears useful for memory problems due to cerebrovascular disease (Chap. 9, Cerebrovascular Disorders). As discussed in Chap. 5 (Cognitive Disorders), donepezil improves the tone of cholinergic systems by inhibiting the breakdown of acetylcholine by acetylcholinesterase. Depression and other psychiatric symptoms in patients with MS reportedly respond well to standard treatments including SSRIs (selective serotonin reuptake inhibitors).[12] (See Chap. 3, Mood Disorders.)

Medical problems tend to develop in patients with MS, and are optimally managed by collaboration between the patient's general clinician and neurologist.[13] Bladder dysfunction is common and brings with it the usual risks of infection and kidney damage. Standard medical treatments are used. A spastic bladder tends to respond to propantheline (Pro-Banthine) or oxybutynin (Ditropan), in conventional doses, with which general clinicians are familiar. Sometimes intermittent or even chronic catheterization becomes necessary. Paralysis raises the risk of bedsores and accompanying infection, as well as of muscle atrophy and other disabilities. Fatigue can be serious in MS although the mechanisms causing it are usually unclear.

Sometimes this symptom benefits from treatment with amantadine (Symmetrel, 100 mg PO at breakfast and lunch) or modafinil (Provigil, Alertec, Vigicier, Modalert, and so on; 200–400 mg/day). Pemoline, which has previously been used for this purpose, has been withdrawn from the market in the United States and Canada.

Rehabilitation

Rehabilitation measures can be helpful, including choice of an appropriate wheelchair if that becomes necessary. Spasticity can be treated with medications or injections of botulinum toxin (see Chap. 9 [Cerebrovascular Disorders] and Chap. 11 [Disorders of Motility]). Sometimes neurosurgery (*thalamotomy*) is resorted to in order to relieve severe and disabling spasticity.

Patients with MS typically need emotional support as well as practical advice about how to deal with their often progressive disabilities. MS is usually a discouraging thing to have or have in one's family.[13] The patient and the family can develop a tendency to play one physician off against the other. The general clinician and neurologist should be closely enough in touch with each other that the patient gets the same advice from both.

OTHER DISORDERS OF MYELIN

A number of other disorders of myelin are common enough that they are likely to be seen by general physicians. A number of rarer disorders are not discussed in this monograph but are well known to neurologists.

Acute Disseminated Encephalomyelitis

This group of illnesses include relatively acute neurological sequelae of infections, rashes (*exanthemas*), or immunizations. They can be divided into two often overlapping forms. One is encephalitic and involves gray matter. It leads to confusion and other symptoms of gray matter disease, and sometimes even to stupor, coma, and decerebrate rigidity. (See Chap. 10, Disorders of Awareness.) The other form typically involves demyelination. As in

MS, the demyelination can be spotty or can be so widespread as to transect the spinal cord functionally (i.e., cause transverse myelitis).

Mechanistically, immune mechanisms seem to mediate this form of acute encephalomyelitis. The mechanism is *medical mimicry*—cross-reaction of an antibody made to a foreign antigen with a normal constituent of the body. Medical mimicry is now thought to play a role in MS itself as discussed above. It has been clearly shown to play a role in most paraneoplastic disorders of the nervous system (i.e., nervous system manifestations of tumors that do not invade the nervous system directly, discussed below).

General physicians should be sensitive to the possible occurrence of relatively acute demyelinating syndromes after apparently innocuous infections or after vaccinations. Differential diagnosis can be difficult particularly when the time relationships are not typical. Neurological symptoms and signs appearing during a febrile illness may reflect direct infection or other damage to the nervous system. Neurological symptoms can appear after an infection so mild that the patient did not notice it. Careful history and clinical course sometimes clarify this situation. Treatment is symptomatic and supportive. Fortunately, these conditions tend to be self-limited in adults. That is not true in children. Children with permanent damage to the nervous system after a bout of measles were not rare until the vaccine against measles became widely available.

Central Pontine Myelinosis

Central pontine myelinosis is typically a complication of other chronic illnesses. The clinical manifestations reflect the pathological lesion, which is dissolution of myelin in the pons and sometimes nearby areas. The seriousness of the condition depends on the amount of demyelination. Sometimes the lesion is a clinically unimportant finding on brain imaging. In severely affected patients, all limbs are paralyzed, and the patients cannot chew, swallow, or speak. In some cases, even the movements of the eyes become abnormal. Severe cases can end up with *locked-in syndrome.* (See Chap. 10, Disorders of Awareness.) Intermediate stages between minimal and terrible disability of course also occur.

The most common condition associated with central pontine myelinosis is severe alcohol abuse. Other recognized causes are cancers, liver failure, and kidney failure with dialysis. The common mechanism is believed often to be nutritional deficiency, particularly of thiamin (vitamin B_1) or niacin (vitamin B_3). In other cases, abnormal regulation of serum sodium has been implicated.

Unfortunately, once the disease has developed, only supportive treatment is available.

MOTOR-SENSORY NEUROPATHIES

Most, but not all, disorders of peripheral nerves lead to problems with both motor and sensory functions.[14] They are discussed below. Neuropathies that tend to be associated with primarily motor difficulties with few or no clinically important sensory abnormalities are discussed in Chap. 11 (Disorders of Motility). Those that tend to be associated with sensory abnormalities with few or no clinically important motor abnormalities are discussed in Chap. 12 (Disorders of Sensation). Neuropathies often involve the autonomic nervous system as well, leading to systemic manifestations such as postural hypotension and poor control of cardiac rhythm. However, the autonomic neuropathies are not discussed in detail here. General clinicians are usually familiar with the treatment of autonomic dysfunction—for instance, of hypotension or hypertension, of cardiac arrhythmias, or of gastrointestinal overactivity or underactivity.

The following discussion focuses on disorders of peripheral nerves that present clinically both with weakness and with either loss of sensation or more often with aberrant and unpleasant sensations (*dysesthesias*). This subject is vast. Only certain high points can be touched on here. In these, as in so many other disorders that affect the nervous system, referral is advisable. Specialists have not only expert knowledge and experience but also access to specialized equipment and techniques that aid in the diagnosis and in following the efficacy of treatment.

Even in specialized centers, the neuropathies in a quarter to a half of the patients receive the final diagnosis of "*idiopathic*." That word is of course medicalese for "we have no idea what's causing this problem." Unfortunately, "idiopathic" is not a good guide to treatment. Sometimes a neuropathy is attributed to a cause whose relation to the clinical illness is not rigorously demonstrable—for instance, exposure years earlier to an industrial solvent or other toxin. In speculating on the possible toxic origin of a neuropathy, it is important not to rouse guilt in the patient or caregiver or make statements that will lead to lawsuits based on speculations for which there is no real biomedical evidence.

Classification and Diagnosis: There are a variety of ways to classify neuropathies, as there are with most neurological diseases and indeed most diseases. There is therefore a variety of sets of diagnostic terms for neuropathies.

Anatomic pathology is the basis of a system of classification much used by neurologists. *Axonal degeneration* refers to the loss of distal parts of these nerve cell processes, with secondary loss of the myelin sheath that had surrounded them. *Segmental demyelination* is loss of the myelin sheath in specific foci, with the nerve processes (axons) preserved. *Wallerian degeneration* is degeneration below and sometimes also above a site of severe damage to a nerve, such as its being cut through. A variety of other types are discussed in specialized texts.

The pattern of nerves involved provides another anatomic (pathoanatomic) classification. *Polyneuropathy* involves several nerves, often starting with the feet and legs. *Mononeuropathy* is damage to a single nerve. *Mononeuropathy multiplex* is serial, often rapid involvement of individual nerves one after the other. *Polyradiculopathy* involves a number of nerve roots, often asymmetrically, in patterns that fit with the distribution of nerve root damage. *Plexopathy* is damage to a nerve plexus, for example, the brachial plexus or lumbosacral plexus.

Signs and symptoms provide another system of classification. For instance, one can divide neuropathies into primarily motor (see Chap. 11, Disorders of Motility), primarily sensory (see Chap. 12, Disorders of Sensation), or combined sensory and motor ("sensorimotor;" the subject of this chapter); into those with or without retained deep tendon reflexes; in those with or without fasciculations; and so on.

Time course provides a diagnostically useful classification:[14] acute, occurring over days; subacute, occurring over weeks; and chronic, lasting months to years. Recurrent neuropathy appears to clear but then recurs. Victor and Ropper[14] recommend a diagnostic approach based on the rate of onset.

Acute onset (within days) most often indicates a vascular, traumatic, or inflammatory cause. The inflammation can be due to an infection, to an immune mechanism, or to a combination of both. Some toxic neuropathies can be relatively acute, although toxic neuropathies are more often subacute or chronic.

Subacute or "early chronic" neuropathies (that develop over weeks to a couple of years) are often due to systemic disease including cancer (*paraneoplastic* syndromes), malnutrition, or toxins. Recognition of the underlying systemic disease tests skill in general medicine as well as neurology. As described in Chapter 11 (Disorders of Motility) and below, occult cancer—particularly of the lung—may announce its presence by causing a neuropathy before the cancer is readily detectable or causes symptoms. It seems reasonable that if suspicion of a paraneoplastic neuropathy is high, newer techniques such as spiral MRI of the lung should be used to search for a tumor. That may, of course, require referral to a center with the necessary specialized equipment. The clinical manifestations of nutritional disease are familiar to general clinicians. Toxins known to cause neuropathies include drugs, heavy metals including arsenic and mercury, industrial solvents, organophosphate insecticides, and a variety of others that typically damage organs other than the nervous system as well (Table 13-3). The manifestations outside the nervous system often reveal the cause of the neuropathy—for instance, basophilic stippling of red blood cells and lead line in lead toxicity.

Chronic neuropathies evolving over a couple of months to a couple of years should encourage the general clinician to search for occult cancer (including of the lung or associated with an abnormal circulating protein) or for undiagnosed diabetes. Recognizing a paraneoplastic syndrome can sometimes save a patient's life, if it leads to a cancer being discovered while it is still curable. Diabetic neuropathy is a common and clinically important form of neuropathy, and diabetes is a common disease. Current data suggest that early and close control of diabetes may slow or prevent the occurrence of the complications of this disease.

Neuropathies evolving over a number of years are often hereditary and sometimes associated with well-studied metabolic diseases (e.g. "inborn errors"). Initial family history does not always reveal the hereditary factor. (For instance, a patient who declares passionately that, "My family has no hereditary taints," although construction of a formal family tree reveals that a maternal uncle and aunt both died in their forties of "some weird thing in their brain.") Examination of close relatives may reveal mild, "unnoticed" deformities like an abnormally high arch. Once the familial nature of the disease is clear, family history often improves. Recognition of the hereditary basis of a disease is valuable for counseling the patient and the family. For some of these conditions, molecular genetic diagnosis is now available through specialized centers.

Etiology is the basis of the classification that provides a powerful guide to effective treatment, in the 50% or so of patients with neuropathies in whom a cause can be determined with reasonable confidence. Table 13-3 lists some of major types of neuropathies by etiology. Though formidable, it is only a truncated list.

The etiologies of peripheral neuropathies can include any of the major categories of disease: i.e., vascular, infectious, autoimmune, degenerative,

TABLE 13–3
Causes of neuropathies

Vascular
- Atherosclerotic
- Cholesterol emboli
- Vasculitis/Collagen-vascular
  - Polyarteritis nodosa
  - Rheumatoid arthritic neuropathy
  - Eosinophilic syndromes
  - Vasculitis of peripheral nerve without systemic involvement
  - Wegener granulomatosis
  - Lupus neuropathy
  - Cryoglobinemia

Infectious
- Lyme disease (can be primarily sensory)
- HIV (human immunodeficiency virus)
- Leprosy (primarily sensory)
- Syphilis (primarily sensory)

Autoimmune
- Sjögren syndrome (primarily sensory, in earlier stages)
- Guillain-Barré syndrome (primarily motor)
- Chronic inflammatory demyelinating polyneuropathy (CIDP; primarily motor)

Inflammatory
- Chronic inflammatory demyelinating polyneuropathy (CIDP)
- Amyloidosis

Endocrine
- Diabetes (often primarily sensory)
- Thyroid insufficiency (rarely)
- Acromegaly/gigantism (entrapment neuropathies)

Nutritional
- Vitamin B_1 (thiamin)
- Other B vitamins

Uremia

Toxic (can be sensorimotor or primarily motor or sensory, depending on the toxin)

Cancer related (paraproteinemias, paraneoplastic syndromes)

Hereditary
- Peroneal muscular atrophy (including Charcot-Marie-Tooth disease I & II)
- Heredopathia atactica polyneuritiformis (Refsum disease)
- Hereditary areflexic dystasia (Roussy-Lévy syndrome)
- Polyneuropathy with hereditary spastic paraplegia
- Abetalipoproteinemia (Bassen-Kornzweig syndrome)
- NARP (ataxia, retinitis pigmentosa, and peripheral neuropathy with normal phytanic acid)
- Others, including diseases first presenting in infancy and early childhood

Severe illness neuropathy (with multiple organ failure)

hereditary, malignant, and so on. Differential diagnosis of neuropathies requires a broad knowledge of Medicine as well as of Neurology. Fortunately, some specific neuropathies can present in typical patterns that aid in the diagnosis, although variant presentations are also common. The conditions discussed here are usually associated with both motor and sensory problems.

Multiple organ failure in sick patients can include a neuropathy. As discussed earlier, attempts to ascribe the failure of peripheral nerves to a specific cause in these patients has not been more fruitful than attempting to identify specific causes of failure of other organ systems.

Diabetic neuropathy is a common complication of a common disease that general physicians treat—or, more accurately, manage. Clinically symptomatic neuropathy occurs in about 15% of older patients with either Type 1 or Type 2 diabetes, but electrophysiological testing reveals abnormalities in about 50% of them. Motor, sensory, autonomic, and cranial nerves can be affected, and mixed syndromes are not rare. Clinically, patients with diabetic neuropathy often complain of unpleasant sensations in their legs. (See Chap. 12, Disorders of Sensation.) The neuropathy can precede recognition of the diabetes, so that testing for diabetes is in order in any patient who has a neuropathy of unclear cause.

Uremic neuropathy results from chronic renal failure.

Porphyria can reveal itself dramatically by the red color of the patient's urine when it has been standing, for instance, in a patient on a respirator with an indwelling catheter and a bag of red urine at the end of the bed. Other diagnostic clues are previous episodes, family history, and precipitation of the syndrome by a barbiturate or other responsible drug. Biochemical and genetic testing reveals the diagnosis.

Nutritional neuropathies typically occur in people who have reasons to be severely malnourished. These include alcoholics; people with eating disorders such as anorexia nervosa or bulimia; those with malabsorption, for instance due to sprue; depressed patients who do not eat; and other conditions well known to internists and general physicians. The nutritional factor widely believed to be responsible for the neuropathy is lack of thiamin (B_1), although some neurologists continue to believe that other B vitamins are also often involved. A convenient blood test for thiamin deficiency is available in specialized clinics or research settings, based on an estimate of the saturation with a thiamin cofactor of an enzyme in red blood cells.

Toxins that cause neuropathies can often be recognized by their actions on other organs than the nervous system. These are known to general clinicians. Consultations with poison centers are advisable if there is any doubt.

A number of medicines in common use can be toxic to peripheral nerves. (Table 13-4 provides a partial list.) Peripheral nerve damage due to *platin* can become clinically manifest weeks after the course of the antineoplastic treatment is over. The *taxol* derivatives tend to produce a more sensory neuropathy while that caused by *vincristine* is more clearly mixed motor and sensory. *Isoniazid* (INH) and *metronidazole* also tend to produce a more sensory neuropathy. (See Chap. 12, Disorders of Sensation.) The neuropathy due to the anti-tuberculosis medications *INH* and *ethionamide* (Trecator), or to the anti-hypertensive drug, *hydralazine*, is prevented by concomitant treatment with vitamin B_6 (pyridoxine) in doses of 150–450 mg/day. Larger doses of this vitamin, in the "mega-dose" range, can themselves cause a disabling neuropathy. *Dapsone* neuropathy can be hard to distinguish from the neuropathy caused by the leprosy this drug is

TABLE 13–4

Medications that cause neuropathies

Anti-tumor agents
Platins
Cisplatin (CDDP; Platinol)
Carboplatin (Paraplatin)
Paclitaxel (Taxol) and docetaxel (Taxotere)
Vincristine (Oncovin)
Antibiotics
Isoniazid (INH; Laniazid, Nydrazid)
Ethionamide (Trecator)
Nitrofurantoin (Furadantin, Macrobid, Macrodantin)
Chloramphenicol (Chloromycetin)
Metronidazole (Flagyl)
Dapsone (DDS)
Stilbamidine (Pentacarinate)
Trichloroethylene (Trilene)
Heart medicines
Amiodorone (Cordarone)
Hydralazine (Alazine, Apresoline, Apresazide)
Others
Disulfiram (Antabuse)
Pyridoxine (vitamin B_1)
Gold salts (Ridaura)
Adulterated L-tryptophan

used to treat. A similar problem exists with *nitrofurantoin*, if it is used to treat a bladder infection in a patient who also has a neuropathy due to renal failure. Gold neuropathy is dose-related and uncommonly seen in patients who have been treated with a total dose of gold of less than 1 g. In general, if a patient who is taking a medication regularly develops a neuropathy, the physician should check whether neuropathy is a known side effect of that medication. Altering medication regimens within the limits of what is necessary for the patient's health can often clarify whether a medicine caused the neuropathy, as well as being appropriate treatment for a neuropathy caused by side effects of a medication. Patients taking medicines they need for their health can, of course, also develop coincident neuropathies.

Ischemia of peripheral nerves from *atherosclerosis*, *cholesterol emboli*, or a *vasculitis* is not rare. Patients with relatively severe, symptomatic damage to the arteries to their legs (*intermittent claudication*) usually have some degree of peripheral nerve damage as well. The abnormalities in peripheral nerves can typically be detected by skilled neurological examination, but the nerve damage is usually relatively unimportant clinically compared to all the other problems these patients are having with their legs. Since diabetes predisposes to atherosclerosis it also predisposes to this kind of combined sensory and motor (sensorimotor) neuropathy.

Collagen-vascular diseases are another cause of peripheral neuropathy, frequently by causing a vasculitis of the relevant small blood vessels. Table 13-3 lists a number of specific syndromes. Internists and other general clinicians are familiar with the diagnosis of these diseases even when they present with atypical signs and symptoms.

Cancer-related neuropathies include those associated with *paraproteinemias*, immune-mediated *paraneoplastic* syndromes, and multiple organ failure in severe late stage disease. *Multiple myeloma* and its variants characteristically cause a sensorimotor neuropathy among many other manifestations. So do "benign" *monoclonal gammopathies*. *Cryoglobulinemia*, *Waldenström macroglobulinemia*, and both inherited and acquired forms of *amyloidosis* are also associated with sensorimotor neuropathies.

In Lambert-Eaton syndrome, the weakness can superficially resemble that of myasthenia gravis (see Chap. 11, Disorders of Motility).

Cancers can damage peripheral nerves by at least two major mechanisms—mechanically and immunologically. These are discussed in Chap. 12 (Disorders of Sensation). Mechanical damage to a peripheral nerve will often damage both motor and sensory fibers. It can occur from primary tumors of a peripheral nerve or from a metastasis pressing on a nerve. Some of the immune-mediated, *paraneoplastic syndromes* can also cause a combined sensory and motor neuropathy.[15] (See Chap. 12, Disorders of Sensation.)

Neurobiology

The above classification by etiology discusses many of the causes of combined sensory and motor neuropathies in the roughly half of these patients in whom a convincing cause can be uncovered. A plausible cause is, of course, not necessarily the most important cause in any specific patient. For instance, diabetics can develop cancers and have neuropathies mediated in large part by "paraneoplastic" immune mechanisms rather than by damage to blood vessels secondary to their diabetes.

In caring for patients with peripheral neuropathies, it is important to remember three characteristics of peripheral nerves. First, their processes (axons) are often long—a meter of more in nerves going from the spinal cord to the foot. Secondly, the cells that form the fatty myelin sheath for peripheral nerves are different than those forming myelin in the central nervous system (Schwann cells rather than oligodendroglia). Third, peripheral nerves have a much greater ability to regenerate than do nerves in the central nervous system. That probably reflects the presence in the central nervous system of molecules such as *Nogo* that prevent the regeneration, rather than a unique capacity of nerve cells with processes in the periphery. Surgical repair of peripheral nerves is often necessary to allow optimal healing. Even then, healing of peripheral nerves is usually time consuming. The long processes of peripheral nerves can have a long way to grow, in terms of biological distances. Unfortunately, healing is also often not complete, and residual abnormal and sometimes uncomfortable sensations (paresthesias) can occur.

Treatment

Treatment of neuropathies varies with the cause of the disease. Unfortunately, neuropathy is not rarely associated with diseases that are fatal, independent of their effect on the peripheral nervous system.

Clinical management of the patient with multiple organ failure in severe, late stage disease is a subject with which internists and general clinicians are familiar. It goes beyond the scope of this manuscript. When the neuropathy in these patients is severe, it can complicate management significantly—for instance, in weaning a patient off a respirator.

Treatment of diabetic neuropathy includes "tight" control of the diabetes to reduce the likelihood of peripheral nerve damage, at least according to currently accepted concepts. Unfortunately, "tight" control of blood glucose levels typically increases the risk of episodes of hypoglycemia, which can themselves damage the brain and lead to cognitive deficits more debilitating than the neuropathy. (See Chap. 5, Cognitive Disorders.)

A first line of treatment for the pain of diabetic neuropathy is usually antidepressants, now more usually one of the newer SSRIs rather than amitriptyline. (See Chap 3, Mood Disorders, and Chap. 7, Pain.) Antiseizure medications sometimes help, particularly with shooting pains. The combination of *gabapentin* (Neurontin) with morphine has been reported to be useful.[16] (See Chap. 10, Disorders of Awareness.) The FDA (U.S. Food & Drug Administration) recently approved an analogue of gabapentin, namely *pregabalin* (Lyrica), for treatment of diabetic neuropathy.[17] A recent report claims that treatment of diabetic neuropathy with an over-the-counter natural remedy, acetyl-L-carnitine, leads to biological as well as clinical improvement.[18]

Porphyria is treated by support including where necessary artificial ventilation. Intravenous hematin (4 mg/kg daily for 3 days to 2 weeks) is believed to be beneficial by a feed-back mechanism on the over expressed enzyme. Glucose is also believed to suppress the responsible gene. Usually pyridoxine is also given because vitamin B_6 (*pyridoxine*) deficiency is assumed. Once the appropriate biochemical or genetic markers have been identified, the rest of the porphyric patient's family should also be tested. Those who carry the predisposition should be carefully instructed in what medications and other substances to avoid so as not to have episodes of this unpleasant and often life-threatening condition.

Treatment of nutritional neuropathies is with good nutrition. Thiamin is given parenterally, typically 100 mg of thiamin hydrochloride. Thiamin and other B vitamins are then given at least daily in therapeutic doses by mouth. Doses of 10 times the recommended daily allowance of B vitamins can be taken safely for indefinite periods, for example, 30 mg thiamin/day. Very large doses of vitamin B_6 should be avoided because they can themselves damage peripheral nerves. A healthy diet should be provided and care taken that the patient is observed to eat it and to retain it. The most nutritious diet in the world does little for a patient who does not eat it or vomits it up.

Treatment of toxic neuropathies is a combination of support, removal of the toxin, and the use of specific antidotes. Clearly, a drug that is suspected to be the cause of a neuropathy should be discontinued if that is compatible with the patient's clinical situation. Sometimes a relatively mild neuropathy may be the price of effective treatment of a cancer or other life-threatening disease. Appropriate medications can sometimes speed the removal of a toxin—for instance, chelators for heavy metals. Depending on the drug, renal dialysis or plasmapheresis is sometimes useful. Antidotes when available can be life-saving. An example is atropine or other cholinergic antagonist for poisoning with an organophosphorus or other cholinesterase inhibitor that leads to the accumulation of harmful levels of acetylcholine. As noted previously, poison centers can be an invaluable resource and are now widely available sources of information. Ischemic disease is treated by a combination of medications well known to general clinicians. Unfortunately, the literature does not provide convincing evidence for the efficacy of a number of otherwise logical treatments for ischemic neuropathy.

Collagen-vascular vasculitis causing neuropathy is treated with steroids and where necessary antimetabolites. Victor and Ropper[14] suggest *methylprednisolone* (1.5 mg/kg) for several days followed by *cyclophosphamide* (1 g/m^2) per month for several months. Alternatives to cyclophosphamide include *azathioprine* and *methotrexate*. Unfortunately, the damage to peripheral nerves tends to persist even when systemic manifestations of the disease are brought under control.

Treatment of neuropathies associated with abnormal circulating proteins (*paraproteinemias*) depends in part on success in treating the underlying disease. That is specifically true for multiple myeloma and its variants. In treating the neuropathy of benign monoclonal gammopathies, a combination of periodic plasmapheresis and immunosuppressants (e.g., chlorambucil, cyclophosphamide, fludarabine) tends to be more effective than plasmapheresis alone. Reports about the effectiveness of treatment of this condition with intravenous immunoglobulin (IVIG) vary. For the distal sensorimotor neuropathies associated with Waldenström macroglobulinemia and with cryoglobulinemia, treatment is usually with a combination of steroids (prednisone), anti-tumor agents (cyclophosphamide, chlorambucil), and plasmapheresis. General clinicians are familiar with these relatively rare conditions and with the medications used to treat them. Treatment of amyloidosis is, unfortunately, still unsatisfactory. That holds for any of the inherited types as well as for the acquired systemic amyloidosis often associated with malignant transformation of plasma cells. Liver transplantation has been reported to cure a patient with one of the inherited forms. The prognosis for the neuropathy associated with the acquired form is dismal.

Paraneoplastic, immune-mediated neuropathies, and other types of damage to the nervous system have been mentioned above. Darnell and Posner[15], who have done extensive studies of these conditions, described 26 different paraneoplastic syndromes and the immune mechanisms involved. The great variability in human antibodies and normal and cancer antigens suggest that new forms of "molecular mimicry" will be identified that lead to as yet undescribed forms of paraneoplastic disorders. The expertise of general clinicians in uncovering systemic cancers may help their neurologist colleagues decipher such syndromes. Darnell and Posner[15] recommend that treatment of paraneoplastic syndromes use three overlapping approaches. One is treatment of the cancer, if possible. Effective removal of the tumor is often an effective treatment of the paraneoplastic syndrome. A second is treatment against the immunological abnormality. They suggest that this be directed against both humeral immunity (antibodies) and cellular immunity (T-cell cytotoxicity), because the precise immunological mechanisms remain unresolved for many of these patients. This type of treatment is well known to general clinicians. Third, supportive and symptomatic treatment is as always important.

Other paraproteinemias and their treatment are alluded to in other parts of this monograph. For instance, Chap. 11 (Disorders of Motility) discusses Lambert-Eaton syndrome and its treatment. Neurologists are trained to recognize these syndromes. Some of them have striking manifestations—for instance, the muscle rigidity of *stiff man syndrome.* Treatments for these conditions also fall within the bailiwick of neurologists.

REFERENCES

1. Jeffery DR. Use of combination therapy with immunomodulators and immunosuppressants in treating multiple sclerosis. *Neurology.* 2004; 63(12 Suppl 6):S41–S46.
2. O'Connor P. Canadian Multiple Sclerosis Working Group. Key issues in the diagnosis and treatment of multiple sclerosis. An overview. *Neurology.* 2002;59(6 Suppl 3): S1–S33.
3. Panitch H, Miller A, Paty D, et al. North American Study Group on Interferon beta-1b in Secondary Progressive MS. Interferon beta-1b in secondary progressive MS: results from a 3-year controlled study. *Neurology.* 2004;63: 1788–1795.

4. Hardmeier M, Wagenpfeil S, Freitag P, et al. European IFN-1a in Relapsing MS Dose Comparison Trial Study Group. Rate of brain atrophy in relapsing MS decreases during treatment with IFNbeta-1a. *Neurology*. 2005;64: 236–240.
5. Weiner HL. Immunosuppressive treatment in multiple sclerosis. *J Neurol Sci*. 2004;223:1–11.
6. Gray O, McDonnell GV, Forbes RB. Methotrexate for multiple sclerosis. *Cochrane Database Syst Rev*. 2004;(2):CD003208.
7. Drachman DB, Brodsky RA. High-dose therapy for autoimmune neurologic diseases. *Curr Opin Oncol*. 2005;17:83–88.
8. Neuhaus O, Stuve O, Zamvil SS, et al. Are statins a treatment option for multiple sclerosis? *Lancet Neurol*. 2004;3:369–371.
9. Stuve O, Prod'homme T, Youssef S, et al. Statins as potential therapeutic agents in multiple sclerosis. *Curr Neurol Neurosci Rep*. 2004;4:237–44.
10. Nicholson LB, Kuchroo VK. Cannabinoids inhibit neurodegeneration in models of multiple sclerosis. *Brain*. 2003;126:2191–2202.
11. Krupp LB, Christodoulou C, Melville P, et al. Donepezil improved memory in multiple sclerosis in a randomized clinical trial. *Neurology*. 2004;63: 1579–1585.
12. Benedetti F, Campori E, Colombo C, et al. Fluvoxamine treatment of major depression associated with multiple sclerosis. *J Neuropsychiatry Clin Neurosci*. 2004;16:364–366.
13. Crayton H, Heyman RA, Rossman HS. A multimodal approach to managing the symptoms of multiple sclerosis. *Neurology*. 2004;63(11 Suppl 5): S12–S18.
14. Victor M, Ropper AH. Diseases of the Peripheral Nerves and Diseases of Cranial Nerves. In: *Principles of Neurology*, 7th ed. McGraw-Hill, NY, 2001, pp. 1370–1445 and 1446–1463.
15. Darnell RB, Posner JB. Paraneoplastic syndromes involving the nervous system. *New Eng J Med*. 2003;349:1543–1554.
16. Gilron I, Bailey JM, Tu D, et al. Morphine, gabapentin, or their combination for neuropathic pain. *N Engl J Med*. 2005;352:1324–1334. Comment in *N Engl J Med*. 2005;352:1373–1375.
17. Richter RW, Portenoy R, Sharma U, et al. Relief of painful diabetic peripheral neuropathy with pregabalin: a randomized, placebo-controlled trial. *J Pain*. 2005;6:253–260. Gabapentin is off patent and must now compete with generic formulations; pregabalin is relatively newly patented.
18. Sima AA, Calvani M, Mehra M, et al. Acetyl-L-Carnitine Study Group. Acetyl-L-carnitine improves pain, nerve regeneration, and vibratory perception in patients with chronic diabetic neuropathy: an analysis of two randomized placebo-controlled trials. *Diabetes Care*. 2005;28:89–94.

CHAPTER FOURTEEN

Disorders of Conduct

Many people have patterns of behavior that interfere with their lives. These people come to the attention of physicians relatively frequently, compared to people whose habits fit comfortably within the social patterns of our species of primate.

The extent to which lifestyles are medical conditions is not clear, nor is the appropriateness of changing them by medications and even surgery. On the one hand, many of these people suffer. Their preferred behavior often makes others suffer—for instance, the women attacked by a man who prefers rape to sex with a willing or eager woman. On the other hand, a number of artists have put forward eloquently the arguments against "medicalization" of unusual behavior. Powerful examples include the play *Equus* or the movie *One Flew Over the Cuckoo's Nest*. In its late spasms, Soviet Communism came up with the psychiatric diagnosis of "Reformist Delusions." Fortunately, that dictatorship did not succeed in throwing a medical mantel over political repression.[1]

Unfortunately, even putatively democratic societies can also label as "sick" behavior, which vocal portions of the society do not like (viz. infra).

LEARNED MALADAPTIVE BEHAVIOR

Some forms of behavior that significantly interfere with life are not due primarily to biological abnormalities in the brain but to lessons the afflicted people would have been better off not learning. In other words, they are primarily problems with software rather than hardware. In previous decades, the term *neurosis* was widely used to refer to these conditions. This term is now out of favor. The index of the current edition of *DSM-IV-RT* (Diagnostic and Statistical Manual of Mental Disorders) does not list it. The use of that word in this section is not because of nostalgia for old-fashioned psychoanalysis but because I don't know of a better term.

Viennese psychiatrists who trained in the larger Freudian group in the 1920s and 1930s taught me a medically useful definition of a neurosis:[2]

A neurosis is a defense mechanism that doesn't work.

If a defense mechanism works, and no one is significantly hurt by it, there is no reason to interfere with it—certainly, no medical reason. In contrast, because they do not work, neurotic defenses can lead to progressively greater disability, as neurotic people are driven to greater and greater extremes of behavior to try to make these unsuccessful psychological mechanisms work. Consider, as an example, a man who derives intense sexual pleasure from women's high-heeled shoes. In its milder forms, this "fetish" is too common to be medicalized. The extended leg is a sign of sexual readiness in many species including chickens. Manolo Blahnik, in New York, at the turn of this century, has become very successful by designing and selling delicate, "feminine" high-heels that put the ankles of the women who wear them at risk orthopedically but not romantically. Even if our hypothetical man cannot come to orgasm, unless the woman to whom he is making love is wearing high heels, that is hardly a problem (unless he is in an emotional relationship with a woman who does not want to wear heels to bed). But consider a more extreme example—a man who prefers buying high-heeled women's shoes to dating real women, and comes to orgasm at home alone by stroking his collection of shoes. According to the definition cited above, his fetish is not usefully thought of as a neurosis, if it works for him. Not having sex with women prevents him from becoming a father, but we do not consider bachelors to be maladjusted by definition—at least, not yet.[3] He can still be a valuable and productive member of the community, a deacon of his church, and a good uncle to his nieces and nephews. His fetish becomes a neurosis when it leads him to behavior that is socially unacceptable or actually harms others. For instance, if it progresses to his upsetting women by dropping his napkin at dinner parties to stare at their high-heeled shoes. Certainly, if he offends them by stroking their shoes or feet. Definitely, if he insists on his wife wearing impractically high heels despite her discomfort and eventual arthritis. What makes behavior neurotic is not the nature of the behavior but its effects on people. As a Viennese psychoanalyst put it, "What is of interest is people's lives, not blow-by-blow accounts of their athletic activities."

Counseling and psychotherapy usually have a more important role than medication in helping people with neuroses. Currently, cognitive-behavioral therapies based on experimental psychology are better supported by clinical trials than are the older psychoanalytic therapies. They appear to have beneficial and lasting effects. Providing cognitive behavioral therapy, like other forms of psychotherapy, requires special training and skills.

Other forms of socially deviant and harmful behavior that require medical evaluation and treatment are discussed below.

SOMATOFORM DISORDERS

People who complain of illnesses beyond what can be explained medically make up a good part of most general medical practices, now as in ancient times. Egyptian and Greek physicians recorded having similar patients. Studies of general practices suggest that 15–50% of the patients seeking medical attention have some form of psychological problem expressed as medical complaints, that is, a *somatization disorder*. Some of these people are not sick at all. Some are not sick enough to explain their complaints. Some intentionally make themselves sick.

Table 14-1 lists the current classification of these somatoform disorders, according to DSM-IV-TR. The current DSM-IV-RT definitions and criteria can differ in significant ways from previous use by nonprofessional or even medical communities. (See Tables 14-1–14-3.) "Hypochondriasis," for instance, now has a precise technical definition (Table 14-2). So does "Conversion Disorder "(Table 14-3). The term Somatization Disorder has replaced the word *"hysteria,"* which is no longer the approved terminology. The precise use of these diagnostic terms according to their current definitions is important in psychiatry and to psychiatrists.

Milder forms of Conversion Disorder (Table 14-3) are extremely common, affecting perhaps a third of the population at some time in their lives. Fortunately, most of these are self-limited. Medically sophisticated people can give convincing histories of an illness they do not have. (See Chap. 6, Anxiety, for an illustrative anecdote about a physician who gave a superb history of increasing angina instead of acknowledging the grief that was really bothering him.)

TABLE 14–1
Somatoform disorders (DSM-IV-TR)

Somatization disorder	Formerly referred to as hysteria or Briquet syndrome
Undifferentiated somatoform disorder	Lasting 6 months but below the threshold for somatization disorder
Conversion disorder	Symptoms suggestive of disease of motor sensory abnormalities of the nervous system
Pain disorder	Primary complaint of pain (see Chap. 7, Pain)
Hypochondriasis	See Table 14-2
Body dysmorphic disorder	Preoccupation with physical defects
Somatoform disorder not otherwise specified	Not meeting criteria for syndromes listed above

Factitious disorders and malingering involve "volitional" acts. In factitious disorders, the patients actually make themselves appear sick in order to be hospitalized. An extreme form is *Munchausen syndrome.* Factitious fever is well known, and is diagnosed by finding an elevated

TABLE 14–2
Criteria for hypochondriasis (DSM-IV-TR)

A. Preoccupation with fears of having, or the idea that one has, a serious disease based on the person's misinterpretation of bodily symptoms.

B. The preoccupation persists despite appropriate medical evaluation and reassurance.

C. The belief in criterion A is not of delusional intensity (as in delusional disorder, somatic type) and is not restricted to a circumscribed concern about appearance (as in body dysmorphic disorder).

D. The preoccupation causes clinically significant distress or impairment in social, occupational, or other important areas of functioning.

E. The duration of the disturbance is at least 6 months.

F. The preoccupation is not better accounted for by generalized anxiety disorder, obsessive-compulsive disorder, panic disorder, a major depressive episode, separation anxiety, or another somatoform disorder.

Specify:
if with poor insight

TABLE 14–3
Criteria for conversion disorder (DSM-IV-RT)

A. One or more symptoms or deficits affecting voluntary motor or sensory function that suggest a neurological or other general medical condition.

B. Psychological factors are judged to be associated with the symptom or deficit because the initiation or exacerbation of the symptom or deficit is preceded by conflicts or other stressors.

C. The symptom or deficit is not intentionally produced or feigned (as in factitious disorder of malingering).

D. The symptom or deficit cannot, after appropriate investigation, be fully explained by a general medical condition, or by direct effects of a substance, or as a culturally sanctioned behavior or experience.

E. The symptom or deficit causes clinically significant distress or impairment in social, occupational, or other important areas of functioning or warrants medical evaluation.

F. The symptom or deficit is not limited to pain or sexual dysfunction, does not occur exclusively during the course of somatization disorder, and is not better accounted for by another mental disorder.

Specify:

with motor symptom or deficit
with sensory symptom or deficit
with seizures or convulsions
with mixed presentation

temperature when the patient is left alone with the thermometer but not when a nurse or other staff stays by the bedside while the temperature is being taken. Patients with somatization disorders may actually make themselves sick. They may inject themselves with insulin or other drugs, or infect their urine with feces, or give themselves wounds, which they then infect with feces or other material. Factitious disorder is a real illness, and patients can die of the illness they induce—for instance, from *septicemia*. "Hospital hobos" with factitious illnesses typically irritate medical staff, who normally assume that their patients are at least trying to tell them the truth. Another broad generalization: the longer one is in practice the more inured one becomes to patients' lies. *Malingering* is faking an illness in order to achieve a specific aim. Sometimes the aim is money, and settling a case financially cures the "compensation neurosis."

Sometimes other gains are sought, as in the following World War II joke.

> A man is drafted into the Navy in 1942. At the base where he is receiving training, he picks up every piece of paper he can find, looks at it, and says, "That's not it." He is referred to psychiatry, where he picks up the papers on the psychiatrist's desk, looks at each one, and says, "That's not it." The baffled psychiatrist gives him a medical discharge. When the sailor sees it, his face breaks into a huge smile, and he says, "That's it!"

From the viewpoint of the country that was engaged in a great and necessary war, the man's behavior was reprehensible malingering. From the strictly medical viewpoint of a human organism preventing its life being put at risk, the behavior was entirely rational—even healthy.[4] The Parisian prostitutes who maintained a warm bed and regular meals by behaving hysterically for Charcot can be thought of as malingerers. They can also be thought of as poor women displaying common sense. Where you stand depends, as usual, on where you sit.

Despite the usefulness of factitious illness and malingering as diagnostic categories, both modern neurobiology and older psychoanalytic insights argue against a clear distinction between "volition" and motivations that people are not aware of. Sperry and Gazanniga[5] have shown the importance of motivations not readily available to the verbal consciousness. LeDoux and coworkers[6] have documented the importance of "emotional learning" in both experimental animals and humans. The psychoanalysts correctly intuited that people can "rationalize" behavior that is in fact driven by desires not readily available to the conscious mind—whatever that is. Particularly in the case of factitious illness, the drive to make oneself sick is likely to arise from "nonvolitional" motivations.

The existence of unrecognized medical illness is an enormous potential pitfall in the diagnosis of somatization disorder, factitious disorder, or malingering. That can be particularly true in disorders with episodic symptoms, such as multiple sclerosis or porphyria. It can also be true for other diseases that can be hard to diagnose in their early stages—for instance, pernicious anemia (vitamin B_{12} deficiency) before manifestations become evident in peripheral blood. Careful diagnostic evaluation is important before a patient is labeled as having a somatization disorder, and the possibility of the concomitant presence of an organic illness that needs treatment should always be kept in mind during follow-up. On the other hand, repeated, unnecessary laboratory tests tend to reinforce the psychiatric condition as well as wasting resources.

Time, as usual, can be the diagnostician's best friend. Sick patients can exaggerate their illnesses or use their illnesses for effect but still need medical treatment.

> A middle-aged woman with salt-sensitive hypertension had an extensive work-up including evaluation by the hypertension service. Her blood pressure was successfully maintained in the normal range with a low salt diet and a mild diuretic. When her regular clinic doctor was not available, she became angry, switched to a diet rich in ham and potato chips, and stopped taking her medicine. She then presented to the clinic with impressively elevated blood pressures, which led the younger physicians who saw her to repeating a "full court press" hypertension work-up. Her 24-hour urinary catechols were measured at least five times by five different doctors. Nevertheless, she did suffer from high blood pressure and did need sustained if relatively mild treatment.

A second diagnostic challenge in patients with somatization disorders and related conditions is recognizing underlying psychiatric disease, most often depression but sometimes other types of psychosis. Delusions including delusions of illness can exist without other manifestations of being mad. Dermatologists and plastic surgeons are well aware of patients with "*body dysmorphic disorder*," who are convinced that a specific physical flaw makes them more or less repulsive. Modern marketing can foster these feelings, for example, the need for breast enlargement to make a woman more attractive. Sometimes getting noses fixed or breasts enlarged ends the associated anxieties. Often it does not.

The limited evidence available suggests that many people with Somatoform Disorders respond well to antidepressants, particularly to SSRIs (selective serotonin reuptake inhibitors). (See Chap. 3, Mood Disorders.) That includes patients with delusions of illness. (Whether the usefulness of antidepressants indicates that these somatization reactions are a form of depression is a matter of terminology rather than biology.) Doses can often be lower than those needed to treat major depressive disorders in younger people, but, as always, the dose needs to be adjusted to the patient. Sometimes floridly psychotic patients with somatization reactions need antipsychotics. (See Chap. 4, Thought Disorders.) As noted above, care must be taken not to miss an organic illness. Throwing up blood is a classic presentation of a stomach ulcer in a schizophrenic complaining of "a hole in my middle." Also, too ready prescription of medication can reinforce the somatization reaction and is to be avoided. Clinical judgment is needed, as always, and even the best clinicians will make treatment decisions that in retrospect will turn out to have been mistakes.

Psychiatric consultation is appropriate when a general clinician suspects a patient of having a somatization disorder. The psychiatrist can make an expert judgment on whether or not the evidence is present for a positive psychiatric diagnosis. Somatoform disorders are hard to treat, and collaboration with a psychiatrist can be very helpful in dealing with these characteristically difficult patients and with the medicolegal issues that these diagnoses can raise, particularly if the general clinician misdiagnoses a "real" medical illness as a somatization reaction.[7]

SEXUAL DISORDERS

People are often concerned about their sexuality, and sometimes they ask general clinicians for advice and help. Drugs such as *sildenafil* (Viagra) are now available to treat impotence due to physical causes such as diabetic neuropathy or after prostatectomy. Other types of medication and mechanical devices are also available. These treatments are part of general medicine and urology, and do not need special discussion here.

The difficulty in discussing sexual problems related to the central nervous system is that the distinction between an acceptable variant of sexual behavior and a medical or psychiatric problem is as much sociological as medical.[8] For instance, for most of the twentieth century, the American Psychiatric Association (APA) defined homosexuality as a disease. More recently, the APA has concluded that homosexuality is not a disease, thereby instantly curing about 5 million Americans of an illness. In a famous letter to a concerned father of an American homosexual, Freud stated clearly that he considered homosexuality a human variant rather than a condition to be cured. Freud offered, however, that if the young man was uncomfortable because of his sexual orientation, psychoanalysis might help with that discomfort. Viennese refugee analysts taught me that while homosexuality was not a disease, there is a tendency for homosexuals to have certain patterns of behavior. My homosexual friends essentially agree. They generally enjoy the company of other homosexuals more than that of straight people. The word "gay" was not chosen carelessly to describe their society.[9] However, some homosexual patterns of behavior can be medically dangerous. "Cruising" now incurs a high risk of contracting and eventually dying from AIDS. In many parts of the United States, men who are openly homosexual are at risk of being discriminated against socially and even of being physically assaulted and sometimes critically injured. The political agitation by gays and lesbians in modern America suggests that many of them are, in fact, still uncomfortable with their sexuality despite their shrill claims of being comfortable with themselves. Some gay and lesbian people may benefit from counseling on this issue.

Table 14-4 lists sexual practices that are described as disorders in the DSM-IV-TR consensus manual on psychiatric disorders, as of 2005. The international classification of disease (ICD-10) does not recognize all of these complaints to be medical problems. English psychiatry does not recognize "female arousal disorder," which according to the Internet affects nearly half of American women.[10] Biologically, women can reproduce the species without having orgasms. Socially, at an earlier time in the United States as in Medieval Europe, "decent" women were not supposed to desire sex. There has been a remarkable flip in attitudes, to now defining inadequate female arousal as an illness. There is no indication that the biology has changed. The classification in Table 14-3 considers masturbation to be a paraphilia, but only if it replaces copulation. The original Freudians did not restrict sexuality to penetration.[11]

Treatment of sexual disorders sometimes involves pharmacology, sometimes counseling and support, and usually non-judgmental common sense. It frequently requires mixtures of all three. An important role for the general clinician is to determine whether a patient's sexual problems are side effects of a non-critical medication. If so, the medicine can be stopped or changed to one without sexual side effects. For instance, an older man with an enlarging prostate and a younger female companion is likely to prefer maintaining his sexual prowess to being able to sleep through the night without getting up to urinate. A patient whose sexuality diminishes during necessary treatment with an SSRI can often be switched to *bupropion* (Wellbutrin), an antidepressant that typically does not impair and often even enhances sexual functioning.

Table 14-5 is a partial list of drugs that can interfere with sexuality. A full list of drugs that have on occasion been linked to impaired sexual functioning would be so long as to be useless. (More complete information is, of course, available on the Internet.) Basically, the general clinician needs to be alert to the possibility that any medication can have sexual side effects, sometimes as an idiosyncratic reaction. The clinician needs to be open to the patient's mentioning those side effects, particularly

TABLE 14–4
Sexual disorders as of 2005 (DSM-IV-TR)

- Hypoactive sexual desire disorder
- Sexual aversion disorder
- Female sexual arousal disorder
- Male erectile disorder
- Female orgasmic disorder (formerly inhibited female orgasm)
- Male orgasmic disorder (formerly inhibited male orgasm)
- Premature ejaculation
- Dyspareunia (not due to a general medical condition)
- Vaginismus
- Sexual dysfunction due to a general medical condition
- Substance-induced sexual dysfunction
- Sexual dysfunction not otherwise specified
  - Female premature orgasm
  - Postcoital headache
  - Orgasmic anhedonia
  - Masturbatory pain
- Paraphilias (abnormal expressions of sexuality)
  - Exhibitionism
  - Fetishism
  - Frotteurism
  - Pedophilia
  - Sexual masochism
  - Sexual sadism
  - Transvestic fetishism
  - Voyeurism
  - Paraphilia not otherwise specified
    - Telephone and computer scatologia
    - Necrophilia
    - Partialism
    - Zoophilia
    - Coprophilia and klismaphilia
    - Urophilia
    - Hypoxyphilia
    - Masturbation in preference to copulation
- Gender identity disorder
- Gender identity disorder not otherwise specified
- Sexual disorder not otherwise specified

TABLE 14-5
Drugs often interfering with sexuality

- Antidepressants
  - SSRIs (fluoxetine, paroxetine, seratraline, citalopram)
  - Tricyclics (imipramine, clomipramine, nortriptyline)
  - MAO inhibitors (parnate, nardil, marplan)
  - Trazodone
  - Buspirone
- Antipsychotics
  - Thioridazine
  - Trifluoperazine
- Antihypertensives
  - β-blockers
  - Other antihypertensives
- Sex hormones
  - Estrogens
  - Antiandrogens
  - Androgens
- Drugs of abuse
  - Opiates
    - Morphine
    - Methadone
    - Heroin
  - Alcohol
  - Barbiturates
  - Cocaine
  - Amphetamines

Abbreviation: MAO, Monoamine oxidase.

after a new medication is started, and to modifying the therapeutic regimen accordingly. For one thing, patients are at risk of not taking medicines that interfere with their sexuality—including older patients and including "decent" women. Some of the drugs listed in Table 14-2 deserve special comment and are discussed in the following paragraphs.

Both mental illness and drugs that treat mental illness can impair sexuality. Depression typically reduces sex drive, but so do many antidepressants. The incidence of reduced desire and increased time to orgasm in patients taking SSRIs has been estimated to be as high as 30–80%. Delay in coming to orgasm can be perceived of as a benefit by a man who ejaculates too fast to please himself and his partner, but it can be a very unpleasant side effect in a woman who finds her lover(s) "too quick." Tricyclic antidepressants can also be important causes of reduced sexuality. Trazodone can cause prolonged and often painful erections (*priapism*). Sometimes they last so long that a patient prefers the nerves to his penis being cut—with resulting impotence—to the permanent erection. Bupropion can be associated with increased sexuality. It is, therefore, sometimes prescribed to patients with depression along with or instead of an SSRI. Prescribing antidepressants in patients in the depressive phase of a bipolar disorder can precipitate mania and the hypersexuality associated with mania. If one regards sexuality as a competitive sport, increased sexuality is a desirable effect—like steroids in baseball players. In certain individuals in certain social situations, however, increase in their sexuality interferes with their lives. Manic sexuality can certainly get people into trouble. People with thought disorders sometimes give problems with sexuality as one of their many reasons for stopping their medications.

Many medicines used to treat medical conditions have sexual side effects. Anti-arrhythmics and anti-hypertensives are well known to decrease sexuality in many patients. β-Blockers are notorious for this effect. Nowadays so many treatments are available for cardiac arrhythmias and for high blood pressure that it is likely that the physician and patient can work together to find a regimen that modifies the disorder without interfering with the patient's sexual relationships. Sex hormones not surprisingly affect desire. Broadly, male hormones (androgens) increase sex drive in both sexes and female sex hormones (anti-androgens) decrease it. (General clinicians are well aware that increased female sexual desire can be the presenting symptom of an otherwise silent androgen-secreting gynecological tumor.) These hormones have other side effects as well. Recent large, tightly structured epidemiological studies have shown that estrogen replacement in women not only does not protect against heart disease but instead appears to shorten life, albeit marginally.

Opiates typically reduce sexual drives. In people addicted to heroin or other opiates, attention to the "rush" associated with drug use tends to replace interest in the "rush" associated with orgasm. Opiate or other drug addiction in prostitutes tends to allow them to have affectless sex. Alcohol, as Shakespeare pointed out, tends to increase desire and reduce ability. So do other sedatives including barbiturates. Cocaine, amphetamine, and other agents that act on dopamine receptors are associated with increased sexuality if taken occasionally but tend to interfere with sexuality if chronically abused. The attempt to increase one's sexuality or prolong and intensify one's orgasms may lead individuals to start to use these agents as recreational drugs.

Sometimes sexual problems are a manifestation of another psychiatric illness that can respond to drug treatment. That is particularly true of depression, and sometimes treatment with antidepressants restores sexuality as well as benefiting other manifestations of a depression that a patient has been less than willing to admit. That is true despite the caveats about antidepressants and sexuality discussed above. As always, clinical judgment is necessary. Rather less often, antipsychotics help with sexual problems. Medications are available to reduce sex drive in people whose sexuality takes socially unacceptable forms—for instance, child molesters. In general, these medications are given by psychiatrists, often within the criminal justice system. The temptation may be great for general clinicians to use such "anti-androgen" drugs to help patients who are tormented by antisocial sexual fixations. Doing so without adequate support from appropriate specialists is, however, risky. Patients can counteract the effects of such drugs with other agents available over the Internet, including Viagra and Cialis. If a person being managed by a general physician commits a sexual felony—specifically including pedophilia—the general physician may have a very hard time mounting a defense if he or she has been acting alone.

Psychiatric treatment of sexual disorders requires expertise which is taught during a psychiatry residency. Often the best thing a general clinician can do is to persuade a person with sexual problems to see a psychiatrist, even if the patient is ashamed or otherwise reluctant to do so. Sometimes, however, all the general clinician needs to do is to convince a patient to lighten up. For patients worried about their performance, encouragement is useful. Treatment with almost anything can allay most sexual anxiety by a powerful placebo effect. With enough mumbo-jumbo, peanut butter can be an aphrodisiac. Sometimes Viagra or Cialis has more important effects on anxiety generated in the central nervous system than on G-protein signaling in the blood vessels of the penis. The mode of action is less important than that the people treated become more comfortable with themselves and their partners. Sometimes people crave reassurance from their doctors that their sexual preferences are not "sick" perversions. That can be particularly true for people who were brought up very strictly. It may reassure them to be told that the medical issue is whether or not anyone is hurt rather than what form sexual athletics take.[12]

PERSONALITY DISORDERS

There are a number of people whose behavior is weird but not sufficiently weird for them to earn the label of psychotic, according to current consensus criteria. The diagnostic classifications for these patients have varied over the years. When the author was a medical student at Columbia in the 1960s, a popular diagnostic label was *pseudoneurotic schizophrenia.* More recently, the work of Otto Kernberg and others has called attention to this group of patients under the heading of *Personality Disorders.* In psychiatry, "personality" is a global term describing both external behavior and subjective experiences. Kornberg's formulation gains empirical support from studies documenting significant genetic as well as environmental determinants of personality and relative stability of personality throughout life. The idea of personality disorders is in one sense a return to the ancient medical concept of "humors." (For instance, medieval physicians would have labeled a person with a depressive personality disorder as having an excess of melancholic humor.)

The DSM-IV-TR general diagnostic criteria for Personality Disorder emphasize behavior that is (1) enduring, (2) interferes with life, and (3) is not better attributed to some other mental illness. Both the American DSM classification and the international ICD-10 classification of disease emphasize that personality disorders lead to variations from socially accepted norms in the patient's society. That implies that the more tolerant the society, the less prevalent the diagnosis of personality disorders is likely to be. However, personality disorders are not simply artifacts of intolerant societies. Extensive studies have documented that patients with personality disorders have brains that on average tend to differ from those of other people, anatomically (by imaging studies) and electrophysiologically.[13] The overlap in neurobiological parameters between "control" and "personality disorder" is too great, however, for such measurements to help with the diagnosis in individual patients.

Personality Disorders, like personality itself, generally have a strong genetic component. For instance, epidemiological studies of *schizophrenia* imply that what is inherited is a tendency toward schizophreniform behavior, which sometimes manifests itself as full-blown, criteria-meeting schizophrenia and sometimes a *schizoid* or *schizotypal personality disorder* (according to current consensus definitions; see also Chap. 4, Thought Disorders). Effects of environment including those of upbringing appear to be strong contributors to which of these disorders develop

TABLE 14-6
Types of personality disorders

Paranoid
Schizoid
Schizotypal
Antisocial
Borderline
Histrionic
Narcissistic
Avoidant
Dependent
Obsessive-compulsive

in people with the genetic predisposition. Psychotherapy to modify the environmental effects is a staple of treatment of these patients.

Table 14-6, based on DSM-IV, lists types of personality disorders. Many of these conditions in their more severe forms are classified as psychoses or as other psychiatric diagnoses. Treatments for the different forms of personality disorder differ enough from each other that each of the various types is best discussed individually.

Schizoid Personality Disorder

This occurs in people who are socially withdrawn and often eccentric but not certifiably crazy. This pattern of behavior is not rare; perhaps 7% of the adult population meet the requirements for this "disorder." If their pattern of life becomes uncomfortable for them, they often benefit from psychotherapy including group psychotherapy and other structured contacts. That is usually true even if they tend not to participate verbally. These people can often make strong emotional attachments to others and others to them, given time and an environment they perceive of as unthreatening. Pharmacological treatment is symptomatic and requires only low doses of the relevant drugs. Antidepressants including SSRIs may help these people be less sensitive to rejection. Benzodiazepines may help them with social anxieties. Antipsychotics may sometimes be necessary, and psychostimulants have been reported to help some of these patients to become more outgoing.

Schizotypal Personality Disorder

This condition falls in the spectrum between schizoid personality disorder and frank schizophrenia. People with this syndrome are really odd. They tend to hold bizarre ideas and frank illusions including ideas of reference. They tend to think magically and to suffer episodes of feeling that familiar surroundings are strange and unreal ("*derealization*"). Sometimes their language is intelligible to others only with difficulty. Not rarely they join cults or other unusual religious groups or dabble in the occult. Challenging their beliefs can threaten them deeply. Current theories suggest that Schizotypal Personality Disorder is the premorbid personality type of schizophrenics. Pharmacological agents are used symptomatically, including antipsychotics when these patients slip into frank insanity. (See Chap. 4, Thought Disorders.) Fortunately, the episodes of full-blown psychosis in these people tend to be brief and generally self-limited.

Borderline Personality Disorder

This may bear a relation to major mood disorder analogous to the relationship that schizoid and schizotypal personality disorders have to schizophrenia. (See Chap. 3, Mood Disorders.) Although the diagnostic category of *borderline personality* was developed by psychoanalysts, more recent twin studies suggest that it has a biological (genetic) component as well as being influenced by upbringing. The genetic vulnerability may reflect problems in the neural mechanisms that normally modulate the regulation of emotion and particularly emotional vulnerability. Current theories propose an interaction between a hereditary vulnerability and a childhood that the patient perceived of as traumatic. (Not necessarily one that outside observers would have considered unusually stressful.) For a time, it was conventional to blame this condition on sexual abuse in childhood, "documented" by the now discredited technique of recovered memory.[14] As usual, the attempt to stereotype psychological problems has been found to be unsound.

Clinically, these patients have problems—often severe—with attachment and separation. Their moods, behaviors, and interactions with other people are characteristically unstable and unsatisfactory. They can easily convert their image of a beloved caretaker to that of a cruel persecutor, and vice versa. This can be difficult and confusing for their parents. Manifestations of depression may become more evident when these patients are in a situation where they feel adequate support is not forthcoming. They are impulsive, and suicide is a real risk.

Treatment of these patients is difficult even for psychiatrists. Special psychoanalytically oriented psychotherapeutic techniques have been developed. Drug therapy can be helpful if the patients take the drugs prescribed in the amounts prescribed. SSRIs and other antidepressants are often useful, and antipsychotic medications are sometimes helpful. Some of these patients respond best to anti-seizure medications, raising the question of whether borderline personality might sometimes be a manifestation of temporal lobe disease. (See Chap. 10, Disorders of Awareness.) The amount of medication prescribed to these patients at any one time should not be too large. These patients are at significant risk of an impulsive suicide or attempt that can turn out fatal.

Narcissistic Personality Disorder

This is characterized by grandiose feelings of self-importance and therefore of entitlement. The relation of narcissistic personality disorder to mania may be analogous to that of schizoid and schizotypal personalities to schizophrenia and of borderline personality to depression.

Narcissistic people often find their lives disappointing. Even if they are very successful, the world around them tends to put a lower value on them than the very high value they put on themselves. That discrepancy can make them angry. People who meet criteria for this condition may also meet criteria for borderline, histrionic, and antisocial personality disorders.

When narcissism interferes severely enough with life to warrant pharmacological intervention, lithium tends to be useful, and sometimes antidepressants are helpful. (See Chap. 3, Mood Disorders.)

Paranoid Personalities

These are characteristically suspicious and tend to project the causes for their problems on others. Bigots including racists and political extremists often have this type of personality. Depending on how one defines it, the disorder is not uncommon and may involve over 2% of the population.[15] Paranoid people, like other people with mental problems, tend to arrange their lives so that events conform to their world view. The psychiatric cliché is that "paranoids really are persecuted."

Modification of this underlying personality type is very difficult. The antipsychotic *pimozide* (Orap) has been reported to help in reducing paranoid ideation. Normal doses of this powerful serotonin-dopamine antagonist are 1–10 mg/day, PO. (See Chap. 4, Thought Disorders.) Antianxiety agents (e.g., benzodiazepines) are sometimes useful in calming the anxieties of paranoid people, and antipsychotics in reducing the intensity of delusions when their thinking becomes seriously deranged. Treatment of paranoid personality disorder should be done by a psychiatrist. Psychotically paranoid people are sometimes dangerous, and they can sometimes hide their psychosis skillfully. Expert judgment that will be recognized as expert in a court of law is necessary in treating them.

Antisocial Personality Disorder

Antisocial personality disorder rather than "psychopath" is the current term for people who pay little or no attention to the norms of behavior in their society. Perhaps three-quarters of the population of prisons meet current diagnostic criteria for antisocial personality disorder (*criminal psychopathy*). Recent studies associate this condition with inadequate formation and/or inadequate function of the frontal lobes, that is, impairment in the part of the brain that mediates "executive functions." These people tend to be glib and successful manipulators, of general clinicians as well as other physicians and other people.[16] Their charm is superficial, however; they characteristically lack real empathy for other people. They may also have concomitant psychiatric conditions including substance abuse and may indulge in utterly unacceptable sexual behavior such as rape—just because they enjoy doing so. Effective treatments for antisocial personality are not available.[17] Psychosurgery or certain conditioning techniques to control their behavior are not politically acceptable in democratic societies, for the obvious reason that they are so open to misuse to silence legitimate dissent.

Histrionic Personality Disorder

This disorder subsumes what was previously called hysteric personality. These people are often charming but their relationships are typically shallow. Their often seductive sexuality is generally more devoted to proving their attraction to the opposite sex than to satisfying their physical drives or expressing physically a deep and long-lasting commitment. People with histrionic personality are characteristically fickle. Under stress, they may develop problems with testing reality (e.g., "Everyone says that I look like I'm still in my twenties.").

Treatment is by psychotherapy, with medications used when necessary to treat symptoms such as depression. Physicians need to maintain a professional relationship with these patients, and not to be seduced by them—emotionally or sexually.

Avoidant Personality Disorder

This occurs when a person is so timid that it interferes seriously with life. (Some of these people have what was once called an "inferiority complex.") Estimates of the prevalence of this condition in the general population run as high as 10%. The popularity of "assertiveness training" suggests that this estimate may not be too high. Pharmacological treatment sometimes includes a β-blocker such as *atenolol* (Tenormin) in standard doses to treat excessive peripheral (*adrenergic*) manifestations of anxiety, such as sweating or rapid heart beat. Sometimes SSRIs or other serotonergic agonists can help these people deal with their negative feelings. (See Chap. 3, Mood Disorders.)

Dependent Personality Disorder

This disorder is diagnosed in people who subordinate their own desires to those of others. Biological factors undoubtedly play a role in this kind of behavior, but classifying it as a disorder deserving medical treatment is largely a sociological phenomenon. In the nineteenth century, handbooks for American women emphasized the virtues of a wife subordinating her desires to those of her husband. (At that time, "decent women" were also supposed to be free of physical sexual desires, as noted earlier.) Dependent personality disorder tends to respond well to psychotherapy by a professional who believes that it needs to be treated. In psychoanalytic terms, the patient's dependency is easily shifted onto the therapist or the "support group." Medications are sometimes used to treat specific symptoms, such as the depression that may be triggered if loss of emotional dependency also leads to loss of financial support—for instance, to a divorce with subsequent degradation of socio-economic status. Patients with this condition can become victims of "therapists" whose political convictions overwhelm a common sense concern for the individual patient.

Obsessive-Compulsive Personality Disorder

This condition is a milder form of *Obsessive-Compulsive Disorder*, which is discussed in Chap. 6 (Anxiety). In its milder forms, this condition is entirely compatible with a life that is personally and professionally fulfilling. The ideal academic physician has been described as a stable hypomanic with a well-compensated obsessive-compulsive neurosis. Compulsiveness and obsessions do, however, deserve treatment when they interfere seriously with life. These patients often recognize their difficulties and ask for help. Treatment is primarily counseling, by trained psychotherapists who can handle the anger these patients easily mobilize in therapy. Medications found useful in anecdotal reports include *clonazepam* (Klonopin) and perhaps other benzodiazepines (see Chap. 6, Anxiety); antidepressants, including SSRIs (e.g., *fluoxetine*, 60–80 mg/day) or the tricyclic *clomipramine* (Anafranil), which are discussed in Chap. 3 (Mood Disorders); and sometimes antipsychotics (e.g., *Nefazodone, Serzone*; see Chapter 4 (Thought Disorders).)

Other Personality Disorders

DSM-IV-TR classifies the following conditions as "Personality disorder, not otherwise specified."

Passive-aggressive people use their passivity in aggressive ways that are often irritating to the people on whom they enable themselves to depend. Treatment is psychotherapy, which can be difficult. These patients can passively refuse to get better. Medications are useful only when clearly indicated. Negativistic personality disorder is a somewhat related category, preferred by psychiatrists who feel that passive aggression is more a description of a defense mechanism than of a personality type. (The difference between those categories is, of course, more theoretical than practical.) Self-defeating personality disorder is now a politically incorrect label, because of concern that women who appear to have this personality type may actually be undergoing physical or psychological abuse. Self-defeating people are, however, skilled at defeating attempts to help them

Depressive personality disorder is a lifelong pattern of gloominess. Psychotherapy can often help, but these people can slip into depressions which need pharmacological treatment. The character of Eeyore in *Winnie the Pooh* exemplifies this type of person.

Sadomasochistic and sadistic personality disorders need not express themselves in a sexual form. Cruelty can manifest itself in many ways.[18] When they do take overtly sexual forms, these disorders overlap with sexual disorders (paraphilia) discussed earlier.

Personality change due to a medical condition is most often due to brain damage, including brain trauma. It is discussed in many other places in this monograph. (See Chap. 3 [Mood Disorders], Chap. 4 [Thought Disorders], Chap. 5 [Cognitive Disorders], Chap. 9 [Cerebrovascular Disorders], and Chap. 10 [Disorders of Awareness].)

ADJUSTMENT DISORDERS AND POSTTRAUMATIC STRESS DISORDER

These conditions occur when people react in unhealthy ways to stressors. Of course, common sense is necessary in deciding what a "healthy reaction" is to a bad situation. As discussed in Chap. 3 (Mood Disorders), debilitating degrees of grief lasting for years after a loved one has died may deserve medical and psychiatric intervention, even though it is hard to classify deep and lasting sorrow at loss of a beloved child or life companion as "sick." Becoming suicidal is clearly unhealthy, as is alcoholism or driving one's car dangerously. On the other hand, attempts to define healthy reactions to stress can become silly—for instance, to define what would have been a "healthy" reaction for prisoners in Nazi death camps. Table 14-7 lists the forms of adjustment disorder recognized by DSM-IV-TR.

TABLE 14–7
Adjustment disorders (DSM-IV-TR)

Adjustment disorders (DSM-IV-TR)
With anxiety
With mixed anxiety and depressed mood
With disturbance of conduct
With mixed disturbance of emotions and conduct
Unspecified
Acute: less than 6 months; chronic: lasting 6 months or longer

Freud recognized that the tendency to develop an adjustment disorder has a "constitutional" basis, and subsequent studies have supported the role of biological factors that predispose to these reactions.

Posttraumatic stress disorder is classified by DSM-IV-TR as a form of anxiety disorder rather than as an adjustment disorder. This condition follows a stress so severe that it causes psychological trauma even to people without a predisposition to adjustment reactions. A classic example is combat; another is being raped. Treatment consists of a mixture of psychotherapy and crisis intervention. Venting to family and friends as well as to paid therapists typically benefits these people. They typically know what the stress that bothers them is, and being allowed to talk about it typically helps. Sometimes medication is appropriate, against excessive anxiety (see Chap. 6, Anxiety), or depression (see Chap. 3, Mood Disorders), or psychotic decompensation (see Chap. 4, Thought Disorders).

IMPULSE CONTROL DISORDERS

Current American psychiatric classification lists a number of disorders that involve impaired impulse control but are distinguished from other psychiatric conditions in which impulse control is impaired. Response to medication in these patients suggests the possibility of changing their diagnoses. In patients who respond to an antiepileptic, the episodic loss of control may be due to undetected seizures. In patients who respond to an antidepressant or an antipsychotic, the episodes may be manifestations of an underlying disorder of mood or thought.

Intermittent Explosive Disorder

This condition characteristically involves discrete episodes of violence, for which the patients are afterwards typically very sorry. Some wife-beaters appear to belong to this group—not that the diagnosis puts their wives at less risk. Anticonvulsants, lithium, and antipsychotics have all been claimed to help individual patients with this dangerous condition. β-blockers have been useful in some patients with explosive rages. These people may very well come to the attention of general physicians, but they should be treated by psychiatrists. These patients, too, can end up in court, as can their doctors.

Kleptomania

Kleptomania is stealing even though the perpetrator does not need and often gives away the object(s) stolen. Their thefts tend to get these people in trouble with the law. Kleptomania may be related to *obsessive-compulsive disorder* or to other psychiatric conditions. These people need psychiatric treatment, including psychotherapy. Anecdotal reports indicate that various drugs can be helpful in individual kleptomaniacs: SSRIs, sometimes other antidepressants, sometimes lithium (Chap. 3, Mood Disorders); sometimes valproate or other antiseizure medications. (See Chap. 10, Disorders of Awareness.)

Pyromania

Pyromania involves setting fires for emotional satisfaction rather than for insurance or other "rational" reason. Effective treatment is not available, although behavior modification is attempted while pyromaniacs are in prison.

Pathological Gambling

Pathological gambling is gambling to an extent that interferes with life. It can be a manifestation of mania as well as of other psychiatric diseases, and there are case reports of successful treatment with lithium. Compulsive gambling has been reported to be a rare complication of dopamine agonist treatment for Parkinson disease. (See Chap. 11, Disorders of Motility.)

Trichotillomania

Trichotillomania is pulling out one's own hair to the point of disfigurement. This can be a reaction to stress; a widely publicized example is an Iraqi prisoner in Abu Ghraib prison who pulled out his hair while chained in an uncomfortable position by his American captors. These patients are best treated collaboratively by a psychiatrist and a dermatologist. SSRIs have been reported to be useful, as have a number of other agents including other antidepressants; lithium; *hydroxyzine* (Vistaril), which has both antianxiety and antihistaminic properties; antipsychotics; the benzodiazepine *clonazepam* (Klonopin); and the opiate antagonist *naltrexone*.

Pathological Shopping

Pathological shopping is not a psychiatric disorder recognized by DSM-IV-TR. Spending money wildly and for things one does not need can be a manifestation of mania. (See Chap. 3, Mood Disorders.)

ADDICTION/SUBSTANCE ABUSE

General clinicians have patients who damage their own lives and often others' lives by overuse of various substances, some legal and some illegal. Some aspects of this behavior are relatively independent of the choice of substance, while others vary with the substance being abused. The mechanisms underlying abuse of various substances are complex, and these patients are typically hard to treat. As usual, consultations with specialists can be critical in providing effective and legally defensible care. Substance abuse has certain general characteristics relatively independent of the specific substance(s) used, as well as specific characteristics for each substance.

General Considerations

The distinction between physical dependence and addiction/abuse is important. The abrupt withdrawal of many drugs that are commonly and appropriately used to treat chronic illnesses can cause severe physical reactions. Steroids normally need to be tapered after chronic use rather than stopped abruptly. Stopping anti-epileptic drugs abruptly can lead to a dangerous increase in the number of seizures. Although both steroids and anti-epileptics can alter mood, there is no point in considering the patients who take these medications chronically to be substance abusers or "addicted" to their medicines. Similarly, there are psychoactive substances that are accepted in common use, such as caffeine. DSM-IV-TR lists diagnostic criteria for caffeine-related disorders and caffeine intoxication, and general clinicians regularly tell patients to cut down or eliminate coffee if it makes them irritable, interferes with their sleep, or upsets their stomachs. Smoking tobacco remains legal in the United States and elsewhere in the world, but the health risks of tobacco use are now well accepted. Nicotine addiction is, however, now accepted as a public health issue, as discussed later in this chapter.

Substance abuse occurs when the desire—the "need"—to obtain the substance twists a person's life out of shape. Typically, the affected people cannot stop taking the abused substance, even if they insist they could stop "any time I want to." They use the substance more than they plan and often more than they admit. They return to it, even after stopping using it for a few days or a week or so. Stopping is usually associated with withdrawal symptoms, which may be limited to mood and energy or may be severe physiological changes. Perhaps most important, abuse of the substance interferes with their functioning—in relations with family and friends, in effectiveness at work, and in other activities they and their societies value. The World Health Organization definition states that drug dependence occurs when the use of a drug or drugs becomes more of a priority for a person than other behaviors that previously had a higher value.

Substance abuse can be a form of self-medication—usually unsuccessful self-medication. A number of substances of abuse are plant products that react with endogenous signal systems in the brain. Morphine and its derivatives act on opiate receptors, cocaine and its analogues on dopamine receptors, and cannabis components on cannabinoid receptors. In theory, it is possible that these plant derivatives are used (abused) to compensate for endogenous deficiency states of the natural transmitter system. Physicians need to become involved in treating substance abuse when self-medication interferes with a patient's life or health. Apparently successful self-medication can still be potentially harmful, because of the risks involved in breaking the law[20] and of using unregulated materials containing potentially toxic contaminants. Medical use of marijuana is now more a political than a medical issue.[21]

Substance abuse and mental illness have a complex relationship. Substance abuse can be a cause or a consequence of mental illness or both. It can mask the manifestations of a psychiatric disease, which appears in more typical form once the patient becomes sober. Most patients with psychiatric illness try to self-medicate with one or another substance, often alcohol and often other drugs.[22] Mood disorder and specifically depression is the mental illness most frequently self-medicated by substance abusers, including alcoholics, and treatment with physician-prescribed anti-depressants may end dependence on a substance of abuse. Sometimes medications for anxiety or antipsychotics are appropriate, depending on the underlying psychiatric problems. For medications that are also drugs of abuse, such as benzodiazepines, barbiturates, or opiates, the lines between "therapeutic use" and "medical addiction" are relatively vague. Current guidelines for pain medication allow prescribing opiates to patients who will go into withdrawal if the opiates are stopped. (See Chap. 7, Pain.) Earlier guidelines discouraged that practice, even with terminally ill cancer patients. A patient who requires large and increasing amounts of Valium or other potential drug of abuse may be receiving the wrong treatment and specifically the wrong medication.

Essentially all drugs of abuse can cause intoxication, and most can cause withdrawal if stopped suddenly in a habituated user. Intoxication and withdrawal are discussed in Chap. 5 (Cognitive Disorders). The discussion below concentrates on the aspects of chronic substance abuse/addiction specific for each of the most relevant substances. Some of these have an anesthetic-like action on brain cells generally, while others act on specific receptor systems. It is important to remember that illegal substances that are abused are often contaminated with other chemicals of which neither the abuser nor the physician is aware. Sometimes the drug pusher knows, sometimes not. The possibility that an unusual reaction is a result of an unrecognized impurity must always be born in mind during treatment of substance abuse, particularly of acute episodes. As emphasized below, it is desirable to obtain a sample of the substance that has been abused for future chemical analysis if unusual and unforeseen complications develop during treatment. That has proven to be critically important in analyzing effects of new "designer drugs."

Alcohol

Ethyl alcohol (ethanol) is the most widely used psychoactive substance in most of the world. It is used even in many Muslim societies that formally forbid it. Ethanol use goes back to the dawn of history. Archeology indicates that agricultural tools and brewers tools made their appearance at about the same time. The argument has been made that people in the Near East domesticated grasses not so much for baking bread as for brewing beer. Attempts to ban the use of alcohol have often been disastrous. The United States attempt at prohibition after World War I is a good example.

Ethanol comes essentially from the diet, although humans produce it in small amounts. Its major action on the brain comes from its ability to dissolve in membranes and thereby alter their properties, an action similar to that of other anesthetics. For many centuries, getting very drunk was the best way available to dim the pain of surgery. Ethanol also has a variety of less dramatic effects. The liver metabolizes about 90% of it, with the rest excreted unchanged. Ethanol is oxidized to acetaldehyde, which is then itself oxidized to acetate. In the liver, these steps rapidly generate a relative excess of materials that can quench free radicals.[23]

In general, people who drink alcohol in moderation live longer than people who totally abstain. The epidemiological evidence to support that statement is overwhelming. On the other hand, excessive use of alcohol or use by people with certain illnesses is harmful and can be deadly. The optimal amount of alcohol intake in normal people appears to be somewhere in the range of 6–36 g of ethanol a day—about the amount found in 1–3 glasses of wine (4 oz glasses). Many studies claim that red wine is the healthiest or the only healthy form in which to ingest ethanol, but other investigators have found that ethanol itself is healthy independent of the beverage in which it is consumed. Cultures that favor the use of red wine tend to consume it daily, with meals, in moderate amounts. That pattern of use may favor its consumption appearing more healthful than other alcoholic beverages consumed in other ways. A specific benefit from red wine may be its contents of polyphenol antioxidants and specifically of resveratrol. Healthy benefits from ethanol itself may also relate to its effect of free radical metabolism.[23] Free radicals are believed to play a part in aging and in many common diseases including atherosclerosis. Regulation of free radical metabolism has therefore been implicated in human health and longevity.

Unfortunately, many people drink too much alcohol. It is the most widely abused substance in Western societies including the United States. A variety of criteria for when alcohol use becomes abuse have been promulgated. The basic criterion, as with other disorders, is significant interference with life and/or health. Unfortunately, many physicians drink more than is good for them and do not make the diagnosis of alcohol abuse in people who drink less than they do.

Some causes of alcohol abuse are relatively common. One is depression. Many people try to find happiness at the bottom of a bottle. When they fail, many of them go on to another bottle. Some estimates are that 40% of alcohol abusers are either frankly depressed or are grieving or otherwise very unhappy (i.e., *dysphoric*). Recognition and treatment of their underlying mood disorder with appropriate medications can often "cure" their alcoholism. (See Chap. 3, Mood Disorders.) Another common cause of alcohol abuse is anxiety, which may or may not be a manifestation of an underlying depression. Alcohol can "steady the nerves" in the short run, but when its effects wear off anxiety can be greater than before taking a drink. More chronic and severe anxiety can lead to more chronic and severe drinking. Yet another common cause of alcohol abuse is social setting. College fraternities and bars near military bases are widely cited examples but are hardly the only ones. There are social and ethnic groups for whom drinking to excess is a proof of masculinity.[24] In general, our society despises drunks but considers people who do not drink at all to be antisocial prigs.[25] There are many "personal" reasons why people abuse alcohol. For instance, someone raised in a family that abhors alcohol abuse may start drinking to express rage at his or her parents. Ultimately there are as many explanations of why people drink too much as there are people who abuse alcohol.

General clinicians are familiar with the direct toxic effects of alcohol on many organs including the liver including inflammations of the liver (*alcoholic hepatitis*). They are also familiar with the complications that can ensue from alcohol abuse, including not only fatty liver and cirrhosis but also heart disease, damage to skeletal muscle, kidney disease, and so on.

Ethanol abuse can damage the nervous system in a variety of ways (Table 14-8). The stages of incapacitation from alcohol relate reasonably

TABLE 14–8

Ethanol-induced disorders of the nervous system

Delirium
Intoxication
Withdrawal (delirium tremens and its complications)
Stupor
Coma
Pathological intoxication
Hallucinosis
Dementia
Nutritional (Wernicke-Korsakoff syndrome)
Other alcohol-related dementias
Peripheral neuropathy (nutritional)
Loss of impulse control/violence

TABLE 14–9
Blood levels of alcohol and symptoms

Blood level mg/dL	Blood level %	Signs and symptoms
10	0.01	Mild disinhibition
30	0.03	Mild impairment of skilled activities, memory, and judgment
50	0.05	Impaired coordination; driving an automobile illegal
100	0.10	Confusion, impaired consciousness
≥400	≥0.40	Stupor, sometimes coma, sometimes death

well to blood levels (Table 14-9). Heavy enough alcohol use in a short enough time can lead to stupor and coma and even death (for instance, in college students who die from acute ethanol overdose during "hazing"). Patients who drink regularly can develop a degree of tolerance to the effects of alcohol, and often claim that they can "hold their liquor." Their conviction that they are "not too drunk to drive" has caused many deaths and injuries, and not only to themselves. Some patients who drink too much develop auditory or visual hallucinations without delirium tremens and without other manifestations of psychosis. In a happily small proportion of them, the hallucinosis becomes permanent. Alcohol abuse can lead to dementia by at least two mechanisms. One is nutritional deficiency, notably deficiency of thiamin (vitamin B_1). The result, Wernicke-Korsakoff syndrome, is discussed in Chap. 5 (Cognitive Disorders). There is a widespread belief but relatively little objective proof that long-standing and severe overuse of alcohol itself leads directly to loss of brain tissue and *alcoholic dementia.* Many alcoholics develop a peripheral neuropathy, which is widely attributed to nutritional deficiency, notably of B vitamins and particularly of thiamin. In "*pathological intoxication,*" one or a few drinks lyse impulse control and precipitate outbursts of violent and destructive rage. The existence of this entity remains controversial, but there is no controversy about the existence of a relationship of alcohol use to violence. Chapter 5 (Cognitive Disorders) discusses alcoholic intoxication, withdrawal, and overdose. Chapter 10 (Disorders of Awareness) discusses stupor and coma.

Much of the violence that occurs in our society is related to alcohol. A conventional estimate is that half of all auto accidents involve someone who has been drinking too much. Certainly alcohol is implicated in bar fights. In the 1970s, the Royal College of Psychiatrists reported that the incidence of rape in the United Kingdom peaked sharply on Friday evenings. Workmen received their pay packets on Friday, spent time in the pub, and arrived home full of beer and looking for "a woman." The relationship between alcohol use and forcible sex is, of course, hardly limited to Great Britain. Drunks can also abuse their children, either actively or passively through neglect.

General clinicians are familiar with the difficulties of finding out about alcohol abuse in their patients. The diagnosis often depends on information from the family or on the appearance of physical stigmata such as signs of liver disease. Alcoholics tend to lie even to themselves about how much they drink and how many problems their drinking causes. Their spouses and families are often ashamed or frightened to admit how much the patient drinks, or are cooperating with the patient's drinking ("enabling"). A mixed smell of alcohol and mouthwash on a patient's breath is a classic tip-off that the patient is drinking more than he or she wants people to know.

Treatment of alcohol abuse involves several simultaneous approaches. One is care of the general health of the patient, particularly nutrition. A problem drinker should at least be taking vitamin pills, including enough vitamin B to ward off Wernicke-Korsakoff disease. The minimal daily requirement for this vitamin in healthy young men is 3 mg/day, but doses 10 or even 100 times as large can be taken without any harm.

A major goal is to persuade the patient to abstain from all alcohol. A variety of psychological modalities are available to help to achieve this laudable but often very difficult goal, including individual and group psychotherapy. Often, the spiritual approach through Alcoholics Anonymous (AA) is the most successful. The cynical psychoanalytic comment is that the patient who regularly attends AA meetings still builds his or her life around alcohol, but now around abstinence instead of use. If alcohol abuse is a complication of depression or other underlying psychiatric disease, antidepressants or other appropriate psychiatric medications can have very gratifying results in regard to the substance abuse as well as for the underlying condition. Lithium can be very useful, but is best started during a hospitalization since the alcohol abuser may simultaneously abuse lithium, with serious and even fatal results. (See Chap. 3, Mood Disorders.) The anti-seizure medication *valproate* can be useful for alcoholics with underlying bipolar disorder who do not have concomitant liver disease. (See Chap. 10, Disorders of Awareness.)

Alcoholism can be thought of as a chronic disease with periodic relapses. Medical care requires maintenance treatment as well as treatment of exacerbations. Analogies have been drawn to the treatment of diabetes. If treatment of alcohol abuse decreases it from chronic use that mangles a patient's and family's life to occasional episodes, allowing a reasonably normal life, that should be considered a therapeutic success. Obviously, complete and permanent cure (abstinence) is better, if it can be achieved.

Disulfiram (Antabuse) is an aversive medication that makes drinking alcohol unpleasant. It is often a helpful adjunct to other treatments of alcoholism. The starting dose of disulfiram is 250–500 mg/day, and the dose can be reduced to 125 mg/day or even less if side effects become troublesome. In patients on Disulfiram, drinking alcohol causes nausea and vomiting, cramps, and flushing. These side effects are due to buildup of acetaldehyde in the body. Enough alcohol combined with Antabuse can lead to vasomotor collapse and is, in fact, a way for alcoholics to commit suicide. There are other problems with using disulfiram to discourage alcohol intake. Perhaps most important is that the alcoholic must continue to take it for it to be effective. If the urge to drink again becomes strong enough, the patient may simply stop the medicine, often lying about compliance to his or her family and physician. Having a spouse or other responsible person administer the Antabuse can sometimes finesse this problem. Common and minor side effects of disulfiram include sleepiness, bad breath, and a skin rash. Impotence is described as a temporary side effect but can easily put a patient permanently off taking the drug. The prescribing physician needs to be sensitive to this complication, which some patients and families may be too proud or embarrassed to bring up. Rare but more dangerous side effects include seizures, neuropathy, blindness (optic neuritis), and psychosis. Disulfiram should not be given to patients with psychosis or significant depression, to women who are at risk of becoming pregnant, to people with disease of the liver (including *esophageal varices*), heart or lungs, or to those with ulcers or other irritation of the stomach or duodenum. Disulfiram can interact with many other medications, including anticoagulants, *phenytoin* (Dilantin), and *isoniazid*. Patients and their families need to be fully informed of the risks of disulfiram treatment before it is initiated, with solid documentation that they were fully informed in the patient's chart.

Alcohol withdrawal syndrome—delirium tremens—is a common and potentially dangerous condition. Even with modern treatment, perhaps 5–10% of patients die during the acute episode. Treatment of the alcohol withdrawal syndrome itself is with benzodiazepines, which have pharmacological cross-tolerance with ethanol. Chapter 6 (Anxiety) discusses these medications in some detail. Treatment with diminishing doses of ethanol itself, orally or intravenously, has no advantages over benzodiazepines if the latter are available. Most but not all clinicians prefer to use repeated doses of a short-acting benzodiazepine such as *oxazepam* (Serax) rather than less-frequent doses of a long-acting form such as *chlordiazepoxide* (Librium). The principle is to start with a low dose, such as 10–15 mg of oxazepam, and increase the dose as needed to bring florid symptoms under control. It is not necessary—indeed, not advisable—to give so much that the tremor and restlessness are completely controlled. Patients can have trouble waking up from too much benzodiazepine, particularly of a long-acting form. Patients with delirium tremens or other withdrawal syndromes also need close attention to their medical care—electrolyte balance, hydration, and nutrition as well as treatment of infection. Probably it is wise to give everyone with delirium tremens vitamins, including 100 mg of thiamin (vitamin B_1) intravenously or intramuscularly. An important question about a patient with delirium tremens is why he or she stopped drinking. Occasionally running out of money to buy drinks is the real reason. More often the patient developed an inter-current illness that made him or her "feel too bad to keep drinking." That can be pneumonia or other infection, pancreatitis, bleeding into the stomach or gut, urinary tract infection, myocardial infarct or other heart disease, or any of a host of other diseases. A good history is characteristically not available from a person with delirium tremens or from the informants who have been with the patient during drinking bouts. As so often in clinical medicine, the physician needs to be a medical detective to take optimal care of these patients.

Chapter 5 (Cognitive Disorders) contains a discussion of alcoholic delirium and a brief discussion of the withdrawal syndrome.

Nicotine

Nicotine is a widely used, legal, addicting drug that is very damaging to human health. Quantitatively, the important source of nicotine for abuse is tobacco. Perhaps a quarter of the population smokes tobacco, in the world as a whole and in the United States. Smoking is very common among psychiatric patients; perhaps as many as 90% of schizophrenics are smokers. General physicians like other people are well aware of the ways tobacco is used, in cigarettes, cigars, pipes, and chewing tobacco. Inhaling tobacco smoke is an effective way to absorb nicotine rapidly, because of the large surface area of the lungs. The most common neurological complication of nicotine abuse is brain damage related to vascular disease and high blood pressure. The general medical complications of smoking are varied, serious, often deadly, and well-known to general clinicians. They include cardiovascular disease, peripheral vascular disease, lung disease including COPD (*chronic obstructive pulmonary disease*), cancers including cancers of the lung, mouth, and throat, and exacerbation of ulcers and other problems of the GI (*gastrointestinal*) tract. Tobacco smoke pollutes the air even for non-smokers, and epidemiological studies have delineated unhealthy effects of "second-hand smoking." The bad health consequences of smoking are not due primarily to nicotine but to other substances in tobacco smoke—the infamous "injurious tars and resins" including substances that cause cancers (*carcinogens*). Major anti-smoking campaigns are a continuing part of the modern American scene and are occurring increasingly in Europe and other countries.

Nicotine is perhaps the most addicting substance known. It is a stimulant that acts directly on nicotine receptors in the brain, which are one of the types of receptors in human brain that are normally stimulated by the endogenous neurotransmitter acetylcholine. Smoking tobacco appears to acutely increase alertness, attention, reaction time, and ability to learn and to solve problems. Many smokers report that smoking lifts their mood and calms them. These mild anti-depressant effects may be the reason that appropriate treatment with anti-depressants can often help smokers quit, as discussed below.

Withdrawal from nicotine is unpleasant—often very unpleasant. The craving for nicotine can be intense. It typically peaks within 1–2 days after quitting smoking but can last for months. Former smokers can develop an intense craving even if they have been without a cigarette for months or years. People who stop smoking typically go through a period that is difficult for them and the people around them. They become tense, irritable, and "snappish." They complain of lack of alertness but have trouble sleeping. Physiologically, their heart rate and blood pressure tend to decrease and their appetite increases. Heavy smokers who stop smoking can easily gain 10 lb or more in weight. However, despite the enormous problem of obesity in the United States, the dangers of smoking are thought to outweigh the dangers of weight gain associated with quitting.

Pharmacological tools to help people stop smoking are available, in addition to a variety of behavioral and psychological techniques.[26] The combined use of pharmacological and behavioral tools together can increase "quit rates" among smokers to as high as 30%. That compares to a quit rate with physician counseling alone of perhaps 10% and from pharmacological agents alone of about 20%. These quit rates are not as discouraging as they may seem, since many smokers will try to stop smoking many times and finally succeed.[27]

One set of these pharmacological tools allow the intake of nicotine without smoking tobacco. These are typically available over the counter. One is in a chewing gum (Nicorette), available in 2 mg strength for people who smoke less than one pack of cigarettes per day and in 4 mg strength for those who smoke more. Its side effects are minor. Some complain of the taste, and others of sore jaws from chewing. Perhaps 20% of smokers who use Nicorette to quit chew it for months, and perhaps 2% for as much as a year or more. In that case, they are still dependent on nicotine, but take it in a much safer form than through smoking tobacco. Nicotine patches are available in a 16-hour slow-release form (Habitrol) and in 16- or 24-hour tapering forms (Nicotrol). Again, side effects are minor—sometimes a rash, sometimes sleeplessness when the 24-hour patch is used. Long term use is not a problem. The patches reportedly improve quit rates, but studies comparing the different patches are scanty. Nicotine nasal spray, available by prescription, leads to higher levels of blood nicotine than gum or patches and can be useful for very dependent smokers. Side effects occur in over two-thirds of users, and include runny nose, watering eyes, and coughing. Abuse of the nasal spray is not a major problem (in contrast to early reports about it). Nicotine inhalers are also available by prescription. These provide a way for former smokers to fuss with their hands in order to take in nicotine. That can be important for some people trying to quit. Pipe smokers, for instance, often enjoy fussing with their pipe almost as much as they do smoking it.

Psychoactive medications can also be an effective aid in quitting smoking. The antidepressant *bupropion* is marketed as Zyban for helping people quit smoking and as Wellbutrin for the treatment of depression. Doses are about the same for both purposes—perhaps 300 mg/day. (See Chap. 3, Mood Disorders.) This drug is reportedly as effective in smokers who do not show signs of an underlying mood disorder as in those who do. Side effects are minor, including mild nausea or difficulty sleeping through the night. The latter is consistent with the proposed mechanism of action of bupropion, which is increasing the efficiency of noradrenalin and perhaps dopamine action in the brain. A tricyclic antidepressant, *nortriptyline* (Pamelor), also appears to help many smokers quit their habit. *Clonidine* (Catapres) appears to help many former smokers get through nicotine withdrawal. It acts on systems that use noradrenalin as neurotransmitter (α-adrenergic systems). Doses are 0.2–0.4 mg/day; side effects can include drowsiness and a fall in blood pressure. Yet another type of psychoactive drug that can help patients quit smoking is benzodiazepines, which can help tense people stay calmer during the difficulties of nicotine withdrawal. (See Chap. 6, Anxiety.)

Cannabis (Marijuana)

Many, many people around the world use cannabis derivatives for pleasure. In the United States, marijuana may be used almost as commonly as alcohol as a recreational chemical and substance of abuse—even though marijuana, unlike alcohol, is at least formally illegal in most jurisdictions. The drug is taken for a calming and euphoric effect, often with alcohol or other psychoactive substances. Undocumented claims have been made that it heightens enjoyment of sex, but as noted earlier, peanut butter can often do that if it is accompanied by enough mumbo-jumbo. The varieties of hemp plant from which the material is derived grow wild in many parts of the world including the United States, as well as being cultivated illegally by producers who then sell the product. In the United States, the most common way to take marijuana is by smoking the crushed, dried plant (mainly the leaves). In other countries, the favored way of taking it is often ingestion. Various forms of cannabis are referred to as marijuana (grass, pot, weed, tea, Mary Jane), charas, bhang, ganja, dagga, and hemp. Acute intoxication with cannabis is discussed in Chap. 5 (Cognitive Disorders); a withdrawal syndrome has never been well-documented.

The pharmacology of cannabis has been extensively studied. The major active component is (-)-Δ9-tetrahydrocannabinol (Δ9-THC), although perhaps 400 other psychoactive chemicals have been found in cannabis extracts. Δ9-THC is a fatty substance that dissolves in body fat where it is stored. That "pharmacokinetic" property can explain some of the peculiarities of cannabis use and addiction.[28] After a single use, the Δ9-THC that has been acting on the brain (itself a tissue rich in fat) is redistributed to peripheral fat stores. In that case, long-term effects of the drug become negligible. With chronic use of cannabis, however, the stores of the active principle in peripheral fat become so large that intoxication becomes essentially constant. Acute use then has relatively little effect on what has become a chronic state of marijuana intoxication. The "a-motivational state" discussed below may be the behavioral result of such chronic intoxication.

The human brain has its own endogenous "cannabinoid" system as it does its own "opiate system." The receptor is well characterized. [29] It is distributed in parts of the brain involving cognition as well as coordination and emotion, including cells which use monoamines as transmitters. (See Chap. 3, Mood Disorders.)

Long-term use of cannabis has a number of serious side effects. One is the carcinogenic and other bad medical effects of smoking anything, including tobacco. There are numerous medical reports and also denials that chronic use of cannabis leads to loss of brain substance (cerebral atrophy), seizures, chromosome damage and birth defects, and sexual difficulties. Whether cannabis itself causes psychosis is argued. Its use can certainly precipitate acute psychotic episodes in schizophrenics who had previously been doing well. A recent report suggests a genetic variation in people in whom cannabis use leads to psychosis—namely, a polymorphism in the *COMT* gene that encodes catechol-O-methyltransferase. Hypomania is not rare in chronic marijuana users. Most pot smokers have had at least one anxiety attack related to using the drug. Flashbacks can also occur, perhaps based in part on the pharmacokinetics discussed above (i.e., Δ9-THC leaching out of a body fat store). It is hard to determine precisely what is responsible for medical and neurological illness in heavy, chronic cannabis users. They are not good historians. They have often taken many drugs, some of which they do not remember and some of which they probably do not know about (i.e., something "slipped to them" during a party).

The existence of an "a-motivational" syndrome in chronic cannabis users is still a matter of controversy. Certainly, people including young people who have previously been achievers often—essentially, characteristically—lose their drive to succeed in a conventional sense after committing themselves to the drug. The generally short and unhappy existence of drug pushers who "work hard" on the streets hardly constitutes contravening evidence. As with use and abuse of any drug, how much of the change of behavior is due to the pharmacological actions of the drug and how much to "volition" is a neurobiologically naïve question.[30] It is better left to the many polemicists on this subject. A number of observers have come to the conclusion that it can take a year or two for a chronic cannabis user to come all the way down—perhaps the time it takes to flush the active principle out of body fat stores.

Cannabis remains formally illegal in the United States, but its use is as integrated into current American life as alcohol—certainly as much as alcohol was during prohibition. It would fly in the face of common experience to say that use of cannabis cannot be integrated into a highly productive life. Cannabis use becomes a problem when it interferes with life, either socially or medically. Again, judgment is necessary by the physician and the patient and family. There is no antidote to cannabis nor a substance that makes its use unpleasant, analogous to disulfiram for alcoholism. A number of social and psychiatric programs are available, including psychiatrists and clinics that specialize in treating addiction.

Medical uses of cannabis include management of pain, nausea, and a variety of aspects of palliative care. At the time this monograph is being written, the United States federal government and a number of state governments are arguing about whether cannabis should be available by prescription. From a purely *medical* viewpoint, it is hard to see why this particular plant extract that acts on an endogenous brain receptor system should not be available for prescription to appropriate patients, when other drugs with equally or greater addictive potential are—for instance, the sedatives and hypnotics.

Cocaine

Cocaine is another widely used recreational drug that is illegal but easy to obtain in the United States. Perhaps 2% of people in the United States use cocaine in any given year, that is, about 5 million people; 10% of the U.S. population has reportedly tried it at least once. Low doses of cocaine have actually been found to improve performance on a variety of tasks, and coca leaf is chewed in the Andes for this purpose. Larger doses of cocaine typically elevate mood, often dangerously, and make judgment deteriorate. Like so many other drugs of abuse, cocaine is said to act as an aphrodisiac (at least for people who believe it does). Cocaine has legitimate medical uses, notably as a local anesthetic in Ophthalmology. There is no legitimate psychiatric use for cocaine.

Cocaine is used recreationally in several forms in the Western world including the United States. Most street cocaine consists of a mixture of the pure powder and cane sugar or other cheap and innocuous substances. Diluting the pure powder as much as the customers will accept is as profitable for the drug pusher as diluting milk is for those who sell that product. The most common way to take cocaine in the United States is "snorting" ("sniffing" or "tooting")—inhaling "a line" of the powder into the nose, where it is rapidly absorbed through the nasal mucosa. Cocaine can also be injected or smoked. "Crack" cocaine is a highly addictive form of the free base that is smoked. Its use has often been associated with intense violence.

The mechanism of action of cocaine is to slow reuptake of the neurotransmitter dopamine, thereby stimulating dopaminergic pathways. These include primary reward centers. They also include the receptors whose relative over-activation is associated with endogenous psychoses. (See Chap. 4, Thought Disorders.) Cocaine changes the balance between adrenergic and cholinergic transmission in the adrenergic direction.

Cocaine can lead to a number of psychiatric syndromes, some of which are frankly dangerous. Relatively higher doses of cocaine, particularly if injected or smoked so that blood levels rise quickly, can induce a manic-like state with inappropriate feelings of control, and ready anger if that sense of control is violated. Cocaine abusers not rarely become frankly psychotic. They can hear voices, see things, and feel abnormal sensations (e.g., "bugs crawling under my skin"). They often become paranoid, and dangerously paranoid. They can become violent to the point of murder. They can become sexually totally inappropriate. Repeated use of cocaine can make a man impotent, which can be another reason for rage. It can induce severe anxiety and sometimes obsessive-compulsive behavior (see Chap. 6, Anxiety, and above.) Cocaine intoxication and withdrawal and more minor degrees of delirium are discussed in Chap. 5 (Cognitive Disorders).

Cocaine can also cause strokes and other forms of brain damage. Typically these are infarctions attributed to the effect of cocaine on constricting blood vessels, but bleeds can also occur. Cocaine is the substance of abuse most commonly associated with seizures, and these can progress to *status epilepticus*. (See Chap. 10, Disorders of Awareness.) Cocaine-induced psychomotor seizures (*partial complex epilepsy*) and specifically psychomotor, partial, or continuous status epilepticus can easily be confused with a cocaine-induced psychosis. Obviously, the treatment is different, and failure to treat status epilepticus can lead to permanent brain damage and death. (See Chap. 10, Disorders of Awareness.)

The general medical complications of cocaine abuse are dangerous and not rarely fatal. Specifically, cocaine can induce fatal heart attacks and *arrhythmias*. The drug-dependent euphoria in these patients can lead them to continue taking cocaine even when they are aware of severe, crushing chest pain or irregularities of their heart beat.

Treatment of cocaine addiction is difficult. Addicts typically think they don't need help until their abuse of the drug interferes grossly with their lives—for instance, by making them physically ill or bankrupting them. Counseling of various forms can be effective but is a matter for specialists, optimally of subspecialists within the field of psychiatry. When cocaine addiction is an attempt to self-medicate an underlying psychiatric illness such as depression, then treatment of the underlying disease with more appropriate medications can be gratifyingly successful. Antipsychotics that block dopamine receptors have been effective in treating animal models of cocaine addiction and its consequences but have been disappointing in treating humans with this addiction.

Amphetamines and Related Compounds

Amphetamines and related compounds are stimulants, as is cocaine. They are synthetic chemical compounds, rather than a natural constituent derived from a plant. There are legitimate medical uses for the amphetamines. They are approved for attention-deficit disorder in children and for narcolepsy. (See Chap. 8, Sleep.) They are sometimes prescribed as adjuncts in the treatment of depressed mood, of obesity, and of chronic fatigue syndrome and *neurasthenia*. The forms of amphetamines used in medicine in the United States include *dextroamphetamine* (Dexedrine), *methylphenidate* (Ritalin), and *methamphetamine* (Desoxyn). Related medicines that have some properties of amphetamines are used to treat nasal congestion in over-the-counter preparations as well as by prescription. They include *ephedrine*, *pseudoephedrine*, and *phenylpropanolamine* (PPA).

Abusers of amphetamines ("speed") usually take them by mouth but sometimes by injection. Methamphetamine ("ice," "crystal meth") is a popular form of amphetamine for abuse. It becomes available primarily through illegal manufacture.[31] Other forms of amphetamine are also made illegally. These include "ecstasy" (MDMA [*3,4-methylenedioxy methamphetamine*], also referred to as XTC or "Adam"), "Eve" (MMDA [*3-methoxy-4,5-methylenedioxyamphetamine*]); STP (DOM [*4-methyl-2,5-dimethoxyamphetamine*]), PMA, and others. In addition to their amphetamine-like effects, these can cause hallucinations. (See discussion below.) MDMA and MMDA are often used by young people. MDMA has been popular in homosexual clubs. Abuse of these agents can be fatal. They release serotonin from nerve endings and can cause permanent damage to the endings of nerves secreting serotonin.

Amphetamines stimulate the activity of dopamine pathways by facilitating the release of dopamine from nerve cells for which it is the neurotransmitter. They thus act on essentially the same neurotransmitter systems as cocaine does, and not surprisingly can have similar effects. Amphetamines can cause a variety of psychiatric syndromes including psychosis. Like cocaine, they are often taken in binges. Even without binging, they can cause intoxication, acute delirium, and a withdrawal syndrome. (See Chap. 5, Cognitive Disorders.) Amphetamines characteristically cause abnormalities of mood. Use is associated with manic-like behavior including euphoria and feelings of power. Withdrawal typically leads to depression and even to ideas of suicide.

A syndrome very much like paranoid schizophrenia can result from either acute or chronic amphetamine use. (See Chap. 4, Thought Disorders.) Behaviorally, amphetamine psychosis tends to be associated with more hyperactivity, hypersexuality, confusion, and incoherence than typical paranoid schizophrenia. Hallucinations tend to be visual rather than auditory, and associations tend not to be as loose as in schizophrenia. However, the differential diagnosis can be very difficult, and schizophrenics can abuse amphetamines. Use or abuse of amphetamines can induce anxiety as can their withdrawal. Manifestations can include panics, phobias, and obsessive-compulsive behavior. Like other drugs of abuse, amphetamine can be taken to enhance sexual performance or pleasure. As with other drugs, high doses and chronic use impair sexual functions and can cause impotence. Amphetamines interfere with normal sleep—one of the reasons some people take them when they want to work all through the night.

Amphetamine abuse, like cocaine abuse, can damage the brain and other organs. Neurological lesions range from twitching to tremor, ataxia, stroke, coma, and death. Infections including brain abscesses and AIDS (*acquired immunodeficiency syndrome*) can be secondary to the use of non-sterile needles and drug preparations. Medical complications of amphetamine abuse include high blood pressure—sometimes dangerously high—as well as heart attacks and cardiac irregularities (arrhythmias) and nausea and vomiting and other gastrointestinal problems. Relative minor effects are on skin color (flushing, pallor, *cyanosis*). Fetuses of pregnant women who abuse amphetamines are likely to be born with low birth weight or other injuries. Amphetamines decrease appetite, which is the reason they are sometimes used to treat obesity. Amphetamine abusers are characteristically thin—sometimes very thin—and at risk of being seriously malnourished.

Amphetamine abusers, like cocaine abusers, tend not to accept treatment until other alternatives are exhausted. Various forms of counseling particularly including counseling by experienced specialists can be useful. Benzodiazepines can help with the anxiety that can accompany decreasing amphetamine use. (See Chap. 6, Anxiety.) The antidepressant bupropion (Wellbutrin) has been suggested to be particularly useful in depression that can accompany cessation of amphetamine use. An underlying depression may, of course, have been the reason that inappropriate self-medication with amphetamines began in the first place. (See Chap. 3, Mood Disorders.) Antipsychotics are useful if there is an underlying thought disorder that needs treatment. Surprisingly, the antipsychotics that block dopamine receptors are not particularly useful in treating amphetamine abuse itself and its consequences in human beings, despite their effectiveness in many animal models.

Opiates

These drugs, which have been known for thousands of years, see wide use in medicine particularly in treating pain. They are plant constituents, from the opium poppy, that act on a transmitter system present in the normal human brain. This endogenous (endorphin) system is a primary reward system as well as involved in decreasing the perception of pain; stimulating with opiates induces pleasant feelings even as it typically impairs judgment. Extensive studies describe the characteristics of this system in detail. Chapter 7 (Pain) discusses the characteristics and mechanisms of action of opiates, and Chap. 5 (Cognitive Disorders) discusses intoxication, delirium, and the withdrawal syndrome associated with their abuse.

The opiate most used for abuse in the United States is a semisynthetic derivative—heroin (*diacetylmorphine*). This drug is not available for medical use in the United States. It is legally available to physicians in other countries such as Britain, notably for the treatment of heart attacks (*myocardial infarcts*). Heroin is more fat-soluble than morphine and therefore appears to enter tissues more rapidly, reputedly providing a greater "rush" than other derivatives do. However, a wide variety of other opiates are also abused, including widely used medications such as morphine and codeine and synthetic or semi-synthetic derivatives originally designed to be "less addicting."

The causes of opiate addiction are complex and continue to be studied intensively. Most people can stop using opiates without great difficulty even if they have become physiologically habituated and even if they have been using the drug for "recreation," as was true for many U.S. soldiers in Vietnam. There is something different about those who become opiate addicts. A clear hereditary (genetic) predisposition to opiate abuse exists, although the responsible gene(s) have not been identified as yet. There is a suspicion that these people have a genetically determined, biological underactivity of the endogenous opioid system in their brains. If so, their use of opiates is as logical as the use of SSRIs in people with depression due to central serotonergic deficiencies or, for that matter, the use of insulin in people with juvenile (insulin-deficient) diabetes. Perhaps nine-tenths of opiate abusers in the United States carry another psychiatric illness as well. Depression or other mood disorders, some form of anxiety disorder, and antisocial personality disorder are particularly common among them, along with other substance abuse disorders. Opioid use can itself precipitate a psychiatric disease, including mood disorders and psychoses. The psychiatric literature contains descriptions of a *heroin behavior syndrome* (Table 14-10). Opiate abuse is found at all economic and social levels, although slums in which heroin is easily available and widely used can foster its abuse. Addiction to opiates can be relatively easy for physicians, nurses, and pharmacists because of their relatively easy access to these drugs. Occasional physicians have integrated opiate use into their lives without apparent problems, so that their drug abuse has not been recognized until after their death.

The illegal use of opiates can lead to serious and life-threatening consequences, even though opiates themselves are relatively safe drugs. Opiates are frequently injected, intravenously or under the skin ("skin popping"). The repeated injections with non-sterile materials can lead to infections. Sometimes these are bacterial—septicemia, abscesses (including brain abscesses), infections of the heart valves (acute and subacute bacterial endocarditis), and many others. Opiate use is a risk factor for AIDS. Pregnant women who abuse opium are at high risk of delivering addicted or otherwise damaged babies. The criminal milieu in which illegal heroin or other opiates are obtained is a risky place. Tolerance to opiates develops readily, so that users may want and sometimes take doses that would incapacitate or kill a naive user. On the other hand, street drugs are rarely pure, and diluting ("cutting") the active drug with sugar or other materials can increase a pusher's

TABLE 14–10
Heroin behavior syndrome

- Underlying depression
  - Agitation
  - Anxiety
  - Fear of failure
  - Feelings of ineffectiveness and powerlessness
- Limited coping strategies
- Impulsiveness
- Difficulty postponing gratification
- Passive-aggressive personality
- Utilization of drugs for social contacts

profits. If a heroin addict doesn't pay his or her dealer or becomes otherwise inconvenient, it is easy for the dealer to provide a dose of relatively purer heroin that then kills the obstreperous customer from an overdose unless adequate medical treatment is given promptly. Fortunately, effective treatment with the opiate-blocking drug naloxone is available. (See Chap. 5, Cognitive Disorders, and Chap. 7, Pain.) Physicians, particularly those in emergency rooms, are generally appropriately sensitive to the need to institute prompt treatment in these patients.

Diagnosis of opiate addiction can be obvious but can also be challenging. General physicians are well aware that people can mimic pain syndromes in order to get opiate prescriptions, and can try to get opiate prescriptions from several doctors at the same time. The presence of pin-point pupils in a person with stupor or coma immediately raises the question of opiate abuse and overdose. So do needle tracts.

The treatment of opiate abuse is difficult and often frustrating. The most successful pharmacological treatment has been switching the addicts to another opiate, methadone, which is provided legally in specialized clinics. Methadone is taken orally and has less of a euphoric effect than heroin. The usual dose is 20–80 mg once a day, but doses as high as 120 mg a day have been used. Methadone use prevents the severe withdrawal syndrome that follows stopping habitual use of heroin or a number of other narcotics. Withdrawal from methadone is relatively mild and easy to perform therapeutically. However, some addicts continue to use methadone for long periods of time. The substitution of a legally available, oral opiate prevents the problems associated with injection of a material obtained in the criminal milieu. From a purely medical point of view, it seems to be effective treatment in some people of the underlying psychiatric disorder that led them to abuse opiates. The use of opiates for psychiatric indications is very controversial, however, in many societies including the United States. Those discussions involve moral and political arguments that are beyond the scope of this monograph.[32] General physicians who try to treat opiate addicts for their addictions put themselves at several types of risk. These patients are not known for their truthfulness when making accusations, including statements about how they got their drugs from doctors.

Benzodiazepines, Barbiturates, and Other Sedatives and Hypnotics

These drugs are widely and appropriately prescribed by physicians but can also become drugs of abuse. They include benzodiazepines, barbiturates, and older and less used medications such as meprobamate (Miltown). Among the many medical uses of these drugs is the relief of excess anxiety and treatment of *status epilepticus* and of acute psychotic breaks. (See Chap. 6, Anxiety; Chap. 10, Disorders of Awareness; and Chap. 4, Thought Disorders.) People who abuse these drugs generally do so for their calming effect. The distinction between the therapeutic use and the abuse of these drugs depends on the judgment of the responsible physician. The admittedly subjective criterion is whether the use of these substances has become "maladaptive." Sometimes it is hard to know whether use of these substances warrants treatment even if the pattern of use is questionable.

> Consider, for instance, a happily married suburban grandmother in her late sixties who has been taking a relatively large amount of meprobamate daily for over 30 years. She has no signs of marrow depression or other physiological side effects. Her personal physician who recently died originally wrote her the prescriptions. The younger doctor who has taken over his practice now continues to write them. At the suggestion that she cut down or eliminate her daily dose of meprobamate, the woman becomes acutely anxious—even panicky. She is almost certainly both physiologically and psychologically habituated to this substance, but she has integrated its use into her "normal," successful life. What is the *medical* point of "curing" her of her "addiction?" What is the *medical* point of delving into the details of her relationship with the dead physician who supported her habit for so many years?

A clearer example of abuse is a person who manages to obtain large amounts of sedatives by getting prescriptions from several different doctors who do not know about each other. Other examples are people who become a risk to themselves or others—for instance, while driving a car or operating other machinery while self-sedated. In this case, prompt intervention is necessary. It is relatively hard to commit suicide with benzodiazepines alone unless something else is taken like large doses of alcohol. It is relatively easy to kill oneself with barbiturates. Reducing the doses and if possible eliminating sedative-hypnotic drugs is not difficult technically. If done gradually, tapering need not be unpleasant for the patient. Getting the patient's cooperation may be a difficult problem even for a psychiatrist who specializes in treating addictions.

The pharmacology of benzodiazepines and barbiturates are discussed in Chap. 6 (Anxiety) and also in Chap. 8 (Sleep). Their mechanisms of action, effects, side effects, and the withdrawal syndromes they can precipitate are discussed there. A medication is available to treat benzodiazepine overdose;

over-titration of this medication can lead to benzodiazepine withdrawal syndrome in a chronic user, as discussed in Chap. 6 (Anxiety). Benzodiazepines are in general safer than barbiturates and are now much more widely prescribed. Older anti-anxiety agents are now seen primarily in patients who have been using them for years, like the lady described above.

Inhalants

Many common organic chemical fluids can become substances of abuse. They include gasoline, airplane glue, paint, and ether. Like alcohol, these chemicals dissolve in membranes and have an anesthetic effect.[33] The usual way of taking in these materials is by breathing them, often from an enclosed container of some sort or from a rag soaked in an organic liquid (i.e., "huffing"). The lung has a large surface area from which these materials can be absorbed, and the altered mental states that result tend to come on quickly and dissipate relatively quickly, in minutes to an hour. Intoxication with gasoline can last for several hours.

Inhalant abuse is dangerous, in part because of the properties of the chemicals themselves and in part because of contaminants that are often mixed with them—for instance, organic derivatives of heavy metals in paint. Neurological complications beyond intoxication include severe delirium, persistent dementia, depression, panic attacks and other forms of anxiety disorder, and psychoses including hallucinations and delusions. Medical complications include depression of respiration, choking with or without aspiration, and irreversible damage to the liver, kidneys, or skeletal muscles including acute necrosis of muscle (*rhabdomyolysis*).

Diagnostic clues to this condition can be a smell of the organic solvent on the patient's person or breath. Other evidence can be rashes or other injuries to the nose, mouth, eyes, or gums.

There is no pharmacological treatment for inhalant addiction, unless it is a manifestation of an underlying psychiatric disorder such as depression or anxiety. Sometimes skilled counseling helps, including with adolescents. Fortunately, occasional users often stop before they maim or kill themselves or others.

Hallucinogens (Psychedelics)

A number of naturally occurring and synthetic chemical substances are capable of inducing hallucinations in both normal people and in people with

TABLE 14–11
Hallucinogens

Name	Source	Typical duration of action
Mescaline	Peyote cactus	6–12 hours
Psilocybin	Mushrooms	4–6 hours
LSD	Synthetic	6–12 hours; flashbacks
MDA	Synthetic	8–12 hours
MDMA	Synthetic	4–6 hours
GHB	Synthetic	3–6 hours
PCP	Synthetic	2–8 hours

Abbreviations: LSD, d-lysergic acid diethylamide; MDA, 3,4-methylenedioxyamphetamine; MDMA, 3,4-methylenedioxy methamphetamine; GHB, γ-hydroxybutyrate; PCP, phencyclidine

underlying psychiatric disorders or predispositions to psychiatric disorders. Table 14-11 lists some now in use in the United States. These are all taken orally. MDA and MDMA are amphetamine derivatives. GHB (γ-hydroxybutyrate) can cause transient amnesia, and is known as a "date rape' drug.

Experiences induced by hallucinogens have been described by users as "mind-expanding" and "religious," but the states induced by these compounds and notably by LSD have also been used as models for psychosis. Perhaps the distinction lies in the eye of the describer. There are religious traditions that have utilized these substances and others that have rejected them.[34] Experiences after taking one of these agents vary considerably, even in the same person (e.g., "good trips" or "bad trips").

The detailed mechanisms of action of these substances remain a subject of research. They have a high affinity for a subtype of serotonin receptor (5-HT_2), and their potency as psychedelics correlates with that binding. Furthermore, their effects can be blocked in animal models by 5-HT_2 receptor antagonists (e.g., *ritanserin*). However, the hallucinogens also bind tightly to a number of other receptors; LSD does so even at very low concentrations (*nmolar*). These multiple binding sites make any attempt to attribute its actions to only one type of receptor risky.

People who use hallucinogens in general do not use them as often as other substances of abuse are taken. In practice, tolerance is therefore not a problem, even though it is a pharmacological property of these drugs.

In addition to the effects the hallucinogens have in common, each of these drugs has, as expected, characteristics that distinguish it from the others.

LSD *(d-lysergic acid diethylamide)* is the most potent hallucinogen known for human beings. Doses of 25–50 μg have behavioral effects, and the usual dose for a psychedelic "trip" is 100–300 μg. Psychological effects of LSD include perceptual abnormalities (hallucinations and illusions), mood changes (elation, depression), often paranoia, and often panic. A "bad trip" typically involves severe panic but can be associated with a suicidal depression. Physical signs of LSD use include dilated pupils, elevated blood pressure and heart rate, salivation and tearing, and increased reflexes.

Hallucinations can recur even long after the original LSD "trip" is over. The official name for these "flashbacks" is *hallucinogen persisting perception disorder* (HPPD). Perhaps half the people who have flashbacks have them repeatedly. Precipitants include the use of other psychoactive materials (marijuana, anti-psychotics) or fatigue or stress. Sometimes simply entering a dark room leads to a flashback.

LSD can have other long-lasting effects. It typically makes schizophrenia worse, and can tip a patient who was managing reasonably well into a psychotic episode. A small number of apparently normal users become and stay psychotic after an LSD trip, particularly after repeated use. Of course, one may wonder how normal people who chose to use LSD repeatedly really were.

In general, people who take LSD do not harm others. However, they can become quite crazy and then do bad things. A famous case that received national publicity some years ago was a mother who cut out the heart of her infant while the mother was on an "acid trip."

PCP *(phencyclidine)* has a different mechanism of action than the other hallucinogens. It blocks a specific type of glutamate receptor, the NMDA receptor, that is involved in learning (more precisely, in *long-term habituation*) as well as in certain types of pathological damage to brain. PCP (angel dust) was originally used as an anesthetic, but its psychic effects have led to its no longer being used therapeutically in humans. In low doses or relatively soon after its ingestion, users tend to become withdrawn sometimes to the point of *catatonia*. (See Chap. 4, Thought Disorders.) Higher doses frequently lead to aggressive behavior including "insane" assaults on other people. These may be in response to hallucinations. At still higher doses, the anesthetic effects take over. Stupor and coma can supervene and last for a week or more, often accompanied by rigid muscles, fevers, and breakdown of muscle (*rhabdomyolysis*). Life support may be necessary for the user to survive.

MDA and MDMA are synthetic amphetamine derivatives. (See above.) High doses are associated with rapid heart beat, dry mouth, muscle aches, and clenching of the jaw. As noted earlier, abuse of these agents can kill the abuser.

GHB is unfortunately a popular drug among young people in certain settings. The initial effect includes euphoria. It has been used by body builders and in "raves." It is utilized as a "date rape" drug, because higher doses cause intoxication and amnesia. Overdose can lead to a complex syndrome that is not rarely seen in emergency rooms. It can include both slow and then fast heart beat (*bradycardia* followed by *tachycardia*), respiratory depression to the point of stopping breathing (*apnea*), low body temperature (*hypothermia*), flushing, sweating, nausea, and vomiting. Behavioral aspects of this syndrome can include CNS (central nervous system) depression, aggressive behavior, seizures, *myoclonus*, and *nystagmus*. Patients can complain of tunnel vision. The GHB withdrawal syndrome resembles that from alcohol or benzodiazepines, except that the physical (autonomic) symptoms are generally milder but the psychotic symptoms are usually worse and last longer. After GHB was banned in 1990, other analogous "designer drugs" have come in to take its place—for instance, butanediol. The preparations of GBH and its analogues that are used recreationally cannot be depended on to be pure. The users often do not know what they have actually taken or what has been "slipped" to them by others.

Treatment

Treatment for people who have taken hallucinogens is supportive and symptomatic. It is often possible to help persons through a "bad trip" simply by staying with them and talking to them. This can be difficult, and runs a risk of the patient having a flare of violence or other inappropriate behavior. The general clinician faced with such a patient is better advised to give an oral dose of a benzodiazepine to calm the patient's anxiety. A number of texts recommend a relatively high dose of 20 mg of *diazepam* (Valium) PO, but the dose and even route of administration may require modification. As always, the best dose is the one that helps the patient without incurring side effects. Other symptomatic medications including antipsychotics can be useful when necessary. The usual choice at the present time is Risperdal or Haldol; older antipsychotics with more cholinergic side effects are avoided. (See Chap. 4, Thought Disorders.)

Designer Drugs

Unfortunately, the creative ingenuity of the drug community continues to lead to the synthesis and use of new "designer drugs." The people synthesizing and purifying them typically do not have the knowledge and attention to detail characteristic of a skilled pharmaceutical chemist. The contaminants in preparations of "designer drugs" can be dreadfully dangerous. The Parkinson-causing drug MTP was discovered as an impurity in such a designer drug. (See Chap. 11, Disorders of Motility.) The young dropout chemist who made it would have died had he not had the good luck to be cared for by a very good neurologist who was able to figure out how to treat the first patient with the then new syndrome of sudden, early onset, very severe parkinsonism.

A relatively new designer drug, which is still uncommon in the United States, is methcathinone ("goob," "crank", "CAT"). Its actions and complications are generally similar to those of amphetamines. It is a synthetic form of the active principle of the leaves of the Khat plant, which is used as a stimulant in the Near East. The synthetic compound, methcathinone, is easily made chemically from ephedrine or pseudoephedrine, which are widely used in over-the-counter cold and allergy remedies.

If possible, samples of the "designer drug"—or for that matter any other drug of abuse—that a person has taken should be obtained for future chemical analysis if necessary. The tools of analytical chemistry are now so powerful that rapid and complete analysis of mixtures of organic compounds is generally reasonably straightforward, by coupling mass spectrometry to chromatographic techniques such as gas-liquid chromatography (GLC) or high pressure liquid chromatography (HPLC). This takes too much time for acute care, but can be critical for a patient who has a new and more or less chronic syndrome (such as the first patient with MPTP-induced parkinsonism).

REFERENCES

1. "Reformist delusions" is discussed in Chap. 4, Thought Disorders. Roughly, the idea was that those who were trying to improve the Soviet system had to be crazy. If they agreed to stop trying to do so after an unpleasant stay in a mental hospital, they were cured. If they again tried to improve the system, they were diagnosed as having a relapse and were re-hospitalized. The Royal College of Psychiatrists in Britain, among others, deserves credit for fighting hard and consistently against this perversion of psychiatry.

2. My parents belonged to this group, many of whom fled from Nazi persecution to New York or London.
3. Without getting anthropological, attitudes on the obligation to procreate vary among cultures and traditions. The first commandment in Genesis is "Be fruitful and multiply." The Gospels celebrate marriage—for instance, Jesus' words and acts at Cana. St. Paul, however, directly contradicted the tradition in which he was raised in his injunction, "It is better to marry than to burn." Paul's statement as well as Gnostic traditions have greatly influenced subsequent Western attitudes, and not only of Christians.
4. Heroism is laudable, but the romanticization of heroism in war raises psychoanalytically interesting issues. TV shows or movies that dramatize the courage of men at war often include episodes in which the hero is grievously wounded and then nursed back to full health and vigor by a beautiful woman. She is often a pneumatic blond whom he has previously rescued or subsequently rescues from some sort of fate worse than death.
5. Gazzaniga MS. Forty-five years of split-brain research and still going strong. *Nat Rev Neurosci.* 2005;6:653–659.
6. Phelps EA, LeDoux JE. Contributions of the amygdala to emotion processing: from animal models to human behavior. *Neuron.* 2005;48:175–187.
7. If a positive misdiagnosis of an organic illness as a somatization reaction is made by a psychiatrist, the general clinician is in a better position to protect himself or herself in legal proceedings if the patient turns out to have had a "real" illness. The documented specialist consultation demonstrates that the general clinician conformed to "standard medical practice" and was not negligent.
8. Consider, for instance, the following example. An internist who went through two divorces retained a strong and continuing sex drive. He had affairs with a variety of women and habitually used prostitutes as well. He died of AIDS. This man's sexual behavior was fully acceptable by current psychiatric criteria and to his "middle-American" background, but it killed him. One does not want to think about how many women he may have infected.
9. The appropriation of the word "gay" for a form of sexual behavior takes a useful word out of common usage. Its original meaning is illustrated in the last line of Yeats' *Lapis Lazuli*: "Their eyes, their ancient glittering eyes are gay."
10. When half the population is said to have a psychiatric disorder, one must raise the question of who defines "normal" and how. The Declaration of Independence did not state that the achievement of orgasm was a self-evident right along with life and liberty.
11. In the 1950s, a nationally prominent minister implied that Freudian psychoanalysis had proven "scientifically" that the maintenance of technical virginity by young women before marriage was a sign of mental health. The

putative biological link between an intact hymen and higher cortical function atrophied after contraceptive pills were introduced.

12. Years ago, a woman wrote to Dear Abby to describe her relationship with her husband. He liked to tie her up when having sex. She did not enjoy that, but wrote that she put up with it because he was a good husband, a good provider, and a good, kind man despite his sexual preferences. She described herself as contented with the trade-off, and signed her letter "Knows the Ropes." Her attitude would have been roundly criticized once the women's liberation movement developed. It is interesting that now, after the successes of the women's movement, a surprising number of articles in "women's magazines" give instructions on how to perform sexual variations so as to delight the man one is "hooking up" with.
13. Irle E, Lange C, Sachsse U. Reduced size and abnormal asymmetry of parietal cortex in women with borderline personality disorder. *Biol Psychiatry*. 2005;57:173–182.
14. Unfortunately, some practitioners still believe in "recovered memories." This is an unsound extension of the basic psychoanalytic techniques of helping people remember things that bother them. "Recovered memories" allow the practitioner to find what he or she is sure had happened irrespective of the experiences of the patient in question—for instance, childhood sexual abuse. This approach has been called *jukebox psychiatry*: "Put in a syndrome, and out comes a pretty little tune. For the same syndrome, out comes the same pretty little tune, irrespective of what is going on in the patient."
15. In the United States in the late twentieth century, white supremacists could still be elected to major elected office including congress. There are times when whole nations appear to become paranoid—for instance, Nazi Germany and Austria.
16. Alcibiades provides an example from ancient times. After he had switched sides from the Athenian to the Spartan side in the Peloponnesian war, he got the wife of the king of Sparta pregnant. He said the king was lucky, since he would have a son of Alcibiades. Whether this gifted ancient Greek had a form of "personality disorder" is up to the reader to decide.
17. Meticulous studies in England in the 1970s showed that criminals jailed in a psychiatrically optimized environment had the same recidivism rate as those sent to ordinary, harsh English jails.
18. A psychoanalytic joke describes a conversation between a masochist and sadist. Masochist: "Hit me!" Sadist: "No!"
19. Physicians are pledged to do what we can to help the people who come to us and want to live longer and as free from disease as possible. However, a persistent and troublesome issue is whether self-destructive behavior can be rational. Footnote 4 above raises this question in regard to heroism in war. Furthermore, our society does not discourage "extreme sports" such as

bungee-jumping, recreational parachuting including periods of free fall, and automobile and motorcycle racing. William Butler Yeats put the argument for allowing risky behavior in powerful verse:

"...I balanced all, brought all to mind,
The years to come seemed waste of breath
A waste of breath the years behind
In balance with this life, this death."
(From *An Irish Airman Foresees His Death*)

20. Converting an addict from heroin to an antipsychotic is considered a therapeutic success, despite the significant side effects of many antipsychotics compared to opiates. That therapeutic attitude reflects the wishes of the larger society, as expressed in legislation and law enforcement. Whether it makes sense *medically* is another question.
21. It is also a somewhat abstract question. Patients can obtain marijuana without much difficulty in states like California where medical use of marijuana was legal until the federal government intervened. Enforcement of the federal law would prevent patients from knowing the purity of the marijuana their physicians advise them to use. That can be a serious risk, since drug dealers sometimes "lace" the pot they sell with more dangerous drugs. (Statement in regard to conflict of interest: The author has never used marijuana and does not intend to. He is too narcissistic about maintaining whatever cognitive abilities he still has.)
22. In the terminology DSM-IV-TR terms, they earn an Axis II as well as an Axis I diagnosis.
23. Specifically, NADH/NADPH, which maintain the chemically reduced state of glutathione and other biological antioxidants.
24. Alcohol abuse has also been suggested to be a mechanism to ward off unwanted homosexual urges. Certainly drinking with his buddies can reassure a man about his own masculinity.
25. This is true even for groups which historically prided themselves on a relatively low incidence of alcohol abuse. If American Jews were forced to emigrate, the countries in which we settled would come to regard Scotch whiskey as a Jewish drink—as people in the United States now regard slivovitz.
26. Evidence exists that at least three behavioral techniques are useful—skills training including behavioral-cognitive techniques, stimulus control, and "oversmoking"—to the point of sickness so that the conditioned response to tobacco smoke is negative. Description of these techniques fall outside the scope of this monograph, which focuses on medications.
27. The author of this monograph has experience in stopping smoking. He quit sixteen times before he finally succeeded on the seventeenth try. (Whether that success was permanent or not remains to be seen, but he has not smoked in over 15 years.)

28. The author is indebted for this analysis of the pharmacokinetics of cannabis to Professor Jan Schuberth of the University of Linköping in Sweden.
29. The receptor has been cloned. It links to an inhibitory G-protein (G_i), which acts to inhibit adenylate cyclase, the enzyme that makes the intracellular signal compound cAMP. "Ananamide" is the material endogenous to human brain that acts on the cannabis receptor. The normal physiological function of this system is not yet known.
30. Changing how our brains work typically changes what we think we decide. The distinction between volition and brain action is philosophical not biological.
31. Crystal meth is reportedly a particularly popular drug of abuse in the central United States, between the Appalachians and the Rocky Mountains. That may be in part because it can be manufactured by local entrepreneurs rather than needing to be imported from South America or Asia.
32. Thank God they are. I am very grateful not to have to stick my head into that ideological caldron.
33. The anesthetic effect of breathing in appropriate organic chemicals such as ether is, of course, widely utilized for surgical anesthesia.
34. Several major mystical traditions teach that "transcendental" experiences induced by drugs are likely to be misleading, certainly compared to the spiritual experiences that can come from rigorous meditation or other spiritual practices. The Jewish statement is, "False messengers outnumber true messengers."

Index

Page numbers followed by *t* denote tables, respectively. Page numbers followed by *n* indicate footnotes.

A

Abulia, 59, 119, 303
ACCP. *See* American College of Clinical Pharmacy
ACE. *See* angiotensin converting enzyme
acetaldehyde, 441
acetaminophen (Tylenol), 182, 198, 199*t*, 201
acetazolamide, 214, 251, 353
acetylcholine, 31, 141
  agonists, 362–363
acetylcholinesterases, 364–365
acetylcysteine, 202
acetyl-L-carnitine, 411
acetylsalicylic acid (ASA), 198, 199, 200, 270
ACTH. *See* adrenocorticotropic hormone
acute abdomen, 186, 197
acute disseminated encephalomyelitis, 401–402
acute inflammatory polyneuropathy, 338–339
  treatment of, 366–367
acute stress disorder, 171–173
acute strokes, treatment of, 271–276
AD. *See* Alzheimer disease
addiction, 438–463
  amphetamine, 454–455
  cocaine, 452–453
  defined, 204
  general considerations of, 438–440
  opiate, 203–205, 455–456
adjustment disorders, 435–436
ADRC. *See* Alzheimer Disease Research Center
adrenocorticotropic hormone (ACTH), 397
adulterated L-tryptophan, 408*t*
Advanced Sleep Phase Disorder, 234–235
affect, 79
aged gait, 330
aging, 130–131, 384
  insomnia and, 228
agoraphobia, 169
agranulocytosis, 49–50, 55, 201
AIDS, 346, 383, 423, 454, 456
akathisia, 55, 92
akinetic mutism, 303, 313
Alazine. *See* hydralazine
alcohol, 117, 354, 407, 425*t*, 426, 440–446, 466*n*24
  delirium and, 138–139
  dementia and, 145, 443

alcohol (*Cont.*):
  insomnia and, 241
  metabolism of, 441
  nervous system disorders induced by, 442*t*
  symptoms of abuse of, 443*t*
  treatment of abuse of, 444–446
  violence and, 443–444
Alcoholics Anonymous, 444
alemtuzumab, 399
ALK1, 267
Allegra. *See* fexofenadine
allergic rhinitis, 227–228
alprazolam (Xanax), 169, 177*t*
ALS. *See* Amyotrophic Lateral Sclerosis
alteplase. *See* tPA
alveolar hypoventilation, 238
Alzheimer Association, 143
Alzheimer dementia, 120–121
Alzheimer disease (AD), 6, 32, 117, 119–122, 160*n*39, 379
  behavioral medication in, 146–148
  diagnosis of, 121
  onset of, 121
  pathophysiology of, 131–133
  treatment of, 148–154
Alzheimer Disease Research Center (ADRC), 154
Alzheimer precursor protein, 152, 153
amantadine (Symmetrel), 359*t*, 363, 401
American College of Clinical Pharmacy (ACCP), 271–272
American Psychiatric Association (APA), 422
aminoglycosides, 285
amiodarone (Cordarone), 408*t*
amitriptyline (Elavil), 52*t*, 54, 172, 212
a-motivational syndrome, 449, 450
amoxapine, 52*t*, 54
amoxicillin, 388
amphetamines, 425*t*, 426, 453–455
  addiction to, 454–455
amyloid, 152
  plaques, 120
  vaccination against, 153
amyloid precursor protein, 132
amyloidosis, 409
Amyotrophic Lateral Sclerosis (ALS), 332, 340
Anafranil. *See* clomipramine
anatomic brain damage, 129–130
androgens, 425*t*, 426
anergia, 59
anesthetics, 11, 17, 116
  local, 214
angiotensin converting enzyme (ACE), 65
anorexia, 298
anosmia, 379
Antabuse. *See* disulfiram
antiandrogens, 425*t*, 426
anticholinergic actions, 54, 93, 115*t*
anticoagulation, 269, 273–275
anticonvulsants, 58, 65, 66–67, 99, 250
  pain and, 213–214
antidepressants, 42–43, 47–48, 175–176, 248, 421
  pain and, 211–213
  tricyclic, 51–57
antiepileptics, 57–58
antihistamines, 116–117, 182, 212, 244–245
antihypertensives, 425*t*, 426
anti-inflammatories, 398
antioxidants, 271, 367, 441
antiplatelet agents, 269
antipsychotics, 65, 67, 87, 104*n*28, 182, 425*t*, 427, 466*n*20
  atypical, 96–99
  side effects of, 87–88, 90–96
  typical, 88–96
antiseizure medications, 65, 297*t*
antisocial personality disorder, 432
anxiety, 163–164, 284
  classification and diagnosis of, 164–173
  general considerations in, 174–175
  generalized, 165–168
  mild, 164–165
  neurobiology, 173–174
  treatments, 174–183
anxious depression, 166–168
APA. *See* American Psychiatric Association
apallic syndrome. *See* persistent vegetative state

aphasia, 257
  ictal, 292
  productive, 292
aplastic anemia, 297
apneustic breathing, 311
apoplexy, 259
apraxia, 324, 342
  gait, 343
  ideational, 324
  ideomotor, 324
  treatment of, 352
Apresazide. *See* hydralazine
Apresoline. *See* hydralazine
Aricept. *See* donepezil
arrhythmias, 54
Artane. *See* trihexyphenidyl
arteriovenous malformations, 260
ASA. *See* acetylsalicylic acid
aspiration, 308, 349
Aspirin. *See* acetylsalicylic acid
asterixis, 325
  treatment of, 354
Atarax. *See* hydroxyzine
ataxia, 64, 327, 395
  hereditary, 397
  sensory, 343, 382
  spinocerebellar, 344
  treatment of, 355–356
atherosclerosis, 409, 441
athetosis, 324, 326
  treatment of, 355
Ativan. *See* lorazepam
atrial fibrillation, 269
autism, 83
autoimmune disorders, 347
automatisms, 293
awareness disorders, 283
  public issues and, 315–316
Axid. *See* nizatidine
axonal degeneration, 404
azathioprine (Imuran), 366

B

Babinski reflex, 342, 343
back pain, 192–193, 219–220
  classification of, 192*t*
back strain, 193–194
baclofen (Lioresal), 350
BAL. *See* British anti-lewisite
ballismus, 327–328, 355
barbiturates, 116, 182–183, 247–248, 425*t*, 457–459
basal ganglia, 342
bedwetting. *See* nocturnal enuresis
behavioral medication, in AD, 146–148
bell palsy, 257*t*
Benadryl. *See* diphenhydramine
benzodiazepines, 68, 98–99, 116, 140–141, 166, 175, 176–178, 203, 219, 220, 243–244, 248, 250, 297*t*, 300–301, 301, 350, 429, 432, 457–459
  dosage of, 180–181
  properties of, 177*t*
  side effects of, 178–182
  as sleep medications, 243*t*
benztropine (Cogentin), 359*t*, 362
β-Blockers, 217, 425*t*, 426
bilateral internuclear ophthalmoplegia, 396
Binswanger disease, 264
bioamine model, 30–32
biogenic monoamines, 57
bipolar disorders, 27*t*, 36
birth defects, lithium and, 62–64
bleeds, brain, 259–261
blood levels, drug, 16
blood pressure, 55
  control of, 268–269
blood sugar, 305*t*
blood ureal nitrogen (BUN), 301
blood-brain barrier, 10, 11–13
  discovery of, 12
  physiological function of, 12
body dysmorphic disorder, 418*t*, 421
bone marrow, 94
borderline personality disorder, 430–431
Botox. *See* botulinum toxin
botulinum toxin (Botox), 350
bradycardia, 462
bradykinesia, 323
bradyphrenia, 124, 323
brain abscess, 306*t*

brain damage, in schizophrenics, 85
brain death, 314–315
brain imaging, 256, 265–266
brain stem, 236
  herniation of, 304, 309–312
  lesions, 381
brain tumor, 306*t*
British anti-lewisite (BAL), 351
bromocriptine (Parlodel), 359*t,* 361
brompton cocktail, 206, 223*n*17
Bufferin. *See* salicylates
BUN. *See* blood ureal nitrogen
bundle branch blocks, 54
Buprenex. *See* buprenorphine
buprenorphine (Buprenex), 210
bupropion (Wellbutrin), 30, 47–48, 48*t,* 423, 448
BuSpar. *See* buspirone
buspirone (BuSpar), 172, 181, 425*t*
butorphanol (Stadol), 210
butyrophenone, 356

C

cabergoline (Dostinex), 359*t,* 361
CAG, 344
Calan. *See* verapamil
calcium channel blockers, 67, 217
cannabinoids, 400
cannabis, 449–451, 467*n*28
  legality of, 450–451
carbamazepine (Tegretol), 67, 99, 171, 192, 213, 297–298, 357
carbidopa, 358
carbon monoxide (CO), 133
carboplatin, 385
carcinogens, 447
carcinoid syndrome, 34
cardiac arrhythmias, 257*t*
carisoprodol (Soma), 220
carotid stenosis, 270–271
casein, 241
cataplexy, 233
Catapres. *See* clonidine
catatonia, 79, 102*n*7, 461
catharsis, 173
CBC. *See* complete blood count
CBT. *See* cognitive-behavioral therapy
CCM1, 267
CCM2, 267
Ceftin. *See* cefuroxime axetil
cefuroxime axetil (Ceftin), 388
Celebrex. *See* celecoxib
celecoxib (Celebrex), 199*t*
central biogenic amine deficiency, 32–34
central deafness, 384
central pain syndromes, 195, 212
central pontine myelinosis, 402–403
central serotonergic deficiency, 31
Centrax. *See* prazepam
cerebellar gait, 327, 330, 343
cerebellar speech, 327
cerebellum, 342
cerebral hemorrhages, causes of, 260*t*
cerebral metabolic rate (CMR), 127, 132
cerebral thromboses, 258–259
cerebrospinal fluid (CSF), 118, 119, 196, 396
cerebrovascular disease, 255
  classification and diagnosis of, 256–266
  neurobiology of, 266–267
  prevention of, 268–271
  treatment of, 267–279
cetirizine (Zyrtec), 212, 245
Charles Bonnet syndrome, 377
chemicals, medications as, 9–10
Cheyne-Stokes respiration, 311
chloral hydrate, 246–247
  side effects of, 247
chlorambucil, 412
chloramphenicol (Chloromycetin), 385, 408*t*
chlordiazepoxide (Librium), 99, 177*t,* 446
Chloromycetin. *See* chloramphenicol
chlorpromazine (Thorazine), 68, 88*t,* 89*t,* 92, 356
cholestatic jaundice, 96
cholesterol emboli, 409
cholinesterase inhibitors, 11, 148–150, 155
  central, 149*t*
  side effects of, 150

chorea, 324, 326
  treatment of, 354–355
choreoathetosis, 326
  paroxysmal, 328
choreoathetotic gait, 330
chronic hepatocerebral degeneration, 336–337
chronic liver disease, 336
chronic obstructive pulmonary disease (COPD), 447
Cialis, 427
cimetidine (Tagamet), 245
circadian rhythm disorders, 234–235
  treatment of, 250–251
circulation, 94–95
circulatory disorders, 262
cisplatin, 385
citalopram, 44*t*
CK. *See* creatine kinase
Claritin. *See* loratadine
clear sensorium, 109
clinical judgment, 5–6
clomipramine (Anafranil), 52*t*, 251, 434
clonazepam (Klonopin, Rivotril), 68, 177*t*, 434, 438
clonidine (Catapres), 448
clonus, 326
clorazepate (Tranxene), 177*t*
clots, 257–259, 269
clotting factor VII, 275
clozapine (Clozaril), 68, 97*t*, 98, 360
Clozaril. *See* clozapine
cluster headaches, 191, 218
CMR. *See* cerebral metabolic rate
cocaine, 425*t*, 426, 451–453
  addiction to, 452–453
  mechanisms of action of, 452
Cochrane database, 19
codeine, 209
Cogentin. *See* benztropine
Cognex. *See* tacrine
cognitive disorders
  classification and diagnosis of, 107–127
  incidence and prevalence of, 106–107
  recognizing, 109–113
cognitive reserve, 120
cognitive-behavioral therapy (CBT), 22, 25
cogwheel rigidity, 324
collagen-vascular disease, 262, 397, 409, 412
coma, 309
  causes of, 305*t*
  classification and diagnosis of, 304–306
  neurobiology of, 306–307
  physiological maintenance in, 308–309
  treatment, 142
  treatment of, 307–309
combined sensory and motor disorders
  neurobiology of, 410
  treatment of, 410–413
combined Systems Disease, 288
Compazine. *See* prochlorperazine
compensation neurosis, 348
complete blood count (CBC), 136
complete transection, 381
compliance, patient, 14
compos mentis, 113
COMT, 450
COMT inhibitors, 359*t*, 362
Comtan. *See* entacapone
conduct disorders, 415
confusion, 93
coning, 304, 307, 309–312
  diagnosis of, 309–311
  neurobiology of, 311
  treatment of, 311–312
consensus conferences, 23*n*2
contraindications, 65
conversion disorder, 417
  criteria for, 419*t*
cooling treatment, 312
COPD. *See* chronic obstructive pulmonary disease
coprophilia, 424*t*
Cordarone. *See* amiodarone
corneal reflex, 310
cortical lesions, 382
Cortical-Basal-Ganglionic syndrome, 336–337, 364
corticosteroids, 312

COX I, 200
COX II, 200, 201
CPR, 133
cranial nerve VII, 257*t*
cranial nerve VIII, 378, 384
creatine kinase (CK), 352
CRH1, 30
criminal psychopathy, 432
cryoglobulinemia, 409
CSF. *See* cerebrospinal fluid
CT, 333
Cushing's disease, 40
cyclophosphamide, 412
cyclosporine, 366
cyclothymia, 37
CYP system, 16, 46, 59, 209, 248, 298

D

daclizumab, 399
Dalgan. *See* dezocine
Dantrium. *See* dantrolene
dantrolene (Dantrium), 94, 350
dapsone, 388, 408, 408*t*
Daranide. *See* dichlorphenamide
Dawson fingers, 396
deafferentation, 294
decerebrate rigidity, 321
de-efferented state, 313
deep tendon reflexes, 342
defense mechanisms, 416
déjà vu, 293
Delayed Sleep Phase Disorder, 234–235
delirium, 54, 105, 157*n*5
  agitated, 79, 108
  alcohol and, 138–139
  apathetic, 108
  causes of, 115
  classification and diagnosis of, 107–108
  confused patients and, 141–142
  dementia v., 105, 113–114
  differential diagnosis of, 114–118
  neurobiology of, 127–131
  nonspecific treatments of, 140–142
  opiates and, 139–140
  treatment of, 136–148
  underlying illness treatment, 136–138
delirium tremens (DTs), 106, 117, 139, 159*n*26, 295, 445–446
Delphic conferences, 23*n*2
delusions, 146–147
dementia, 14, 107, 278
  alcohol and, 145, 443
  Alzheimer, 120–121
  classification and diagnosis of, 108–109
  delirium v., 105, 113–114
  differential diagnosis of, 118–127
  frontotemporal, 125, 340
  mixed, 122–123
  neurobiology of, 127–131
  parkinsonian, 125
  pathophysiology of, 131–136
  treatment, 142–148
  vascular, 122–124, 264
dementia pugilistica, 118
Demerol. *See* meperidine
demyelination, 396
Depakene. *See* valproate
Depakote. *See* valproate
dependence, opiate, 203–205
Deprenyl. *See* selegiline
depression, 26–35, 75, 204, 265, 441–442
  anxious, 166–168
  classification and diagnosis of, 26–28
  clinical course of, 34–35
  insomnia and, 228
  maintenance therapy, 59–60
  medication for, 42–60
  neurobiology of, 28–32
  post-stroke, 278–279
  psychotic, 29
  reactive, 29
  somatic signs of, 34
  suicide and, 41
  treatment, 43
  treatment-resistant, 71
  unipolar, 43
depressive diathesis, 29
depressive disorders, 27*t*
depressive equivalents, 27
depressive personality disorder, 434–435

depressive reaction, 29
depressive syndromes, 32
derealization, 430
dermatomyositis, 322, 347
desipramine, 52*t,* 54, 56
Desoxyn. *See* methamphetamine
Desyrel. *See* trazodone
Dexedrine. *See* dextroamphetamine
dextroamphetamine (Dexedrine), 453
dezocine (Dalgan), 210
diabetes, 205, 305*t,* 384–385
diabetic neuropathy, 384, 407
  treatment of, 388, 411
diagnosis, 1
diathesis, 35
diazepam (Valium), 99, 177*t,* 179, 462
dichlorphenamide (Daranide), 386
diffuse Cerebral Sclerosis, 395
diffusion-weighted MRI imaging (DWI), 263
digitalis, 17, 23*n*6, 116
Dilantin. *See* phenytoin
diphenhydramine (Benadryl), 244*t,* 359*t,* 362
diplopia, 374, 375, 395
dipyridamole, 269
DISC1, 82
DISC2, 82
disseminated encephalomyelitis, 397
disseminated Lupus, 261–262, 397
disseminated sclerosis, 393
distribution, drug, 15
  physiological volume of, 15
disulfiram (Antabuse), 408*t,* 445
diuretics, 353
dizocilpine. *See* MK–801
dizziness, 378
  classification and diagnosis of, 284–286
d-lysergic acid diethylamide. *See* LSD
DMD, 344
DNA, 19, 82
  sequencing, 7*n*4
docetaxel (Taxotere), 408*t*
donepezil (Aricept), 11, 141, 148, 150, 155, 240, 400
dopamine, 86, 155
dopamine receptor antagonists, high and low potency, 88*t*
dopaminergic agonists, 360–361
Dopergin. *See* lisuride
dorsal ganglion disease, 381
dosage, 18
Dostinex. *See* cabergoline
doxepin (Sinequan), 52*t,* 54, 175, 212
doxycycline, 388
dRD4, 1
dreams, 236–237
drug abuse. *See* substance abuse
drug action, human variation and, 18–20
drug therapy, 20–22
DSM (Diagnostic and Statistical Manual of American Psychiatric Association), 78, 100
  IV, 79
  IV-R, 227
  IV-RT, 416
  IV-TR, 165, 166, 423, 428, 466*n*22
dTNBP1, 2
DTs. *See* delirium tremens
duloxetine, 212
DWI. *See* diffusion-weighted MRI imaging
dynorphin, 203
dysarthria, 395
dysdiadochokinesia, 327
dysesthesias, 382, 403
dyskinesia tardive, 356
dysmetria, 327
dystonia, 91, 328, 356–357
  paroxysmal, 328

E

ECGs, 276
Ecotrin. *See* salicylates
ecstasy. *See* MDMA
ECT. *See* electric shock treatment
edrophonium (Tensilon), 337
EEG, 64, 92, 230, 294, 315
Effexor. *See* venlafaxine
Ehlers-Danlos syndrome, 195
Eisdorfer's rule, 144

Elavil. *See* amitriptyline
electric shock treatment (ECT), 71, 101, 171
electrolytes, 301
electromyography, 322, 333, 338
elementary operations, 76
emboli, 258
emotional learning systems, 173
encephalitis, 85, 103*n*18, 119, 345
encephalitis periaxialis diffusa, 395
encephalomyelitis
  acute disseminated, 401–402
  disseminated, 397
endocrine effects, 95–96
endoglin, 267
endorphins, 196, 203
engrams, 237
enkephalins, 203
entacapone (Comtan), 359*t*
environmental influences, 19
  schizophrenia and, 84–85
eosinophilia, 55
ephedrine, 453
epidural bleeding, 260
epilepsy, 57–58, 379. *See also* fits; seizures
  behavioral manifestations of, 301–302
  Grand Mal, 291–292
  partial complex, 452
  Petit Mal, 290
  surgical treatment of, 302
  visual, 316*n*3
epileptic personality disorder, 294
episodic demyelination, 393
ergotamine, 217, 218
erythrocyte sedimentation rate (ESR), 195
erythromycin, 388
escitalopram (Lexapro), 44*t*, 175
esophageal varices, 445
ESR. *See* erythrocyte sedimentation rate
estrogens, 425*t*
eszopiclone (Lunesta), 246
État criblé, 264
ethionamide (Trecator), 408
ethopropazine (Parsidol), 357
ethosuximide (Zarontin), 296
ethyl alcohol. *See* alcohol
euthymia, 36
Exelon. *See* rivastigmine
exhibitionism, 424*t*
extra neural expression, 11
eyes, 96
  disorders of, 374*t*
  movements of, 309–310

F

factitious disorder, 419–420
fainting, 286–289
  causes of, 286, 287*t*
  seizures and, 292*t*
  treatment of, 289
famotidine (Pepcid), 245
fasciculations, 328, 340
  common causes of, 332*t*
  treatment of, 357
female arousal disorder, 423, 424*t*
female orgasmic disorder, 424*t*
female premature orgasm, 424*t*
fetishes, 416
fexofenadine (Allegra), 245
fibromyositis, 187, 194–195, 220–221
field cuts, 376
fits, 289–303. *See also* epilepsy; seizures
  classification and diagnosis of, 290–294
  focal, 292–293
  generalized, 291–292
  neurobiology of, 294–296
  treatment of, 296–302
flares, 35
flooding, 170
fludarabine, 412
fludrocortisone, 55
flumazenil, 180
fluoxetine (Prozac), 44*t*, 46, 47, 175, 434
fluphenazine (Prolixin), 88*t*, 89*t*, 356
flurazepam, 232
folie à deux, 79
foot-drop, 329
free radicals, 441
Friedreich's ataxia, 344
frontal gait, 330

frontal lobotomy, 71
frontotemporal Dementias (FTDs), 125, 340
  pathophysiology of, 134
  treatment of, 155
frotteurism, 424*t*
FTDs. *See* Frontotemporal Dementias
fulminant hepatitis, 298
Furadantin. *See* nitrofurantoin

G

GABA, 31, 174, 176–177, 178, 246, 350, 364
gabapentin (Neurontin), 67, 213, 297*t*, 300, 411
gait apraxias, 343
gait disorders, 329–331, 342
  aged, 330
  cerebellar, 330, 343
  choreoathetotic, 330
  foot-drop, 329
  frontal, 330
  magnetic, 330, 343
  paretic, 329
  parkinsonian, 330, 343
  steppage, 343
  tabetic, 343
  waddling, 329, 343
  wide-based, 343
galactorrhea, 55
galantamine (Reminyl), 148, 150
gall bladder, 207
gambling disorders, 437
gas-liquid chromatography (GLC), 462
gastrointestinal effects, 150
gating, 196, 197
gegenhalten, 324
gender identity disorder, 424*t*
gene defects, 2
gene expression, 23*n*3
gene-environment interactions, 29–30
generalized anxiety disorder, 165–168
  diagnostic criteria for, 167*t*
genetic predispositions, for schizophrenia, 81–84
Gerstmann syndrome, 123
GHB, 462
giant cell arteritis. *See* temporal arteritis
glaucoma, 373, 386
  acute, 373
  chronic, 373
GLC. *See* Gas-liquid chromatography
gliosis, 132
glossopharyngeal neuralgia, 192
glucose, 133, 301, 411
glutamate, 151
glutamatergic excitotoxicity, 151
glutamatergic NMDA receptors, 128
glutathione, 466*n*23
glycerin, 312
gold salts (Ridaura), 408*t*
gout, 35
Grand Mal epilepsy, 291–292
Guillain-Barré syndrome, 313, 333
gynecomastia, 55

H

habit spasms, 328–329
habituation, 179
  opiate, 203–205
Halcion. *See* triazolam
Haldol. *See* haloperidol
hallucinations, 146–147, 302, 359–360
  hypnagogic, 233–234
  olfactory, 379
  visual, 377
hallucinogen persisting perception disorder (HPPD), 461
hallucinogens, 459–462
  treatment for, 463–464
haloperidol (Haldol), 69, 88*t*, 89*t*, 97, 141, 356, 357, 360, 462
halothane, 11, 23*n*2
hamartomas, 295
Hashimoto encephalopathy, 355
HD. *See* Huntington disease
headaches, 46–47, 222*n*6
  classification and diagnosis of, 187–192
  cluster, 191, 218

headaches (*Cont.*):
pain and, 215–220
tension, 189
hearing disorders, 377–380
treatment of, 387
heart damage, 54
heart rate, 310–311
heat stroke, 306*t*
hemiballismus, 324
hemiparesis, 322
hemiplegia, 321
Heredopathia Atactica Polyneuritiformis, 378
herniated nucleus pulposus, 193
heroin, 140, 211, 425*t*, 426, 455, 466*n*20. *See also* opiates
behavior syndrome, 456*t*
heroism, 464*n*4
HEXA, 1
high pressure liquid chromatography (HPLC), 462
hippocampal sclerosis, 126
idiopathic, 125–126, 135
treatment of, 155
hippocampus, 158*n*18
histrionic personality disorder, 432–433
homosexuality, 422–423
hormonal effects, 55
housekeeping enzymes, 11
HPLC. *See* high pressure liquid chromatography
HPPD. *See* hallucinogen persisting perception disorder
huffing, 459
human variation, drug action and, 18–20
Huntington disease (HD), 126, 333, 344
pathophysiology of, 136
treatment of, 156
hydralazine (Alazine, Apresoline, Apresazide), 408*t*
hydroxyzine (Atarax, Vistaril), 182, 244*t*, 438
hypercarbia, 234
hyperemesis gravidarum, 126
hypermania, 35
hyperpathia, 382
hypersexuality, 35
hypersomnia, 229
neurobiology of, 237–238
treatment of, 249–250
hypertension, 14, 55, 421
hypertensive retinopathy, 375
hyperthyroidism, 346–347
hyperventilation, 284, 312
hypnagogic hallucinations, 233–234
hypnic starts, 230
neurobiology of, 238
hypoactive sexual desire disorder, 424*t*
hypoalgesia, 185
hypocarbia, 284
hypochondriasis, 417
criteria for, 418*t*
hypocretin, 236, 239
hypoglycemia, 138
hypokinesia, 323
hypomania, 35, 36, 450
hypomimia, 323
hypoparathyroidism, 347
hyposmia, 379
hypotension, 287–288, 289
hypothalamus, 33
hypothermia, 312, 462
hypotonia, 324, 351
hypoxia, 136, 234, 305*t*
hypoxia-ischemia, 123
hypoxyphilia, 424*t*
hysteria, 288, 368*n*1, 417

I

ibuprofen (Motrin), 199*t*
ice cream, 145
ICP. *See* Intracranial pressure
imipramine (Tofranil), 52*t*, 54, 172, 175, 212
Imitrex. *See* sumatriptan
immunosuppressants, 398–400, 412
immunosuppression, 207
impulse control disorders, 436–438
Imuran. *See* azathioprine
inactivation, drug, 15
indomethacin, 199*t*, 201, 218
infectious hepatitis, 29

inhalants, 459
insomnia, 73*n*14, 226–228
  aging and, 228
  alcohol and, 241
  causes of, 227–228
  defined, 227
  depression and, 228
  neurobiology of, 237
  treatment of, 228, 240–249
intention tremor, 327
intercurrent disease, 345–348
interferon Beta–1a, 397–398
  side effects of, 399*t*
intermittent claudication, 409
intermittent explosive disorder, 436–437
intoxication, 440
intracranial pressure (ICP), 311
intravenous immunoglobulin (IVIG), 412
involutional melancholia, 28
involutional psychosis, 28
ischemia, 123
isoniazid, 385, 408*t*, 445
Isoptin. *See* verapamil
isosorbide, 312
IVIG. *See* intravenous immunoglobulin

J

jamaisvu, 293
jargon, 3
jukebox psychiatry, 465*n*14

K

Kandel, Erik, 76
kernicterus, 357
ketone bodies, 157*n*14
kidney problems, 63
Kleine-Levin syndrome, 231
kleptomania, 437
Klonopin. *See* clonazepam

L

lacunar states, 264
lacunar strokes, 259
Lambert-Eaton syndrome, 338, 365, 409
Lamictal. *See* lamotrigine
lamotrigine (Lamictal), 67, 213, 297*t*, 299–300
lassification, 1
latanoprost (Xalatan), 386
lateral hypothalamic area, 33
LBD. *See* Lewy Body Dementia
L-DOPA (Sinemet), 92, 358–361, 359*t*, 363, 364
learned maladaptive behavior, 415–417
Lennox-Gastaut syndrome, 290
leprosy, 385, 388
leucopenia, 55
leukin 6, 267
leukoaraiosis, 264
leukocytosis, 55
Lewy bodies, 335
Lewy Body Dementia (LBD), 124–125
  pathophysiology of, 134
  treatment of, 154–155
Lexapro. *See* escitalopram
lhermitte sign, 396
light, 236
light-headedness, 284
Lioresal. *See* baclofen
lisuride (Dopergin, Revanil), 361
lithium, 58, 61–66, 98, 444
  birth defects and, 62–64
  blood levels, 64
  dosages, 65–66
  drug interactions and, 65
  side effects of, 62, 64
  toxicity, 64
liver, 96
  chronic disease of, 336
  failure, 305*t*
liver flap, 325
locked-in syndrome, 313, 378, 402
locus ceruleus, 32
loratadine (Claritin), 212, 245
lorazepam (Ativan), 68, 69, 177*t*, 178
Lou Gherig disease. *See* Amyotrophic Lateral Sclerosis (ALS)
LSD, 460, 461
Luminal. *See* phenobarbital
Lunesta. *See* eszopiclone

lung failure, 306*t*
lupus, 35, 262
Lyme disease, 31, 85, 383
  treatment of, 388
Lyrica. *See* pregabalin

M

Macrobid. *See* nitrofurantoin
Macrodantin. *See* nitrofurantoin
Macugen. *See* pegaptanib
macular degeneration, 375–376, 384
magnetic gait, 330, 343
major strokes, 256–257
male erectile disorder, 424*t*
male orgasmic disorder, 424*t*
malingering, 419–420
mania, 26, 35–36, 53, 69, 75
  medications for, 60–68
  neurobiological causes of, 35
manic-depressive disease, 26, 36–38
  classification and diagnosis of, 37
  medications for, 60–68
  neurobiology of, 38
mannitol, 312
MAO inhibitors. *See* monoamine oxidase inhibitors
maprotiline, 52*t*
marijuana. *See* cannabis
masturbation, 423, 424*t*
masturbatory pain, 424*t*
Maxalt. *See* rizatriptan
MDMA, 453, 462
Mebaral. *See* mephobarbital
medical mimicry, 402
medications as chemicals, 9–10
  classifications of, 10–11
medroxyprogesterone, 251
melatonin, 242–243
Mellaril. *See* thioridazine
memantine (Namenda), 150–152
Ménière disease, 285–286, 378
meninges, 260
meningitis, 119, 306*t*, 377–378
Mental Status Questionnaire (MSQ), 110
mental status worksheets, 111*t*–112*t*
meperidine (Demerol), 209
mephobarbital (Mebaral), 300
meprobamate, 458
Merck Manual, 118
mesencephalon, 229
mesial temporal sclerosis, 295
mesoridazine (Serentil), 88*t*, 89*t*
Mestinon. *See* pyridostigmine
metabolic encephalopathies, 127–129
metabolism, drug, 15–16
metachromatic leukodystrophy, 82
methadone, 210, 425*t*, 457
methamphetamine (Desoxyn), 453
methazolamide (Neptazane), 386
methcathinone, 463
methotrexate, 187
3,4-methylenedioxy methamphetamine. *See* MDMA
methylphenidate (Ritalin), 59, 453
methylprednisone, 397
metronidazole, 385, 408*t*
microtubule-associated proteins, 134
midazolam, 301
migraines, 189–191, 257*t*
  basilar, 190
  causes of, 190
  classic, 189
  common, 189
  hemiplegic, 190
  ophthalmic, 190
  treatment of, 216
Miltown. *See* meprobamate
mind-altering drugs, 140–142
minimally conscious state, 313–314
minor strokes, 263–265
Mirapex. *See* pramipexole
mirror focus, 295
mirtazapine (Remeron), 48*t*, 49, 212, 216
mitochondrial myopathies, 333
mixed dementia, 122–123
mK–801 (Dizocilpine), 151
MMSE, 110
modafinil (Provigil), 250, 401
molecular mimicry, 393
monoamine oxidase (MAO) inhibitors, 31, 55, 57, 171, 181, 359*t*, 362, 425*t*
monoclonal antibodies, 399

monoclonal gammopathies, 409, 412
monogenetic disorders, 2
mononeuropathy, 404
monoplegia, 321
mood disorders, 75
mood episodes, 27*t*
morphine, 18, 203, 205, 208–209, 210, 425*t*
motility disorders
causes of chronic, 343–344
classification and diagnosis of, 320–341
diagnostic considerations for, 331–341
hereditary, 344
injuries and, 345
intercurrent diseases and, 345–348
medical causes of, 334
neurobiology of, 341–348
treatment of, 348–368
motor effects, 55
motor neuron disease, 339–340
treatment of, 367
motor system
primary, 341–342
secondary, 342–343
motor-sensory neuropathies, 403–410
anatomic pathology of, 404
classification and diagnosis of, 403–404
etiology of, 405–410
signs and symptoms of, 404
time course of, 404–405
Motrin. *See* ibuprofen
MPTPs, 15
MRI, 33, 85, 153, 333, 396
MSQ. *See* Mental Status Questionnaire
multiple sclerosis, 375, 392–401
clinical manifestation of, 394
complications of, 400–401
differential diagnosis in, 397
etiology of, 393–394
neurological examinations in, 395
pathology of, 394–397
rehabilitation, 401
risk factors for, 393–394
Münchausen syndrome, 418
muscle disease
drugs causing, 347*t*
treatment of, 352–353
muscular dystrophies, 344
myasthenia gravis, 337–338, 347, 375
drugs or toxins exacerbating, 339*t*
treatment of, 364–366
mycotic aneurysms, 266
myelin, disorders of, 392*t*
myoclonus, 326, 462
treatment of, 355
myotonic dystrophy, 322–323
Mysoline. *See* primidone

N

nalbuphine (Nubain), 210
naloxone (Narcan), 140, 211
naltrexone, 211, 438
Namenda. *See* memantine
naproxen, 199*t*
Narcan. *See* naloxone
narcissistic personality disorder, 431
narcolepsy, 232–233
neurobiology of, 239–240
treatment of, 250
Nardil. *See* phenelzine
natalizumab, 399
National Institute of Aging (NIA), 143
Navane. *See* thiothixene
necrophilia, 424*t*
nefazodone (Serzone), 48*t*, 176, 434
neocortical death. *See* persistent vegetative state
neostigmine (Prostigmin), 337, 364
neovascularization, 376
Neptazane. *See* methazolamide
nerve root disease, 382
nervous system disorders, 3
neurocardiac syncope, 286
neuroleptic malignant syndrome, 93–94
neurological disease, 4
neuromuscular junction, 347
Neurontin. *See* gabapentin
neuropathy, 213. *See also* diabetic neuropathy; motor-sensory neuropathies
causes of, 406*t*, 408*t*

neuroses, 172–173
neurosis, 416
neurotransmitters, 31
  agonists, 18
  antagonists, 18
  schizophrenia and, 86
  systems, 17–18
newton, Isaac, 158*n*20
NIA. *See* National Institute of Aging
niacin, 402
nicorette, 448
nicotine, 204, 446–449, 466*n*26
  withdrawal, 447
night terrors. *See* sleep terrors
nightmares, 233
Nitoman. *See* tetrabenazine
nitrofurantoin (Furadantin, Macrobid, Macrodantin), 408*t*, 409
Nitsch, Roger, 153
nizatidine (Axid), 245
NMDA blockers, 150–152
NMDA receptors, 160*n*35
nociceptive stimuli, 195
nocturnal enuresis, 230
  neurobiology of, 238
nocturnal paroxysmal dystonia, 231
  neurobiology of, 238–239
  treatment of, 250
nogo, 410
nonphamacological treatment, 70–71
non-steroidal anti-inflammatory agents (NSAIDs), 152, 198–202, 216, 218, 219, 221, 244, 252*n*11. *See also specific types*
  side effects of, 201
norepinephrine, 30
nortriptyline (Pamelor), 52*t*, 56, 448
NRG1, 2, 84
NSAIDs. *See* non-steroidal anti-inflammatory agents
Nubain. *See* nalbuphine
nutrition, 144–146
nutritional neuropathies, 407
  treatment of, 411
nystagmus, 310, 327, 375

O

obsessive-compulsive disorder (OCD), 170–171, 434
occult cancers, 405
OCD. *See* Obsessive-compulsive disorder
oculocephalic reflex, 309
ointments, 214
olanzapine (Zyprexa), 68, 97*t*, 98
old-wives potions, 241
oligemia, 123
oligoclonal bands, 396
Ondine's curse, 234, 239
ophthalmoplegia, 257*t*
opiates, 202–211, 220, 425*t*, 426, 455–457. *See also* heroin; specific types
  addiction to, 203–205, 455–456
  antagonists, 211
  delirium and, 139–140
  habituation, dependence and addiction, 203–205
  respiratory depression in, 205–206
  side effects of, 206–207
  types of, 207–211
optic chiasm, 76, 376
optic neuritis, 387, 394
Orap. *See* pimozide
orbitofrontal cortex, 31
orgasmic anhedonia, 424*t*
orthostatic hypotension, 51, 54–55
osteoarthritis, 186
overdoses, 21
  SSRI, 47
oxazepam (Serax), 177*t*, 178, 446
oxcarbazepine (Trileptal), 213
oxycodone, 210
oxygen free radicals, 132

P

paclitaxel, 385
pain
  anticonvulsants and, 213–214
  antidepressants and, 211–213

classification and diagnosis of, 185–195
headaches and, 215–220
neurobiology of, 195–197
treatment, 197–221
pain disorder, 418*t*
pain receptors, 185
paired helical filaments (PHF), 132
palliative care, 186
Pamelor. *See* nortriptyline
panic, 169
paralysis, 321–322
flaccid, 321, 350–351
periodic, 323
sensory, 321–322
spastic, 321, 349–350
treatment of, 349–351
paraneoplastic neuropathy, 405
treatment of, 413
paraneoplastic syndromes, 346, 385
treatment of, 388
paranoid personalities, 431–432
paraphilias, 424*t*
paraplegia, 321
paraproteinemias, 409, 412, 413
parasomnias, 229–234
neurobiology of, 238–239
paraventricular nucleus, 33
paresis, 322
spastic, 342
treatment of, 349–351
paresthesias, 382
paretic gait, 329
Parkinson disease (PD), 124, 230, 334–341, 346, 348
hereditary, 344
medications for, 359*t*
treatment of, 358–363
Parkinsonian dementia, 125
pathophysiology of, 134
treatment of, 154–155
Parkinsonian gait, 330, 343
Parkinsonism, 91–92
Parlodel. *See* bromocriptine
paroxetine (Paxil), 44*t*, 169, 175
paroxysmal choreoathetosis, 328
paroxysmal dystonia, 328
pars compacta, 15
partialism, 424*t*
passive-aggressive people, 434
pathognomonic, 207
pathological gambling, 437
pathological inattentiveness, 302–303
pathological shopping, 438
patient compliance, 14
Paxil. *See* paroxetine
PCP (phencyclidine), 151, 461–462
PD. *See* Parkinson disease
PDR (physicians' desk reference), 14, 23*n*5, 117–118
pedophilia, 424*t*, 427
PEG tubes, 308
pegaptanib (Macugen), 376
pemoline, 401
penicillamine, 351
penicillin, 17, 388
Pentacarinat. *See* stilbamidine
pentazocine (Talwin), 210
pentobarbital, 301
Pepcid. *See* famotidine
percocet, 210
pergolide (Permax), 359*t*, 361
perhexiline, 385
peripheral nerve disease, 382
Permax. *See* pergolide
pernicious anemia, 420
perphenazine (Trilafon), 89*t*
persistent vegetative state (PVS), 314
personality disorders, 428–435
antisocial, 432
borderline, 430–431
depressive, 434–435
histrionic, 432–433
narcissistic, 431
paranoid, 431–432
passive-aggressive, 434
sadomasochistic, 435
schizoid, 429
schizotypal, 428, 430
types of, 429*t*
PET, 33
Petit Mal epilepsy, 290
"Phantom limb" pain, 186

pharmacodynamics, 13–18
  defined, 13, 16–17
pharmacogenetics, 18
pharmacokinetics, 13–18
phencyclidine. *See* PCP
phenelzine (Nardil), 171, 172
Phenergan. *See* promethazine
phenobarbital (Luminal), 297*t,* 300
phenothiazine, 356
phenylpropanolamine (PPA), 453
phenytoin (Dilantin), 213, 297*t,* 298–299, 357, 445
  chronic side effects of, 299*t*
PHF. *See* paired helical filaments
phobias, 169–170, 284
  types of, 170*t*
photosensitivity, 96
physical therapy, 220
physicians' desk reference. *See* PDR
physostigmine, 149, 160*n*30
Pick disease, 125
Pickwickian syndrome, 234
pimozide (Orap), 88*t,* 89*t,* 432
placebo effects, 147
plantar flexion, 310
plasmapheresis, 398
platin, 408
plexopathy, 404
polyiomyelitis, 345
polymyositis, 322, 347
polyneuropathy, 404
  acute inflammatory, 338–339, 366–367
polyphenols, 441
polyradiculopathy, 404
porphyria, 407
  treatment of, 411
postcoital headache, 424*t*
post-herpetic neuralgias, 212
postsynaptic nerve cells, 18
post-traumatic stress disorder, 171–173, 435–436
postural tremor, 63–64
posture, abnormal, 310, 323
  treatment of, 351–352
potassium, 353
pramipexole (Mirapex), 359*t,* 361
prazepam (Centrax), 177*t*
prednisone, 397
pregabalin (Lyrica), 411
pregnancy, 95
premature ejaculation, 424*t*
priapism, 50, 176, 426
primary lateral sclerosis, 340
primary motor system, 341–342
primidone (Mysoline), 300, 354
prochlorperazine (Compazine), 89*t*
progressive bulbar palsy, 340
progressive muscular atrophy, 340
Progressive Supranuclear Palsy (PSP), 336, 343, 364
Prolixin. *See* fluphenazine
promazine (Sarine), 89*t*
promethazine (Phenergan), 182, 244*t,* 285
propantheline (Pro-Banthine), 400
propranolol, 217
proprioception, 381
prostaglandin F2α, 386
prosthetic valves, 269
Prostigmin. *See* neostigmine
prostitution, 6–7, 8*n*8
protriptyline, 52*t,* 251
Provigil. *See* modafinil
Prozac. *See* fluoxetine
pseudo angina, 28
pseudoephedrine, 453
pseudoneurotic schizophrenia, 78–79, 428
pseudotumor cerebri, 188
PSP. *See* Progressive Supranuclear Palsy
psychedelics. *See* hallucinogens
psychiatric disease, 4
psychogenic stressors, 33
psychoses
  classification of, 78–81
  endogenous, 80
  exogenous, 80
  neurobiology of, 81–86
  nonpharmacological treatments of, 100–101
  treatment of, 86–99
psychosis, acute, 87
  treatment of, 69–70, 99–100

psychostimulants, 59
psychosurgery, 101
psychotic depression, 29
psychotic disorders, 28
psychotomimetic reactions, 211
ptosis, 337, 374, 375
public issues, awareness disorders and, 315–316
pupils, 375
PVS. *See* persistent vegetative state
pyridostigmine (Mestinon), 364, 365
pyridoxine, 385, 408, 408*t*, 411
pyromania, 437

Q

quaaludes, 117
quadriplegia, 321
quetiapine (Seroquel), 68, 97*t*, 98

R

ramelteon (Rozerem), 246
ranitidine (Zantac), 245
raphe nuclei, 32, 236
rashes, 55
reactive depression, 29
reboxetine, 50
recovered memories, 430, 465*n*14
red wine, 441
reduced movements, 321
Reformist Delusions, 5, 415, 463*n*1
Refsum disease, 387
relative ischemia, 295
religion, 317*n*17
REM sleep disorder, 230, 236
  neurobiology of, 238
  treatment of, 250
Remeron. *See* mirtazapine
Reminyl. *See* galantamine
remission, 35
remyelination, 396
Requip. *See* ropinirole
reserpine (Serpasil), 356
respiratory depression, 205–206
restless legs syndrome, 231
  neurobiology of, 238
reticular activating system, 306
retina, 375
  disorders of, 376*t*
retinitis pigmentosa, 96
Revanil. *See* lisuride
rhabdomyolysis, 459, 462
ridaura. *See* gold salts
rigidity, 324
Risperdal. *See* risperidone
risperidone (Risperdal), 68, 97*t*, 141, 147, 155, 360, 462
Ritalin. *See* methylphenidate
ritanserin, 460
rituximab, 399
rivastigmine (Exelon), 148, 150
Rivotril. *See* clonazepam
rizatriptan (Maxalt), 216, 217
rofecoxib (Vioxx), 199*t*
roman Catholics, 39
ropinirole (Requip), 359*t*, 361
Rozerem. *See* ramelteon

S

sadomasochistic personality disorder, 435
salicylates (Bufferin, Ecotrin), 199*t*, 269. *See also* acetylsalicylic acid
salves, 214
Sarine. *See* promazine
schizoaffective disorder, 37, 75
schizoid personality disorder, 429
schizophrenia, 7*n*5, 35, 37, 69, 75, 77, 104*n*27, 428
  brain damage and, 85
  defined, 79
  environmental influences on, 84–85
  genetic predisposition for, 81–84
  neurotransmitter disorders in, 86
  phenomenon in, 80
  proposed genes for, 83*t*
  pseudoneurotic, 78–79
schizotypal personality disorder, 428, 430
Schwann cells, 410

sciatica, 382
scintillating scotoma, 190
seasonal affective disorder, 70
second degree blocks, 54
sedation, 53, 92–93
segmental demyelination, 404
seizures, 55, 92, 257*t*, 284. *See also* epilepsy; fits
  complex partial, 290, 293–294
  energy demands in, 295
  faints v., 292*t*
  generalized, 291*t*
  Grand Mal, 290
  international classification of, 291*t*
  partial, 291*t*
  special epileptic, 291*t*
  treatment of, 296–302
  versive, 292
selective serotonin reuptake inhibitors (SSRIs), 10, 30, 43, 44–47, 144, 155, 170, 217–218, 279, 400, 421, 425*t*, 429, 434
  absorption of, 45
  choice of, 44–45
  overdoses on, 47
  side effects of, 45–46
  suicide and, 47
selegiline (Deprenyl), 58, 359*t*
self-medication, 438–439
senile dementia, 120
sensation disorders
  abnormal, 382
  classification and diagnosis of, 371–372
  losses, 381–382
  lost, 382–383
  neurobiology of, 383–385
  of special sensations, 371–383
  treatment of general, 387–388
  treatment of specific, 385–387
sensory modalities, 380*t*
sensory paroxysms, 230–231
  neurobiology of, 238
sensory root disease, 381
septicemia, 419
Serax. *See* oxazepam
Serentil. *See* mesoridazine
Seroquel. *See* quetiapine
serotonin, 30, 86, 174, 241, 460
  homeostasis, 34
  measurements of, 33
Serpasil. *See* reserpine
sertraline, 44*t*
serum hepatitis, 29
Serzone. *See* nefazodone
sexual aversion disorder, 424*t*
sexual disorders, 422–427
  drugs as cause of, 425*t*
  DSM-IV-TR, 424
  psychiatric treatment of, 427
sexual function, 46
sexual masochism, 424*t*
sexual sadism, 424*t*
sexually dimorphic nucleus, 33
shock, 306*t*
shopping, pathological, 438
Shy-Drager syndrome, 335
side effects, 16
  of antipsychotics, 87–88, 90–96
  of benzodiazepines, 178–182
  of chloral hydrate, 247
  of cholinesterase inhibitors, 150
  of interferon, 399*t*
  lithium, 62, 64
  NSAIDs, 201
  of opiates, 206–207
  of phenytoin, 299*t*
  physiological, 11
  SSRIs, 45–46
  TCAs, 53–56
sildenafil, 46
Sinemet. *See* L-DOPA
Sinequan. *See* doxepin
Sjögren syndrome, 262, 385
skin reactions, 96
sleep apneas, 234
  neurobiology of, 239
  treatment of, 251
sleep automatisms, 232
  treatment of, 250
sleep disorders
  classification and diagnosis of, 226–235
  neurobiology of, 235–240
  sleep patterns and, 225

sleep paralyses, 231
treatment of, 251
sleep terrors, 233
sleepwalking, 231–232
neurobiology of, 238
slow-wave sleep, 235–236
smell disorders, 379–380
treatment of, 387
social management treatment, 100–101
social phobias, 169–170
Soma. *See* carisoprodol
somatic signs, of depression, 31
somatization disorder, 418*t*
somatoform disorder, 165–168, 417–422
diagnostic criteria for, 168*t*
somatosensory cortex, 196
somnambulism. *See* sleepwalking
Sonata. *See* zaleplon
spasticity, medications for, 349*t*
SPECT, 33, 127
spinal cord, transection of, 381
spinocerebellar ataxias, 344
SSRIs. *See* selective serotonin reuptake inhibitors
st. John's Wort, 58–59
Stadol. *See* butorphanol
status epilepticus, 294, 452, 458
treatment of, 301
Stelazine. *See* trifluoperazine
steppage gait, 343
steroids, 214, 352, 397
Stevens-Johnson syndrome, 300
stilbamidine (Pentacarinat), 408*t*
streptomycin, 285
stress disorders, 171–173
striate cortex, 76
striatonigral degeneration, 335–336
strokes, 284, 305*t*
chronic care after, 277–279
depression and, 278–279
genetic predisposition to, 267
predisposing medical conditions to, 261
recovery from, 275–276
rehabilitation, 276–277
surgical treatment of, 275
treatment of acute, 271–276
stupor, 303
treatment of, 142, 307–309
subarachnoid bleeding, 260
subdural bleeding, 260
substance abuse, 438–463
alcohol, 440–446
amphetamines, 453–455
barbiturates, 457–459
benzodiazepines, 457–459
cocaine, 451–453
general considerations of, 438–440
hallucinogens, 459–462
inhalants, 459
nicotine, 446–449
opiates, 455–457
substance-induced sexual dysfunction, 424*t*
substantia nigra, 15
suicide, 21, 38–42, 56, 72*n*12–73*n*12, 202
depression and, 41
occurrences of, 38
planning, 40
rationality and, 42
risk factors for, 38–39, 41
SSRIs and, 47
sumatriptan (Imitrex), 216, 217
suprachiasmatic nucleus, 33
susceptibility genes, 29
sweating, 55
syncope, 286
syncytium, 17
syndrome of the bits, 126–127
syphilis, 85, 345–346, 383, 389*n*4, 389n5, 397
treatment of, 388
syringomyelia, 333

T

tabes dorsalis, 382
tabetic gait, 343
tachycardia, 462
tacrine (THA, Cognex), 149, 150
Tagamet. *See* cimetidine
talk therapy, 20–22, 25
Talwin. *See* pentazocine

tangles, 120
tardive dyskinesia, 90–91
Tasmar. *See* tolcapone
taste disorders, 379–380
  treatment of, 387
tauopathies, 125
Taxol. *See* paclitaxel
Taxotere. *See* docetaxel
Tay-Sachs disease, 82, 84
Tegretol. *See* carbamazepine
temporal arteritis, 191, 257*t*, 373, 386
temporal lobe, 293–294
Tensilon. *See* edrophonium
tension headaches, 189
tetrabenazine (Nitoman), 355, 356
THA. *See* tacrine
thalamus, 196, 197
  disease of, 382
  lesions of, 381
therapeutic effects, 16
therapeutic index, 17
therapeutic window, 17
therapy
  cognitive behavioral, 22, 25
  drug, 20–22
  talk, 20–22, 25
thermodynamics, 206
theta waves, 236
thiamin, 138, 156, 308, 346, 355–356, 402, 411, 446
  deficiency, 305*t*
thiamine pyrophosphate (TPP), 135
thioridazine (Mellaril), 88*t*, 89*t*, 96, 425*t*
thiothixene (Navane), 68, 88*t*, 89*t*
Thorazine. *See* chlorpromazine
thought broadcasting, 80
thought disorders, 75
  classification and diagnosis of, 78–81
  neurobiology of, 81–86
  nonpharmacological treatment of, 100–101
  treatment of, 86–99
thrombolysis, 266
thromboses
  cerebral, 259
  venous, 259
thyroid-stimulating hormone (TSH), 63
TIAs. *See* transient ischemic attacks
tic douloureux, 191–192
tics, 328–329
  treatment of, 357–358
Tigan. *See* trimethobenzamide
timolol, 386
tinnitus, 285, 378
titubation, 327
tizanidine (Zanaflex), 350
Todd's paralysis, 292
Tofranil. *See* imipramine
tolcapone (Tasmar), 359*t*
Topamax. *See* topiramate
topiramate (Topamax), 67, 213, 218, 297*t*, 300
Tourette's syndrome, 6, 329, 357
toxic neuropathy, 407–408
  treatment of, 412
toxicity, 16
toxoplasmosis, 346, 352
tPA (Alteplase), 272–273
  inclusion and exclusion criteria for, 274*t*
TPP. *See* thiamine pyrophosphate
tramadol (Ultram), 209
transcranial magnetic stimulation, 101
transient epileptic amnesia, 293
transient ischemic attacks (TIAs), 258, 263–265, 272
transverse myelitis, 395
transvestic fetishism, 424*t*
Tranxene. *See* clorazepate
trauma, 257*t*
trazodone (Desyrel), 48*t*, 50–51, 155, 172, 176, 249, 425*t*, 426
Trecator. *See* ethionamide
tremors, 324, 325
  action, 325
  emotional, 325
  essential, 324, 325, 353–354
  familial, 325, 353–354
  hysterical, 325
  orthostatic, 325, 354
  senile, 325
  treatment of, 353–354
triazolam (Halcion), 177*t*, 179, 243
trichinosis, 345, 352

trichloroethylene (Trilene), 408*t*
trichotillomania, 437–438
tricyclic antidepressants, 51–57, 212, 425*t*
  advantages of, 53
  dosages of, 56–57
  mechanisms of action of, 51–52
  side effects of, 53–56
trifluoperazine (Stelazine), 88*t*, 89*t*, 425*t*
triflupromazine (Vesprin), 89*t*
trigeminal neuralgia, 213
triglycerides, 267
trihexyphenidyl (Artane), 357, 359*t*, 362
Trilafon. *See* perphenazine
Trilene. *See* trichloroethylene
Trileptal. *See* oxcarbazepine
trimethobenzamide (Tigan), 285
trimipramine, 52*t*, 54
triptans, 218
trypanosomiasis, 229
tryptophan, 241–242
TSH. *See* thyroid-stimulating hormone
Tylenol. *See* acetaminophen

U

UARS. *See* sleep apneas
Ultram. *See* tramadol
undifferentiated somatoform disorder, 418*t*
unipolar depression, 43
unoprostone, 386
upper airways resistance syndrome (UARS). *See* sleep apneas
urea, 312
uremia, 305*t*
uremic neuropathy, 407
urophilia, 424*t*

V

V Leiden mutation, 259
VaD. *See* vascular dementia
vagus nerve, 71
Valium. *See* diazepam
valproate (Depakene, Depakote), 67, 99, 171, 297*t*, 298, 444
Valsalva maneuver, 288
vascular dementia (VaD), 122–124, 264
  pathophysiology of, 133–134
  treatment of, 154
vascular stenoses, 271
vasculitis, 261–262, 397
vasogenic attacks, 286
venlafaxine (Effexor), 48*t*, 49, 171, 176
venous thromboses, 259
verapamil (Calan, Isoptin), 218
vertical gaze paralysis, 336
vertigo, 285, 395
Vesprin. *See* triflupromazine
vestibular rehabilitation, 285
Viagra, 427
vibration, 384
vincristine, 408, 408*t*
violence, 147
  alcohol and, 443–444
Vioxx. *See* rofecoxib
vision disorders, 373–377
  treatment of, 385–387
Vistaril. *See* hydroxyzine
visual agnosias, 376–377
vitamin deficiencies
  B_{12}, 356
  pathophysiology of, 135–136
von Economo encephalitis, 229
voyeurism, 424*t*

W

waddling gait, 329–330, 343
Waldenström macroglobulinemia, 409, 412
wallerian degeneration, 404
walnut brain, 121
weakness, 322–323
Wegener granulomatosis, 374
weight gain, 54, 95
Welander dystrophy, 322
Wellbutrin. *See* bupropion

Weltschmerz, 26
Wernicke-Korsakoff syndrome, 126, 137, 355, 443
  pathophysiology of, 135
  treatment of, 156
west syndrome, 290
wide-based gait, 343
Wilson Disease, 357
withdrawal, 140, 179, 203, 354, 439, 440. *See also* delirium tremens
  nicotine, 447

X

Xalatan. *See* latanoprost
Xanax. *See* alprazolam

Z

zaleplon (Sonata), 245
Zanaflex. *See* tizanidine
Zandac. *See* ranitidine
Zarontin. *See* ethosuximide
Zeldox. *See* ziprasidone
ziprasidone (Zeldox), 68, 97*t*, 98
zolmitriptan (Zomig), 216, 217
Zoloft, 46, 146
zolpidem (Ambien), 245
Zomig. *See* zolmitriptan
Zonegran. *See* zonisamide
zonisamide (Zonegran), 213
zoophilia, 424*t*
Zyprexa. *See* olanzapine
Zyrtec. *See* cetirizine

www.ingramcontent.com/pod-product-compliance
Lightning Source LLC
Chambersburg PA
CBHW060423220326
41598CB00021BA/2267
* 9 7 8 0 0 7 1 4 4 0 3 6 3 *